A Remarkable Life
A Remarkable Journey

A Remarkable Life
A Remarkable Journey

"A Wellness Companion for Glyconutrient and Meridian Support"

T. Aristotle, D.C., L.Ac.

Pathways to Health Publishing
P.O. Box 457
Brookport, Illinois 62910

Library of Congress Number: (cataloging in progress)

ISBN: 0-9770984-0-0

There is one whose rash words are like sword thrusts,
but the tongue of the wise brings healing.

~ Proverbs 12:18

**A man too busy to take care of his health
is like a mechanic too busy to take care of his tools.**

~ Spanish Proverb

TABLE OF CONTENTS

Introduction

Most diseases are the result of medication
which has been prescribed to relieve and take away a
beneficent and warning symptom on the part of Nature.
- Elbert Hubbard

Getting Started:

This is a "how-to" textbook on the use of nutrition and meridian point application. This book is intended to be used by those wanting assistance in supporting the body using basic cell communication molecules – utilizing glyconutrients as well as meridian system support.

Alphabetically listed are over 355 specific health challenges. These methods are neither medical treatment nor advice for health conditions. Always consult your own health professional for specific health conditions.

The nutritional ingredients shown under the "daily nutritional program" headings are listed as general products.
The following letters are used:

GlycoN (Adv)	Cata	MC	SkZone
PhytoN	ImmS	GIPro	EM
PreH	Sp	GIZyme	GlycoAO
GEssentials	Clean	CB	

You will need to determine the definition for the products for each health challenge. Simply turn to the "Product Definitions" in the Appendix A on page 381. If you have more than one condition, determine the number one health challenge and address it first.

A common question arises: Why do I need to take GlycoN *with* the GlycoAO? It is necessary to combine the core product (GlycoN) with the GlycoAO because of the dosage requirements. Just taking the AO by itself without the Glyconutrient (GlycoN) is not enough for the body to harmonize during illness. If you are interested in the dosages without GlycoAO, only with the GlycoN, I suggest purchasing the first book; "In Search of Manna".

Abbreviations found in the conditions section are as follows:
- tsp = teaspoon
- tabs = tablets
- caps = caplets

Serving sizes listed in this book are for adults. Servings for children up to 12 years old can be found by calling the company listed in the Appendix.

The section, "Tips for Meridian Support", is an overview on how to begin balancing the meridian system as an adjunct to the nutritional menus. The meridian points listed have historical significance and many are based upon the successful clinical results by the author.

If your condition is not found, please refer to Section II on page 377, "Health Challenges Not Listed".

Welcome to "Life Care not "Sick Care"

Having observed the miraculous healings of the human body, once all systems are balanced and in harmony, has been a wonderful opportunity for being grateful. In the book, "A Course of Miracles", it states that miracles are expressions of "miracle-mindedness and miracle-mindedness means right-mindedness." Please remember, "To observe true healing, we must not inject the emotion of fear into the already weakened and fearful patient". Rather, supporting the patient's release of fear, the mind and body are then able to work together as the healing process unfolds.

My purpose in completing this text, just as it was in the previous book, "In Search of Manna" is to forward the healing process worldwide. Whether this book sits next to a loved one in a hospital bed or at home on a nightstand, it will both educate and serve as a reference companion to those in need who are experiencing health challenges.

When including glyconutrients and meridian therapy as an adjunct to treatment or prevention of dis-ease, I know in my heart that all will have the opportunity to heal more than they would have previously. I implore you to share the knowledge you gain, remembering that many of the meridian points listed date back almost 5,000 years with a historical track record of clinical success.

You may have heard of the saying, "Many are called but few are chosen." By endeavoring to gain the knowledge shared in this book, I will assume you are "one of the chosen" that wishes to participate in the healing process and ease the pain of the many individuals that are suffering needlessly. Illness tempts us to become detached; therefore, we must be reconnected to The Source. I applaud you in your decision to help yourselves and those you love.

Now, with Quantum Physics, we are beginning to explore through science the power of intention and how it affects the world around us. If you have not seen the film, "What The Bleep Do We Know!?", I suggest you take a look. How would you change your thinking if you knew of your ability to influence your surroundings by a simple thought? (As stated in Proverbs, "As a man thinketh in his heart so is he.").

Ask yourself, what is in your heart and what is in your consciousness? I refer to a story shared with me: There was a man walking through a busy construction site. He casually walked up to the first worker and asked, "What are you doing?" The worker responded, "I'm doing my job and putting in my time." A second worker was asked the same question, this next worker responded, "I'm building a stone wall". Finally, the man encountered a third worker and asked, "What are you doing?" This worker looked up and said, "I am building God's house". Same stone wall. Same project. Different consciousness.

4

Since the release of "In Search of Manna," I have received countless e-mails, letters and phone calls sharing personal success stories surrounding the use of glyconutrients and meridian therapy. Who holds the secret to this healing? We have all heard of people being referred to as "a true healer" or as having "healing hands." I would suggest that we modify our thinking here. The thread that is woven throughout us all is that we facilitate the healing process. The key to this lies within the following thought; I do not believe it is us that does the healing. We facilitate it. Alternatively, I suggest using the term "Healing Facilitator". Many marketing experts would probably agree in labeling this as a "Unique Selling Proposition" or USP. Regardless of the term used, if we as "healing facilitators" detach from our egos and release our judgments, we will truly strengthen the expression of the body's ability to heal and re-connect to The Source.

"And they departed and went through the villages, preaching the gospel and healing everywhere".   ~ Luke 9:6

I welcome you to A Remarkable Life, A Remarkable Journey.

Dr. Aristotle

Acute and Wellness Program Definitions

In Section I: Health Challenges, specific challenges are shown with daily recommendations. You will find the following terms and general definitions. To define each term below, simply turn to the "Product Definitions" in the Appendix A on page 381.

GlycoN with AntiO:
Glyconutrients (and advanced) with Anti-Oxidants – Establishes cell to cell communication. Correct amounts permit cells to communicate more efficiently. These nutrients support the immune system and antioxidant levels in cells. Examples of immune system challenges include lupus, allergies, cancer, asthma and delayed healing of wounds.

PhytoN:
Phytonutrients – There are over 10,000 in number known to date. Phytonutrients are found in vegetables and fruits. Phytonutrients are crucial in heart disease prevention and cancer fighting activity. Phytonutrients include free radical scavengers and anti-oxidants. They are synergistic with the glyconutrients.

PreH:
Phytosterols – Correct cell function requires molecules that support proper endocrine function. This includes over a variety of seventy hormones for body regulation including; DHEA, progesterone, testosterone etc. Considerable benefit is observed with intake of a standardized wild yam.

GEssentials and Cata:
Minerals and Vitamins (Established Nutrition) – Absorbing nutrients as close to the food form as possible is most beneficial to the body. Also, completing a Dietary Needs Assessment is suggested for identifying which combination of foods (proteins, fats, and carbohydrates) you should consider for intake. The two types of minerals, vitamins and antioxidants complexes recommended. GEssentials, which contain the standard or basic amounts of minerals, vitamins and anti-oxidants. Cata is a term for the vitamin, mineral and anti-oxidant complex that contains essential nutrients and anti-oxidants. This is generally considered for more severe symptoms or health problems.

Clean:
Intestinal Support with Flora: Supporting intestinal health and the cleansing mechanisms of the body is important for the natural ecology of the intestines, regularity and general colon health. Absorption of nutrients from food and supplementation may be compromised if the intestines ability to absorb is inhibited. Proper cleansing protocols are a necessary component of a balanced and healthy regimen. Clean is the term for the formula that supports intestinal health and adds the beneficial flora.

CB:
Cardiovascular Balancing: Nourishing and nutritionally supporting the cardiovascular system is necessary in order to maintain healthy arterial walls, heart muscle and cholesterol levels. The human body contains 60,000 miles of blood vessels. Maintaining balanced circulation throughout this network is extremely important.

ImmS
Immune System Balancing: The immune system plays a vital role in the healing process. The immune system protects us from the cold and flu, as well as a variety of other infectious diseases, and strives to get us well again when we become ill. Our immune system, like every other system in the body, is coordinated and controlled by the nervous system. ImmS is important in that it assists in the removal of toxins, foreign substances and optimizes the immune system.

MC
Vitamin C: Vitamin C is needed for the formation of collagen, the "glue" that strengthens many parts of the body, such as muscles and blood vessels. Vitamin C derived from acerola is a powerful antioxidant and plays important roles in wound healing and as a natural antihistamine. This vitamin also supports the immune system to combat viruses and to detoxify alcohol and other substances. MC is a unique herbal blend and natural source of vitamin C.

GstroP
Gastro-Intestinal Flora: Healthy bacteria and microorganisms in the intestines are known as probiotics. While present in the digestive system, they help keep it running smoothly and support digestion. The body's immune system is supported when you provide enough beneficial bacteria.
GstroP provides the support needed in a healthy intestine.

GstroZ
Gastro-Intestinal Enzymes: Proper food breakdown is essential for maximum absorption of nutrients in the digestive tract. At times, the body's ability to breakdown ingested material is not functioning at its' maximum level. Enzymes assist in the digestive process which results in healthy nutrient absorption. GstroZ provides support for the enzymatic process in the body.

SP
Sporting/Athletic Recovery: Athletic exertion can lead to muscle fatigue and/or breakdown of muscle tissue. A formula that works in harmony with the body to support its' natural recovery from physical stress and burning of fat is important. SP is designed to assist in athletic recovery and support lean tissue development.

SkZone
Skin Care: The skin is the largest organ of the body and yet most of us don't do enough to maintain our skin's health. SkZone is an aloe gel that protects the skin and alleviates roughness.

Healing Reactions (Cell Memory and Retracing)

In addition to health improvement, what occurs as we begin to replace the lower grade nutrition with superior nutrition? A healing crisis or retracing.

When beneficial nutrients are taken and the use of stimulants such as coffee, tea, chocolate or cocoa is suddenly stopped, headaches are common, and a healing crisis occurs. This is due to the elimination, by the body, of toxins which are removed from the tissues and transported via the blood stream. Before the toxins arrive at their final destination for elimination, these "irritants" register in our system as pain or more commonly as a mild or splitting headache.

Usually, within three to five days, the symptoms vanish and we feel stronger due to the recuperation that follows. To a lesser extent, the same process occurs when we abandon lower quality processed foods and replace them with better whole organic foods.

The initial healing crisis is followed by an increase of strength, a feeling of diminishing stress and great well-being.
During the initial healing crisis you may experience symptoms of a prior illness such as fever, rash, hives, bowel gas, stuffy or runny nose, headaches, insomnia, increased thirst, weakness, lethargy, loss of appetite, nausea, diarrhea, fever blisters, constipation, dizziness, nervousness, as well as various body aches and pains similar to a cold or flu. Please understand that these are corrective reactions.

When you experience a healing reaction, be assured your body is making positive changes toward an improved state of health. Understand that these short-lived reactions are an integral part of your healing process. This is a small price to pay for long-lasting health benefits.

How To Support Healing Reactions

1. To help flush out toxins and assist your body in the natural cleansing process, drink enough water that equals half of your body weight in ounces per day. For example, if you weigh 120 pounds then you should drink 60 oz. per day (120 divided by 2 equals 60). Water quality is crucial. Drink room temperature, non-carbonated water in glass bottles (plastic containers leach toxic polycarbons into the water and your system has to then detoxify them). If you have a heart or kidney problem, please check with your healthcare provider.

2. Increase your intake of vegetables and whole grains. Purchase a vegetable juicer and juice vegetables at least 3 times per week. This can help accelerate the removal of toxins of any type.

3. Move your body. Walking, jumping, and bicycling for at least 25 minutes a day is a good start.

4. Apply the meridian points during your detoxification and healing process. As symptoms of healing reactions appear, simply stimulate the points indicated on the meridian charts that are specific to your condition.

5. When bathing, use a loofa, scrubbing bath brush or a rough sponge to assist in the removal of dead skin cells.

6. Depending on the amount of toxins that are eliminated from your body and if you feel that your healing reaction is interfering with your daily routine, you can reduce your recommended program for a few days, and then gradually increase to the recommended amounts.

Your Health and a Few Notes

During a disease process, if you decide to improve your nutrition while on medication, your requirements for medications may diminish. It is important that you work with your health care provider and ask if your medication can be reduced. If he/she is not willing to discuss your options, I suggest finding an alternate practitioner.

Please note that the suggestions and programs in this book are not recommendations for therapy and do not substitute for diagnosis and treatment by your own doctor. For conditions not listed, general guidelines can be found in Section II, "Health Challenges not listed".

These wellness programs are goals. You can work up to the larger amounts if you are unable to tolerate the healing reaction. Start small by cutting the amounts in half and increase every 3 to 5 days to the goal amount. Be patient with your body. It was patient with you during many years of neglect and is simply in need of healing.

Once you experience the desired effect, it will be possible to reduce the amounts by following the same rules as above.

A Note Regarding AdvGlycoN (see appendix A on page 381 for definition)

If you decide to include the **AdvGlycoN,** <u>without</u> the GlycoAO, simply use the same serving as shown for the GlycoN. For example, if the shown serving for GlycoN is 4 teaspoons, then you would use 4 teaspoons of AdvGlycoN. (without the AO)

If you decide to include the **AdvGlycoN** <u>with</u> the GlycoAO, simply use ½ (half) the serving as shown for the GlycoN. For example, if the shown serving is 4 teaspoons, then you would use 2 teaspoons of AdvGlycoN with the shown serving of GlycoAO.

A Few Words On Hospitals

Stimulating meridian points and offering glyconutrients to loved ones in a hospital setting is an efficient method of supporting the healing process. Some hospitals have rules that regulate the intake of proper nutrition. Many times, to administer the necessary nutrients that the body needs to heal, the attending physician may require that he/she authorizes its use so that drug interactions can be avoided. Side effects are not a problem with meridian point stimulation as it will not interfere with medication. Please remember it is your responsibility to inquire about other options and other treatment protocols with your doctor. It is best to work with a doctor that has a background in nutrition and can make the proper recommendations.

Unfortunately, some hospitals will not allow nutrition to be given by family members. This can result in diminished healing of the patient. Try to schedule a meeting with your doctor or the nurse caring for your loved one. Ask how you can help to make sure the food supplements are administered.

The administration of glyconutrients and meridian support for patients in the intensive care unit (ICU) can be a sensitive issue. At times a patient is not able to voluntarily chew food or drink liquid. In this case, a feeding tube is used. Occasionally, feeding tubes are not used and patients are fed through an intravenous (IV) route. Currently, there are no IV products available for the glyconutrient use.

An NG (naso-gastric) tube can also be used to transfer nutrients directly into the stomach when a patient cannot take food or drink by mouth. If using an NG tube it is important to dilute the glyconutrients so they do not block the tube. Typically, use 1 tablespoon of glyconutrient powder with 8 oz. of bottled water, or tube feeding solution, every 2 hours. Be sure the mixture is mixed thoroughly and then placed through the tube. Be sure to flush bottled (use glass bottles) spring water through the tube to clear the mixture (this helps prevent clogging). Remember, it will be your responsibility to monitor the administration of nutrients.

Apply meridian point stimulation at least three (3) times a day in the ICU. Stimulated points with finger pressure, soft laser or tei shein application. These are all non-invasive and application is simple. Please refer to tips for meridian support on the following page.

Tips for Meridian Support

The meridian points shown are for one half the body (unilateral) for simplicity. Be sure to stimulate both sides of the body. For example: a point shown on the left leg will also exist on the right leg and needs stimulation; a point on the right side of the chest also exists on the left side (mirror image) and must be stimulated. Points that are midline have no duplicate (mirror image) points. If a meridian point is tender to the touch, this is a good indication for extra stimulation. Be sure to "browse" the area of the point to locate the tender spots. The meridian points are about the size of a quarter. Products are available at www.tarisproducts.com or your local health and wellness store.

Scar tissue on the body reduces the flow of meridians and can inhibit the healing process.   As a general rule, always stimulate scar tissue, including scars from prior surgeries over one month and injuries. Soft laser application can be started three days after surgery. Acceptable methods of general scar tissue stimulation are soft laser, gentle massage or teishein. Stimulate old scars at least once a day for 30 seconds.

Acupressure: Finger pressure is applied to the skin directly on the meridian point. Use a firm technique without causing discomfort. Rub the meridian point for 30 to 45 seconds. If in a crisis situation, rub three times a day. For chronic problems, perform only once a day.

Teishein (*tay-sheen*): Gently tap the meridian point 20 times. The non-invasive teishein is a classic acupressure non-piercing needle. Its use is worldwide, found in clinics, hospitals and research institutes throughout the world. It is a favorite of health care practitioners. Perform in a crisis situation three times a day. For chronic problems, perform only once a day.

Soft laser: Hold the laser tip (the end of the laser) approximately ½ to 1 inch from the meridian point or desired area. Stimulate with the laser 30 seconds to 1 minute per point. A clockwise circular motion is recommended. Perform in a crisis situation three times a day. For chronic problems, perform only once a day.

Section I: Health Challenges

Abdominal Pain

Daily Nutritional Crisis Program	Daily Nutritional Wellness Program
GlycoN*:2 ½ tsp & GlycoAO: 3 caps	GlycoN*:1/2 tsp & GlycoAO: 2 caps
PhytoN: 1/4 tsp	PhytoN: 1/4 tsp
PreH: 3 tabs	PreH: 3 tabs
GEssentials: 4 tabs	GEssentials: 4 tabs
GstroP: 3 caps	GstroP: 1 cap
GstroZ: 2 caps before meals	GstroZ: 1 cap before meals

*For Adv.GlycoN see page 10. Product definitions are in Appendix A on page 381.

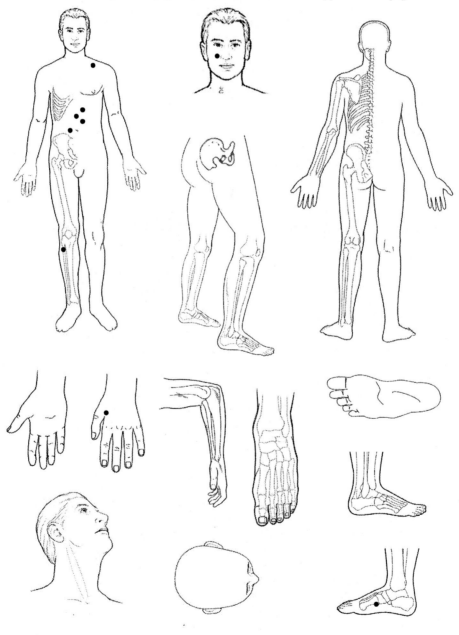

Abscess, Skin

Daily Nutritional Crisis Program	Daily Nutritional Wellness Program
GlycoN*: 1 ½ tsp & GlycoAO: 3 caps PhytoN: 1 tsp PreH: 3 tabs GEssentials: 4 tabs ImmS: 4 tabs MC: 4 caps	GlycoN*: ½ tsp & GlycoAO: 2 caps PhytoN: 1/4 tsp PreH: 3 tabs GEssentials: 4 tabs ImmS: 2 tabs MC: 2 caps

*For Adv.GlycoN see page 10. Product definitions are in Appendix A on page 381.

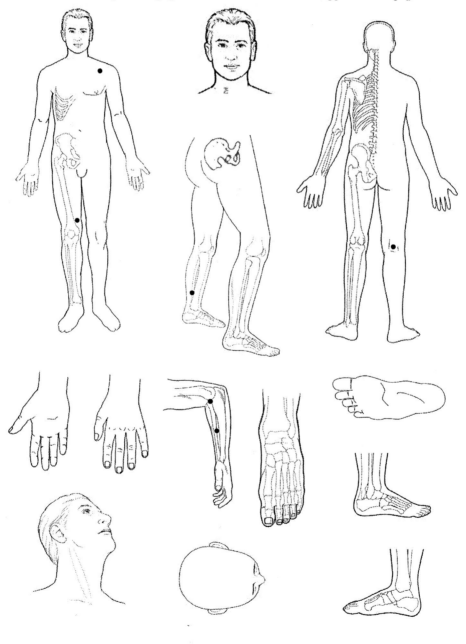

Acne
(soft laser on affected areas)

Daily Nutritional Crisis Program	Daily Nutritional Wellness Program
GlycoN*: 1 ½ tsp & GlycoAO: 3 caps PhytoN: ½ tsp PreH: 3 tabs GEssentials: 4 tabs Clean: 3 caps twice a day (2 weeks)	GlycoN*: ½ tsp & GlycoAO: 2 caps PhytoN: ½ tsp PreH: 3 tabs GEssentials: 4 tabs Clean: 1 cap twice a day

*For Adv.GlycoN see page 10. Product definitions are in Appendix A on page 381.

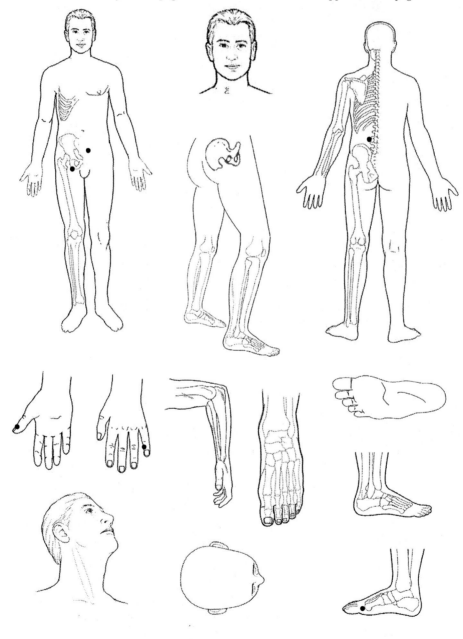

Actinic Keratosis

Daily Nutritional Crisis Program	Daily Nutritional Wellness Program
GlycoN*: ½ tsp & GlycoAO: 2 caps PhytoN: ½ tsp PreH: 3 tabs Cata: 4 tabs MC: 4 caps	GlycoN*: ½ tsp & GlycoAO: 2 caps PhytoN: ½ tsp PreH: 3 tabs Cata: 4 tabs MC: 2 caps

*For Adv.GlycoN see page 10. Product definitions are in Appendix A on page 381.

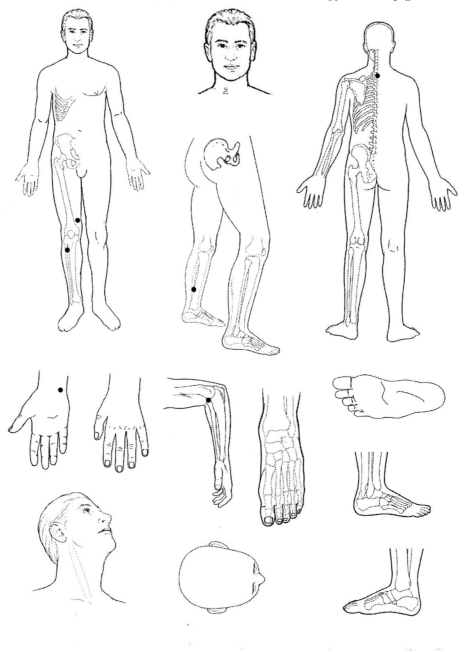

ADD w/Hyperactivity

Daily Nutritional Crisis Program	Daily Nutritional Wellness Program
GlycoN*: 2 ½ tsp & GlycoAO: 3 caps PhytoN: 1 tsp PreH: 4 tabs Cata: 4 tabs	GlycoN*: 1 ½ tsp & GlycoAO: 3 caps PhytoN: 1 tsp PreH: 3 tabs Cata: 4 tabs

*For Adv.GlycoN see page 10. Product definitions are in Appendix A on page 381.

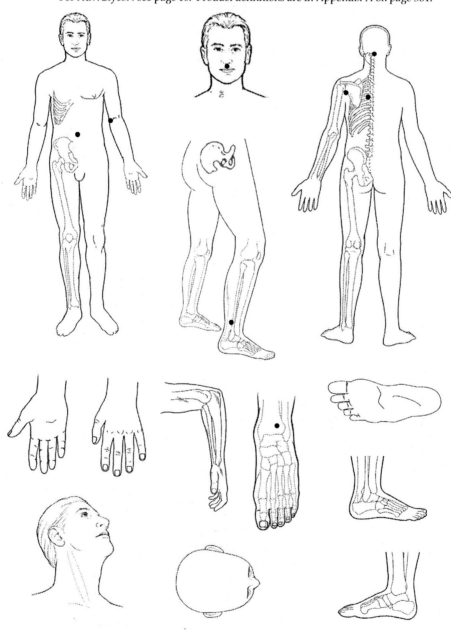

Addiction

Daily Nutritional Crisis Program	Daily Nutritional Wellness Program
GlycoN*: 2½ tsp & GlycoAO: 3 caps PhytoN: 1/4 tsp PreH: 3 tabs Cata: 6 tabs	GlycoN*: 1½ tsp & GlycoAO: 3 caps PhytoN: 1/4 tsp PreH: 3 tabs Cata: 6 tabs

*For Adv.GlycoN see page 10. Product definitions are in Appendix A on page 381.

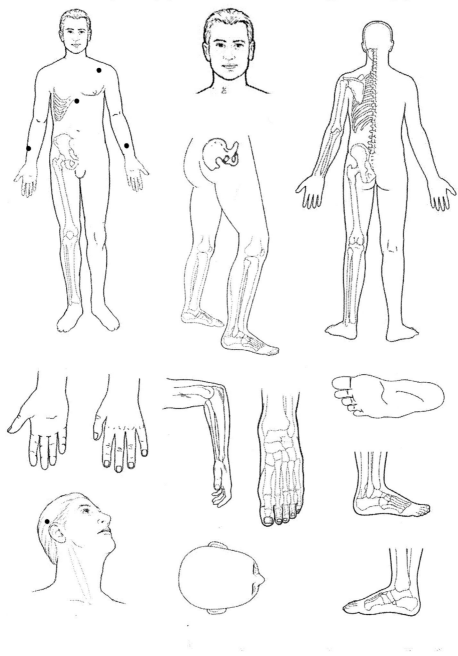

Adrenal Exhaustion

Daily Nutritional Crisis Program	Daily Nutritional Wellness Program
GlycoN*: 3½ tsp & GlycoAO: 3 caps PhytoN: 1 tsp PreH: 6 tabs Cata: 6 tabs ImmS: 4 tabs SP: 4 caps	GlycoN*: 1½ tsp & GlycoAO: 3 caps PhytoN: 1/4 tsp PreH: 3 tabs Cata: 4 tabs ImmS: 3 tabs SP: 3 caps

*For Adv.GlycoN see page 10. Product definitions are in Appendix A on page 381.

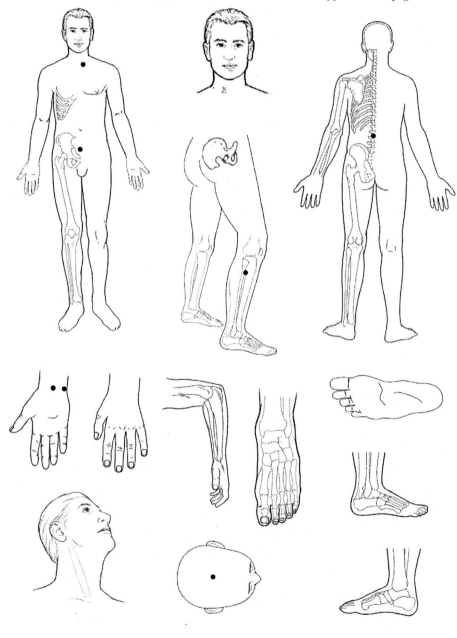

Adrenal Insufficiency (Addison's Disease)

Daily Nutritional Crisis Program	Daily Nutritional Wellness Program
GlycoN*: 3½ tsp & GlycoAO: 3 caps PhytoN: 1 tsp PreH: 6 tabs Cata: 6 tabs ImmS: 4 tabs SP: 4 caps	GlycoN*: 1½ tsp & GlycoAO: 3 caps PhytoN: 1/4 tsp PreH: 3 tabs Cata: 4 tabs ImmS: 3 tabs SP: 3 caps

*For Adv.GlycoN see page 10. Product definitions are in Appendix A on page 381.

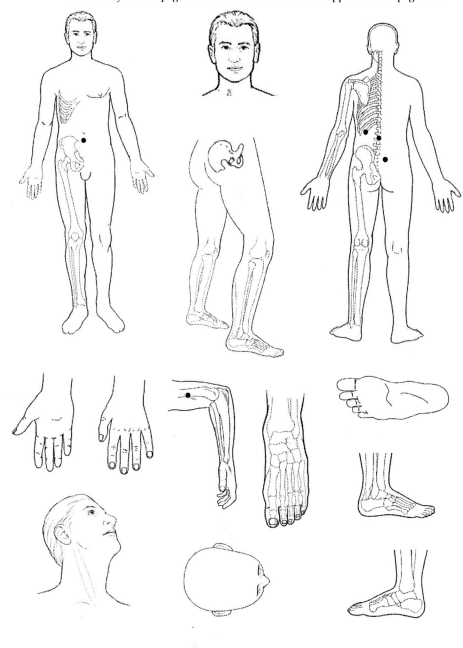

21

Adult Respiratory Distress Syndrome (ARDS)

Daily Nutritional Crisis Program	Daily Nutritional Wellness Program
GlycoN*: 10 ¾ tsp & GlycoAO: 6 caps PhytoN: 2 tsp PreH: 3 tabs Cata: 6 tabs MC: 4 caps	GlycoN*: ½ tsp & GlycoAO: 2 caps PhytoN: 1 tsp PreH: 3 tabs Cata: 4 tabs MC: 2 caps

*For Adv.GlycoN see page 10. Product definitions are in Appendix A on page 381.

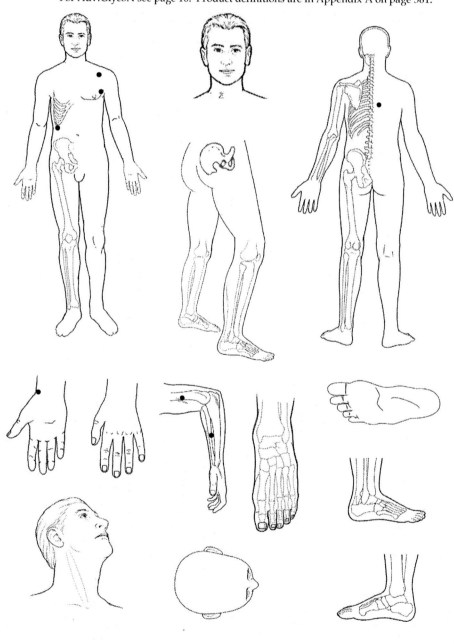

AIDS

Daily Nutritional Crisis Program	Daily Nutritional Wellness Program
GlycoN*: 10 ¾ tsp & GlycoAO: 6 caps PhytoN: 2 tsp PreH: 6 tabs Cata: 6 tabs ImmS: 6 tabs MC: 4 caps	GlycoN*: 2 ½ tsp & GlycoAO: 3 caps PhytoN: 1 tsp PreH: 3 tabs Cata: 6 tabs ImmS: 3 tabs MC: 2 caps

*For Adv.GlycoN see page 10. Product definitions are in Appendix A on page 381.

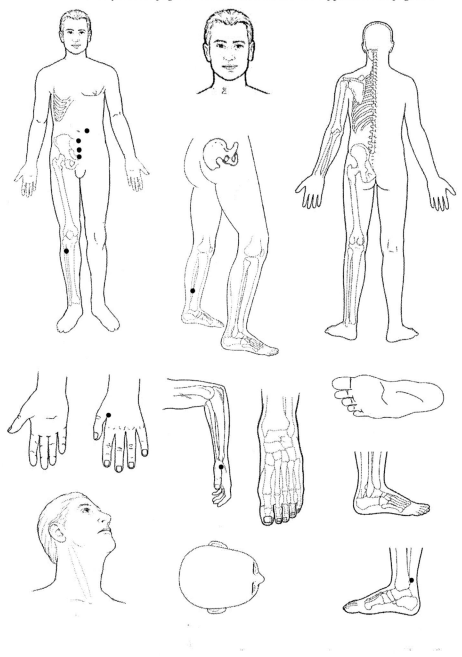

Alcohol Abuse

Daily Nutritional Crisis Program	Daily Nutritional Wellness Program
GlycoN*: 5 ¼ tsp & GlycoAO: 4 caps PhytoN: 1 tsp PreH: 6 tabs Cata: 4 tabs MC: 4 caps ImmS: 4 tabs	GlycoN*: 1 ½ tsp & GlycoAO: 3 caps PhytoN: 1/4 tsp PreH: 4 tabs Cata: 4 tabs MC: 2 caps ImmS: 2 tabs

*For Adv.GlycoN see page 10. Product definitions are in Appendix A on page 381.

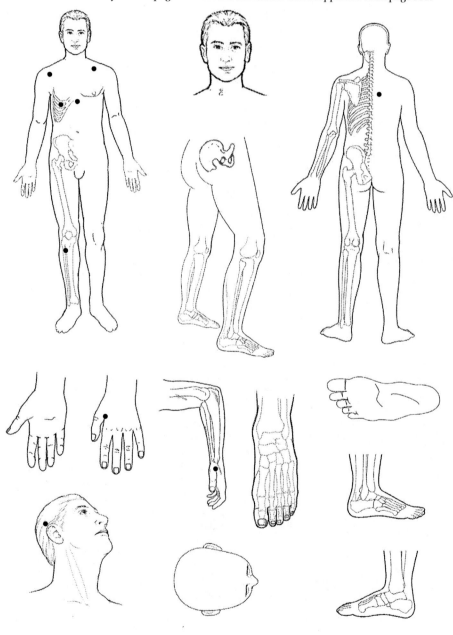

Allergic Rhinitis

Daily Nutritional Crisis Program	Daily Nutritional Wellness Program
GlycoN*: 2 ½ tsp & GlycoAO: 3 caps PhytoN: 1/4 tsp PreH: 3 tabs GEssentials: 4 tabs MC: 4 caps	GlycoN*: ½ tsp & GlycoAO: 2 caps PhytoN: 1/4 tsp PreH: 3 tabs GEssentials: 4 tabs MC: 2 caps

*For Adv.GlycoN see page 10. Product definitions are in Appendix A on page 381.

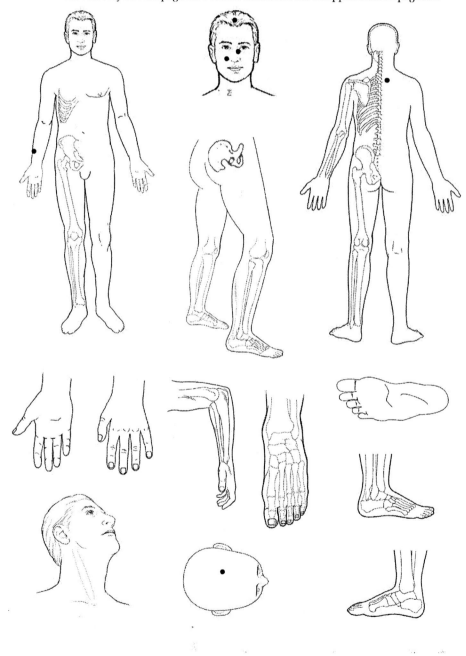

Allergy

Daily Nutritional Crisis Program	Daily Nutritional Wellness Program
GlycoN*: 2 ½ tsp & GlycoAO: 3 caps	GlycoN*: ½ tsp & GlycoAO: 2 caps
PhytoN: 1/4 tsp	PhytoN: 1/4 tsp
PreH: 3 tabs	PreH: 3 tabs
GEssentials: 4 tabs	GEssentials: 4 tabs
Clean: 3 caps twice a day (2 weeks)	Clean: 1 cap
MC: 4 caps	MC: 4 caps

*For Adv.GlycoN see page 10. Product definitions are in Appendix A on page 381.

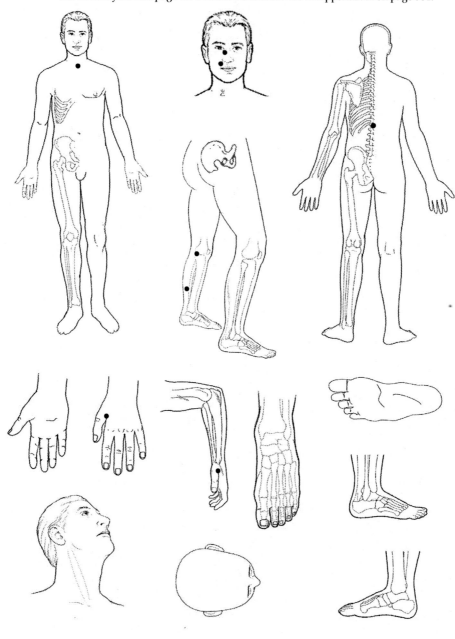

Alopecia

Daily Nutritional Crisis Program	Daily Nutritional Wellness Program
GlycoN*: 2 ½ tsp & GlycoAO: 3 caps PhytoN: 1 tsp PreH: 6 tabs GEssentials: 4 tabs	GlycoN*: ½ tsp & GlycoAO: 2 caps PhytoN: 1/4 tsp PreH: 3 tabs GEssentials: 4 tabs

*For Adv.GlycoN see page 10. Product definitions are in Appendix A on page 381.

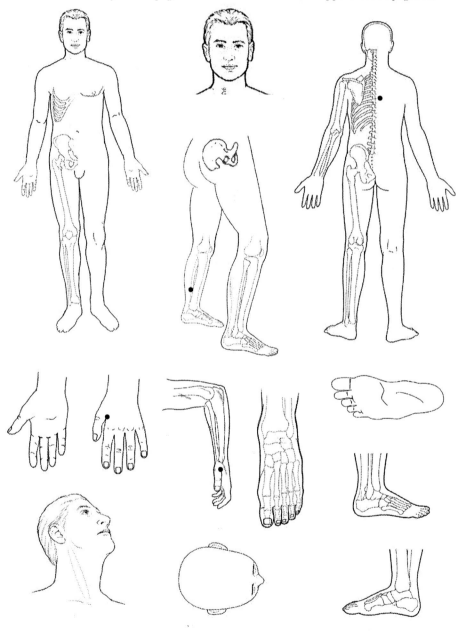

ALS (Amyotrophic Lateral Sclerosis)

Daily Nutritional Crisis Program	Daily Nutritional Wellness Program
GlycoN*: 10 ¾ tsp & GlycoAO: 6 caps PhytoN: 3 tsp PreH: 6 tabs Cata: 6 tabs MC: 4 caps ImmS: 4 tabs	GlycoN*: 5 ¼ tsp & GlycoAO: 4 caps PhytoN: 1 tsp PreH: 4 tabs Cata: 6 tabs MC: 3 caps ImmS: 3 tabs

*For Adv.GlycoN see page 10. Product definitions are in Appendix A on page 381.

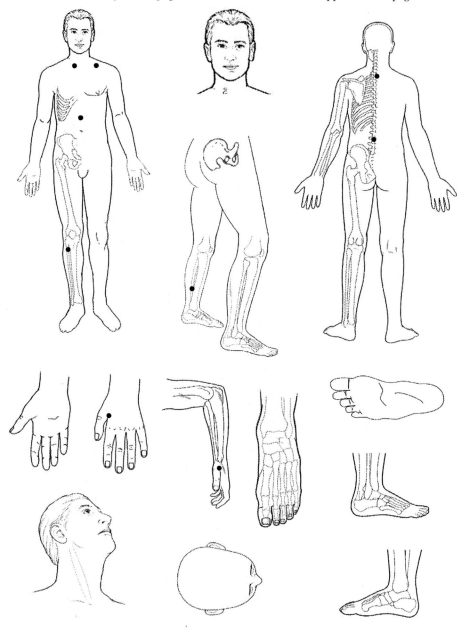

Alzheimer's (Dementia)

Daily Nutritional Crisis Program	Daily Nutritional Wellness Program
GlycoN*: 10 ¾ tsp & GlycoAO: 6 caps	GlycoN*: 5 ¼ tsp & GlycoAO: 4 caps
PhytoN: 1 tsp	PhytoN: 1 tsp
PreH: 6 tabs	PreH: 6 tabs
Cata: 6 tabs	Cata: 6 tabs
ImmS: 4 tabs	ImmS: 2 tabs
Clean: 3 caps twice a day (2 weeks)	Clean: 1 cap

*For Adv.GlycoN see page 10. Product definitions are in Appendix A on page 381.

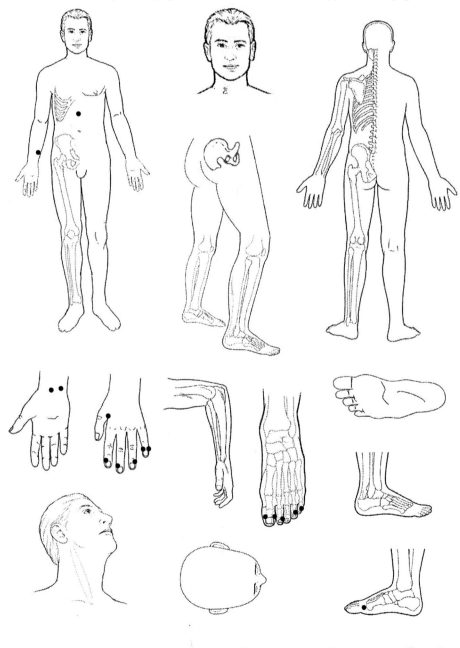

Amalgam Toxicity

Daily Nutritional Crisis Program	Daily Nutritional Wellness Program
GlycoN*: 5 ¼ tsp & GlycoAO: 4 caps PhytoN: 1 tsp PreH: 3 tabs Cata: 6 tabs Clean: 3 caps twice a day (2 weeks) ImmS: 4 tabs	GlycoN*: 1 ½ tsp & GlycoAO: 3 caps PhytoN: 1/4 tsp PreH: 3 tabs Cata: 6 tabs Clean: 1 cap ImmS: 2 tabs

*For Adv.GlycoN see page 10. Product definitions are in Appendix A on page 381.

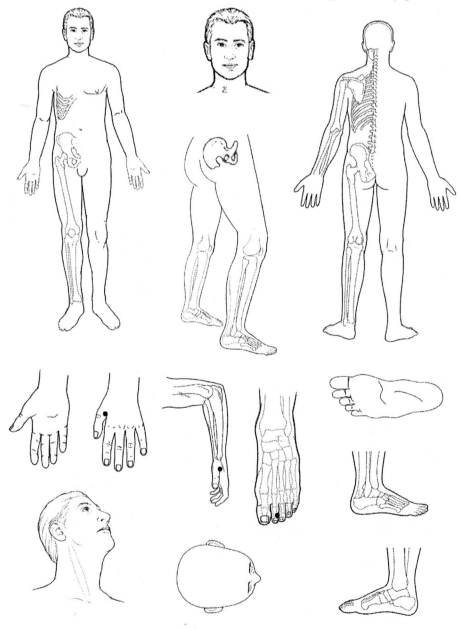

30

Amenorrhea

Daily Nutritional Crisis Program	Daily Nutritional Wellness Program
GlycoN*: 2 ½ tsp & GlycoAO: 3 caps PhytoN: 1 tsp PreH: 6 tabs Cata: 4 tabs	GlycoN*: 1 ½ tsp & GlycoAO: 3 caps PhytoN: 1/4 tsp PreH: 4 tabs Cata: 4 tabs

*For Adv.GlycoN see page 10. Product definitions are in Appendix A on page 381.

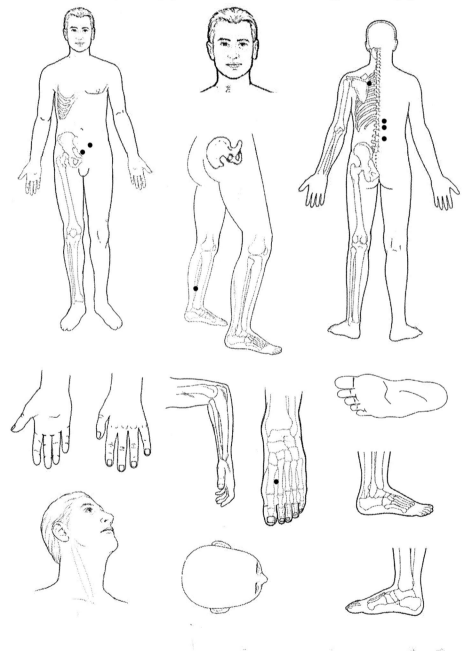

Amyotrophic Lateral Sclerosis (ALS)

Daily Nutritional Crisis Program	Daily Nutritional Wellness Program
GlycoN*: 10 ¾ tsp & GlycoAO: 6 caps PhytoN: 1 tsp PreH: 6 tabs Cata: 6 tabs	GlycoN*: 5 ¼ tsp & GlycoAO: 4 caps PhytoN: 1 tsp PreH: 4 tabs Cata: 6 tabs

*For Adv.GlycoN see page 10. Product definitions are in Appendix A on page 381.

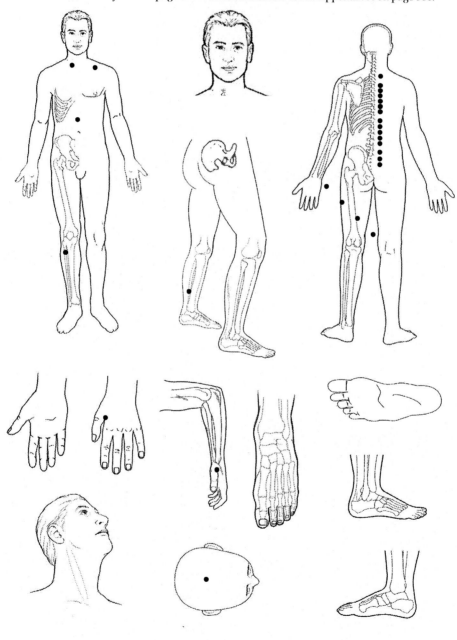

Anemia

Daily Nutritional Crisis Program	Daily Nutritional Wellness Program
GlycoN*: 2 ½ tsp & GlycoAO: 3 caps PhytoN: 1 tsp PreH: 3 tabs GEssentials: 4 tabs MC: 3 caps	GlycoN*: 1 ½ tsp & GlycoAO: 3 caps PhytoN: 1 tsp PreH: 3 tabs GEssentials: 4 tabs MC: 2 caps

*For Adv.GlycoN see page 10. Product definitions are in Appendix A on page 381.

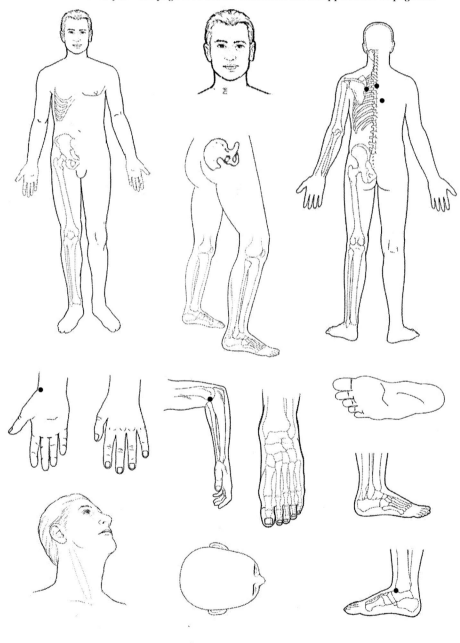

Anemia, Sickle Cell

Daily Nutritional Crisis Program	Daily Nutritional Wellness Program
GlycoN*: 2 ½ tsp & GlycoAO: 3 caps PhytoN: 1 tsp PreH: 3 tabs GEssentials: 4 tabs MC: 3 caps	GlycoN*: 1 ½ tsp & GlycoAO: 3 caps PhytoN: 1 tsp PreH: 3 tabs GEssentials: 4 tabs MC: 2 caps

*For Adv.GlycoN see page 10. Product definitions are in Appendix A on page 381.

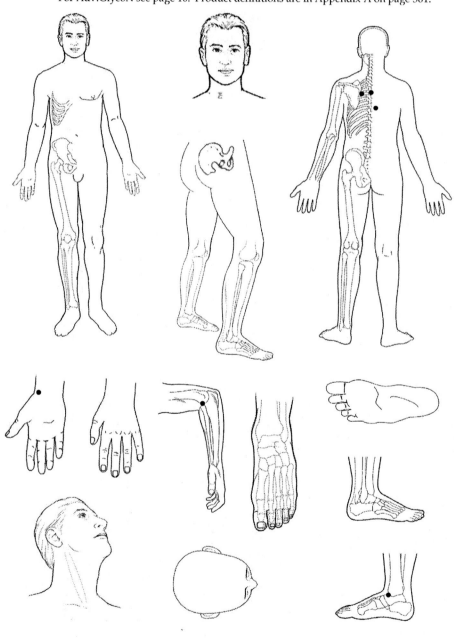

Aneurysm (Aortic)

Daily Nutritional Crisis Program	Daily Nutritional Wellness Program
GlycoN*: 5 ¼ tsp & GlycoAO: 4 caps PhytoN: 2 tsp PreH: 4 tabs GEssentials: 4 tabs MC: 4 caps	GlycoN*: 2 ½ tsp & GlycoAO: 3 caps PhytoN: 1 tsp PreH: 3 tabs GEssentials: 4 tabs MC: 2 caps

*For Adv.GlycoN see page 10. Product definitions are in Appendix A on page 381.

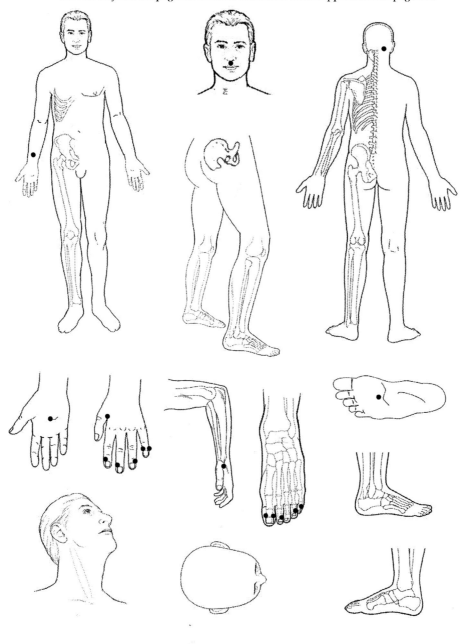

35

Angina Pectoris

Daily Nutritional Crisis Program	Daily Nutritional Wellness Program
GlycoN*: 5 ¼ tsp & GlycoAO: 4 caps PhytoN: 1 tsp PreH: 4 tabs Cata: 6 tabs CB: 6 caps	GlycoN*: 1 ½ tsp & GlycoAO: 3 caps PhytoN: 1 tsp PreH: 3 tabs Cata: 6 tabs CB: 4 caps

*For Adv.GlycoN see page 10. Product definitions are in Appendix A on page 381.

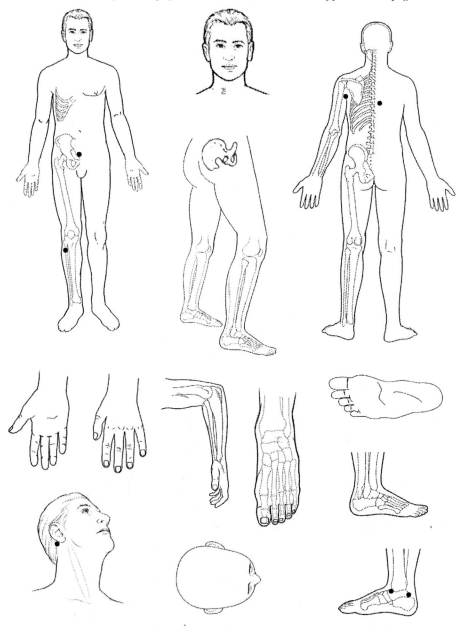

Angioneurotic Edema

Daily Nutritional Crisis Program	Daily Nutritional Wellness Program
GlycoN*: 5 ¼ tsp & GlycoAO: 4 caps PhytoN: 1 tsp PreH: 4 tabs Cata: 6 tabs MC: 3 caps	GlycoN*: 1 ½ tsp & GlycoAO: 3 caps PhytoN: 1 tsp PreH: 3 tabs Cata: 4 tabs MC: 2 caps

*For Adv.GlycoN see page 10. Product definitions are in Appendix A on page 381.

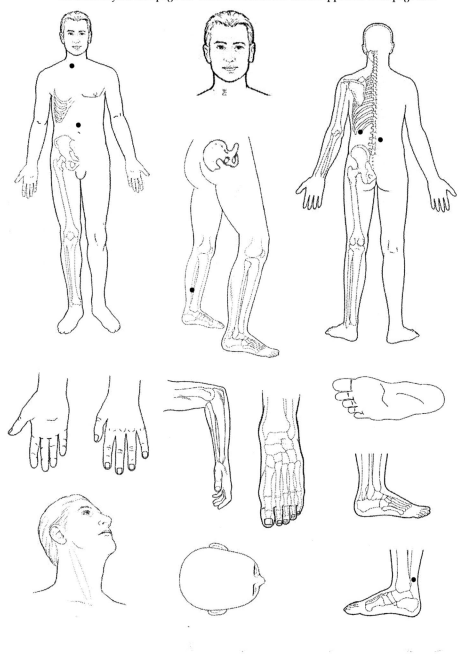

Ankylosing Spondylitis (AS)

Daily Nutritional Crisis Program	Daily Nutritional Wellness Program
GlycoN*: 1 ½ tsp & GlycoAO: 3 caps PhytoN: 1/4 tsp PreH: 6 tabs GEssentials: 4 tabs MC: 4 caps	GlycoN*: 1 ½ tsp & GlycoAO: 3 caps PhytoN: 1/4 tsp PreH: 3 tabs GEssentials: 4 tabs MC: 2 caps

*For Adv.GlycoN see page 10. Product definitions are in Appendix A on page 381.

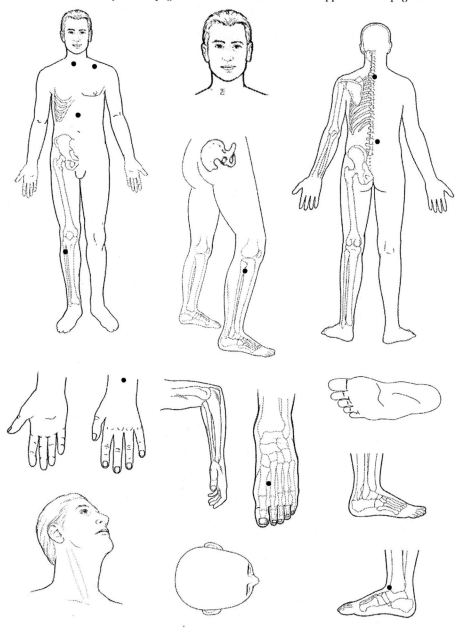

Anorexia

Daily Nutritional Crisis Program	Daily Nutritional Wellness Program
GlycoN*: 3 ½ tsp & GlycoAO: 3 caps PhytoN: 1 tsp PreH: 6 tabs GEssentials: 4 tabs GstroP: 3 caps ImmS: 4 tabs	GlycoN*: 1 ½ tsp & GlycoAO: 3 caps PhytoN: 1 tsp PreH: 4 tabs GEssentials: 4 tabs GstroP: 2 caps ImmS: 2 tabs

*For Adv.GlycoN see page 10. Product definitions are in Appendix A on page 381.

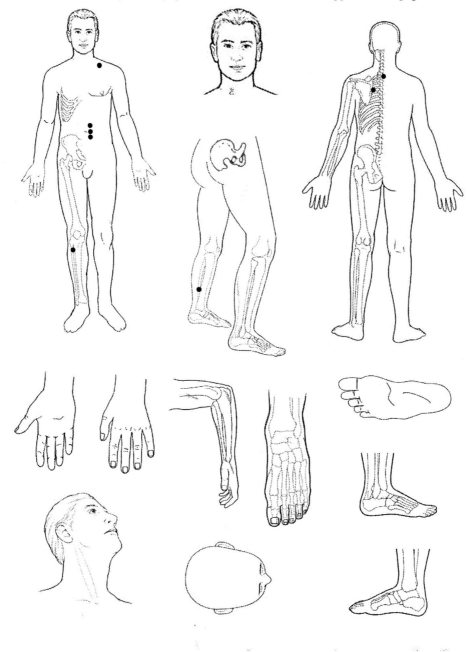

Anorexia Nervosa

Daily Nutritional Crisis Program	Daily Nutritional Wellness Program
GlycoN*: 3 ½ tsp & GlycoAO: 3 caps PhytoN: 1 tsp PreH: 6 tabs GEssentials: 4 tabs GstroP: 3 caps ImmS: 4 tabs	GlycoN*: 1 ½ tsp & GlycoAO: 3 caps PhytoN: 1 tsp PreH: 4 tabs GEssentials: 4 tabs GstroP: 2 caps ImmS: 2 tabs

*For Adv.GlycoN see page 10. Product definitions are in Appendix A on page 381.

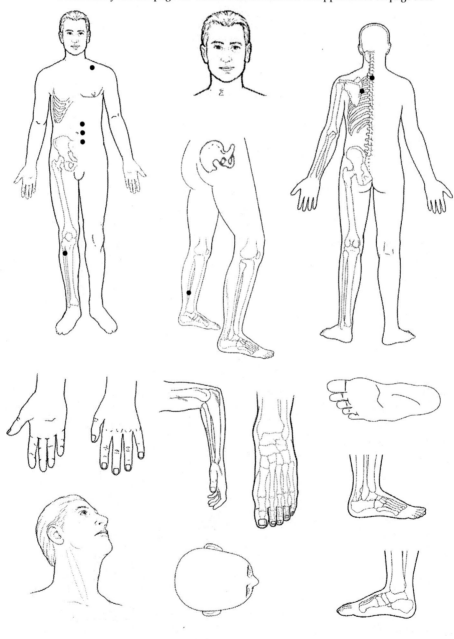

Antihistamine

Daily Nutritional Crisis Program	Daily Nutritional Wellness Program
GlycoN*: 1 ½ tsp & GlycoAO: 3 caps	GlycoN*: ½ tsp & GlycoAO: 2 caps
PhytoN: 1 tsp	PhytoN: 1/4 tsp
PreH: 4 tabs	PreH: 3 tabs
GEssentials: 4 tabs	GEssentials: 4 tabs
Clean: 3 caps twice a day (2 weeks)	Clean: 2 caps
MC: 5 caps	MC: 3 caps

*For Adv.GlycoN see page 10. Product definitions are in Appendix A on page 381.

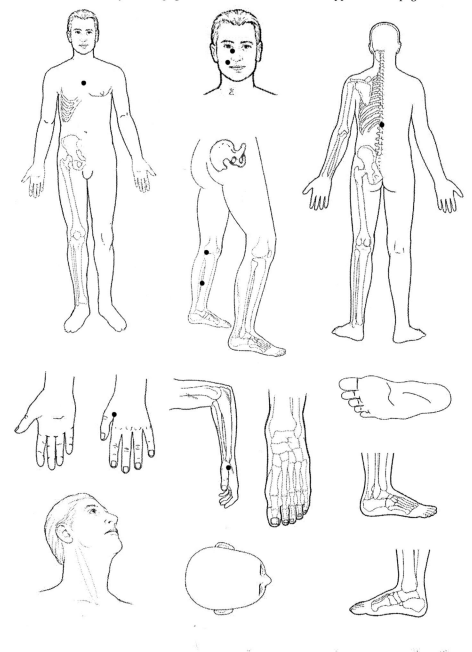

Anxiety

Daily Nutritional Crisis Program	Daily Nutritional Wellness Program
GlycoN*: 2 ½ tsp & GlycoAO: 3 caps PhytoN: 1 tsp PreH: 6 tabs GEssentials: 4 tabs SP: 4 caps	GlycoN*: ½ tsp & GlycoAO: 2 caps PhytoN: 1/4 tsp PreH: 3 tabs GEssentials: 4 tabs SP: 2 caps

*For Adv.GlycoN see page 10. Product definitions are in Appendix A on page 381.

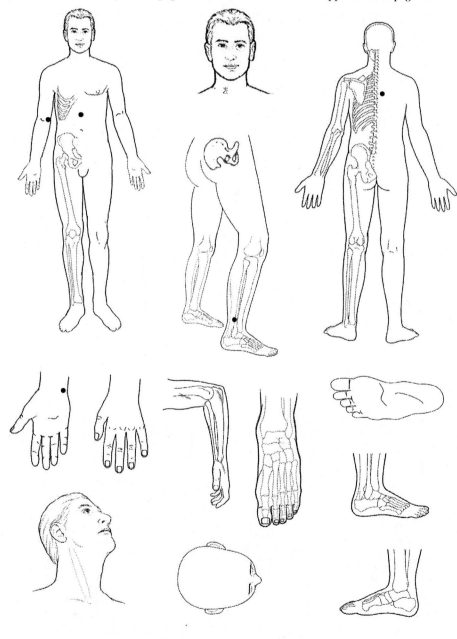

Aphthous Ulcer (Canker Sore)

Daily Nutritional Crisis Program	Daily Nutritional Wellness Program
GlycoN*: 2 ½ tsp & GlycoAO: 3 caps PhytoN: 1/4 tsp PreH: 4 tabs GEssentials: 4 tabs ImmS: 5 tabs MC: 4 caps	GlycoN*: ½ tsp & GlycoAO: 2 caps PhytoN: 1/4 tsp PreI I: 3 tabs GEssentials: 4 tabs ImmS: 3 tabs MC: 2 caps

*For Adv.GlycoN see page 10. Product definitions are in Appendix A on page 381.

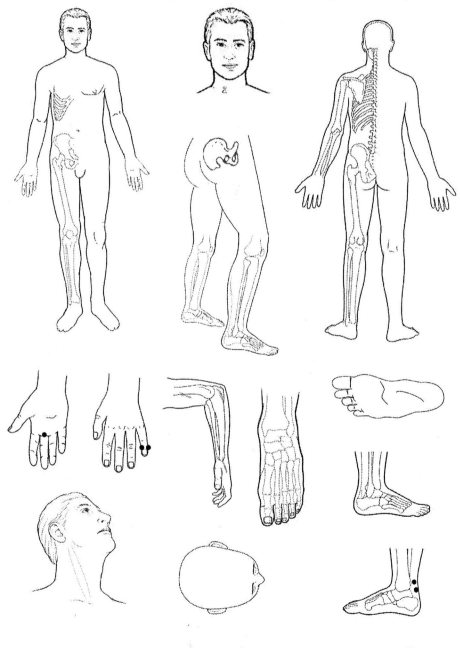

Arrhythmia

Daily Nutritional Crisis Program	Daily Nutritional Wellness Program
GlycoN*: 5 ¼ tsp & GlycoAO: 4 caps PhytoN: 1 tsp PreH: 4 tabs Cata: 6 tabs CB: 6 caps	GlycoN*: 1 ½ tsp & GlycoAO: 3 caps PhytoN: 3/4 tsp PreH: 3 tabs Cata: 6 tabs CB: 3 caps

*For Adv.GlycoN see page 10. Product definitions are in Appendix A on page 381.

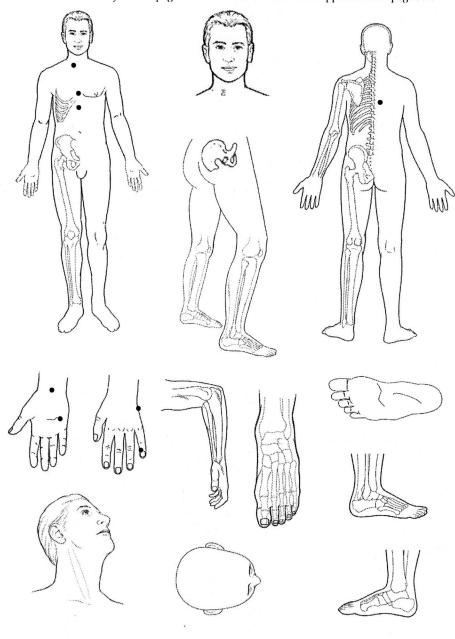

Arterial Insufficiency

Daily Nutritional Crisis Program	Daily Nutritional Wellness Program
GlycoN*: 5 ¼ tsp & GlycoAO: 4 caps PhytoN: 1 tsp PreH: 6 tabs Cata: 6 tabs MC: 4 caps	GlycoN*: 1 ½ tsp & GlycoAO: 3 caps PhytoN: 3/4 tsp PreH: 3 tabs Cata: 6 tabs MC: 2 caps

*For Adv.GlycoN see page 10. Product definitions are in Appendix A on page 381.

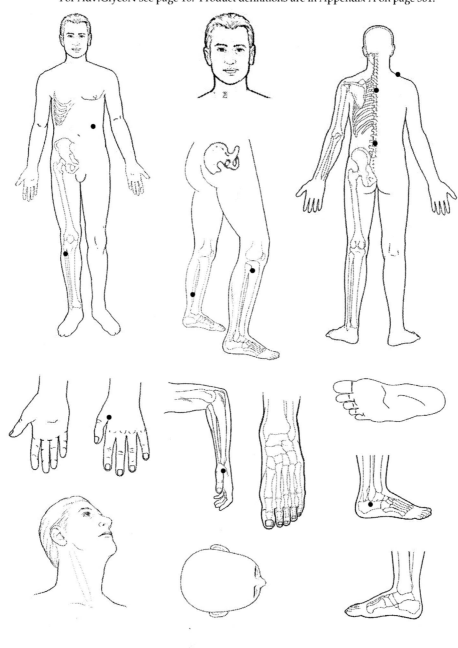

Arthralgia

Daily Nutritional Crisis Program	Daily Nutritional Wellness Program
GlycoN*: 5 ¼ tsp & GlycoAO: 4 caps PhytoN: 1 tsp PreH: 6 tabs Cata: 6 tabs SP: 3 caps Clean: 3 caps twice a day (2 weeks)	GlycoN*: 1 ½ tsp & GlycoAO: 3 caps PhytoN: 3/4 tsp PreH: 4 tabs Cata: 6 tabs SP: 2 caps Clean: 1 cap

*For Adv.GlycoN see page 10. Product definitions are in Appendix A on page 381.

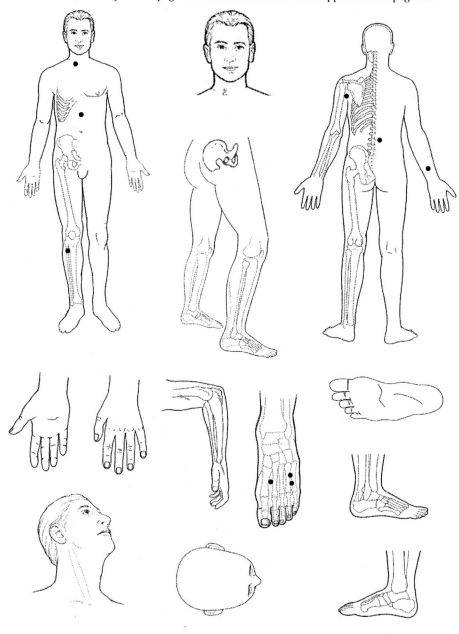

Arthritis

Daily Nutritional Crisis Program	Daily Nutritional Wellness Program
GlycoN*: 5 ¼ tsp & GlycoAO: 4 caps PhytoN: 1 tsp PreH: 6 tabs Cata: 6 tabs Clean: 3 caps twice a day (2 weeks) MC: 4 caps	GlycoN*: 1 ½ tsp & GlycoAO: 3 caps PhytoN: 3/4 tsp PreH: 4 tabs Cata: 6 tabs Clean: 1 cap MC: 2 caps

*For Adv.GlycoN see page 10. Product definitions are in Appendix A on page 381.

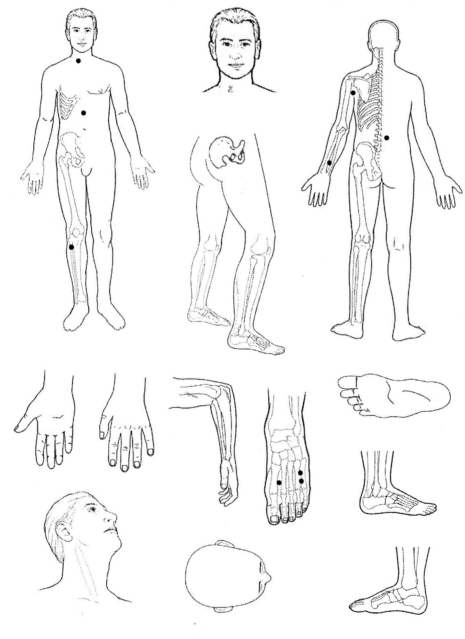

AS (Ankylosing Spondylitis)

Daily Nutritional Crisis Program	Daily Nutritional Wellness Program
GlycoN*: 1 ½ tsp & GlycoAO: 3 caps PhytoN: 1/2 tsp PreH: 6 tabs Cata: 4 tabs MC: 4 caps	GlycoN*: 1 ½ tsp & GlycoAO: 3 caps PhytoN: 1/4 tsp PreH: 3 tabs Cata: 4 tabs MC: 2 caps

*For Adv.GlycoN see page 10. Product definitions are in Appendix A on page 381.

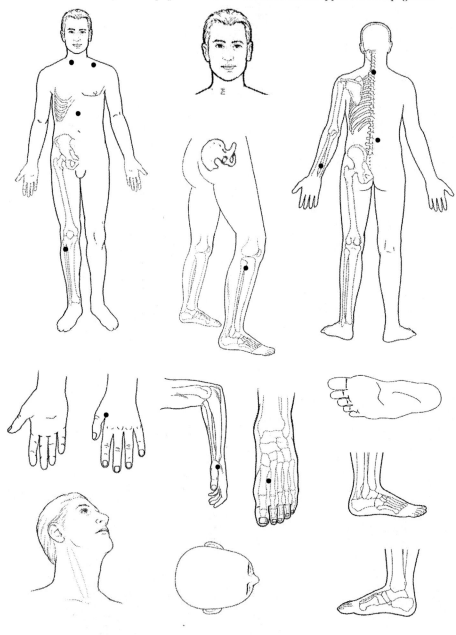

ASHD/CAD (Atherosclerotic Heart Disease)

Daily Nutritional Crisis Program	Daily Nutritional Wellness Program
GlycoN*: 5 ¼ tsp & GlycoAO: 4 caps PhytoN: 2 tsp PreH: 4 tabs Cata: 4 tabs CB: 5 caps	GlycoN*: 1 ½ tsp & GlycoAO: 3 caps PhytoN: 1 tsp PreH: 4 tabs Cata: 4 tabs CB: 3 caps

*For Adv.GlycoN see page 10. Product definitions are in Appendix A on page 381.

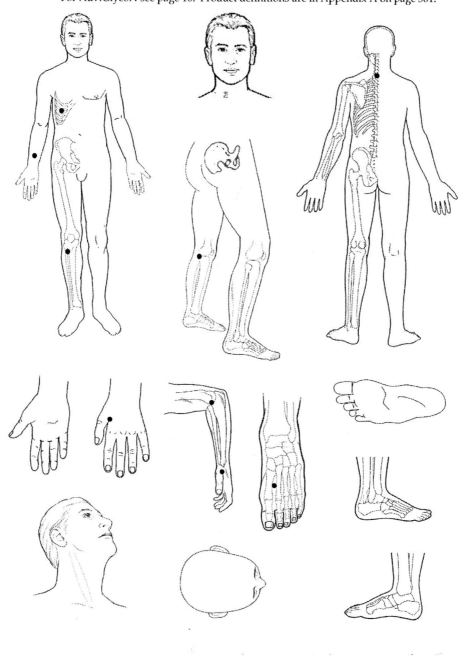

Asthma w/o Status Asthmaticus

Daily Nutritional Crisis Program	Daily Nutritional Wellness Program
GlycoN*: 5 ¼ tsp & GlycoAO: 4 caps PhytoN: 1 tsp PreH: 4 tabs Cata: 4 tabs Clean: 3 caps twice a day (3 weeks) ImmS: 5 tabs	GlycoN*: 1 ½ tsp & GlycoAO: 3 caps PhytoN: 3/4 tsp PreH: 3 tabs Cata: 4 tabs Clean: 2 caps ImmS: 3 tabs

*For Adv.GlycoN see page 10. Product definitions are in Appendix A on page 381.

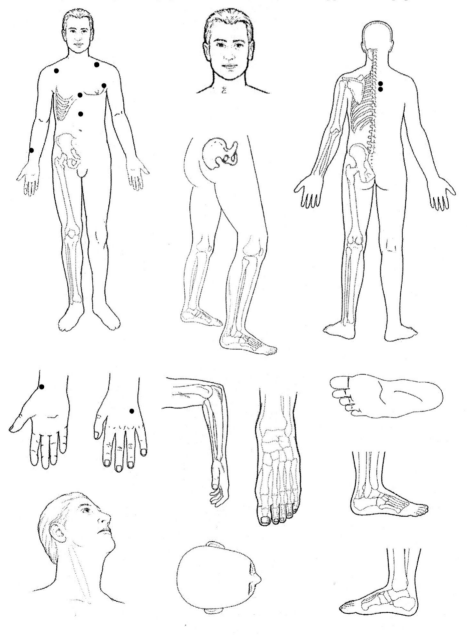

Athlete's Foot

Daily Nutritional Crisis Program	Daily Nutritional Wellness Program
GlycoN*: 1 ½ tsp & GlycoAO: 3 caps PhytoN: 1/2 tsp PreH: 3 tabs GEssentials: 4 tabs Clean: 3 caps twice a day (2 weeks) ImmS: 4 tabs	GlycoN*: 1/2 tsp & GlycoAO: 2 caps PhytoN: 1/4 tsp PreH: 3 tabs GEssentials: 4 tabs Clean: 1 cap ImmS: 2 tabs

*For Adv.GlycoN see page 10. Product definitions are in Appendix A on page 381.

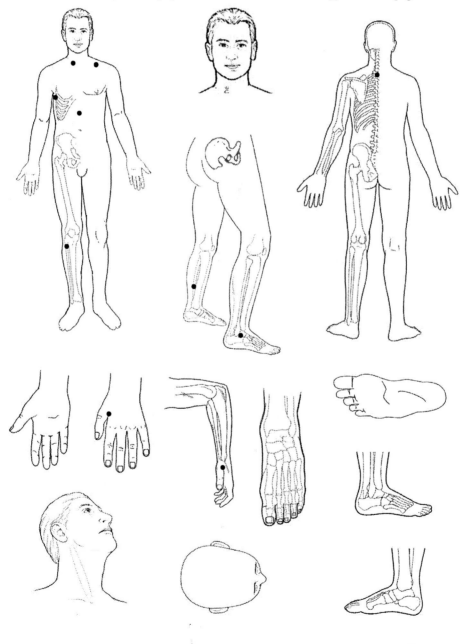

Atrial Fibrillation

Daily Nutritional Crisis Program	Daily Nutritional Wellness Program
GlycoN*: 5 ¼ tsp & GlycoAO: 4 caps PhytoN: 1 tsp PreH: 3 tabs Cata: 6 tabs CB: 6 caps	GlycoN*: 1 ½ tsp & GlycoAO: 3 caps PhytoN: 3/4 tsp PreH: 3 tabs Cata: 6 tabs CB: 4 caps

*For Adv.GlycoN see page 10. Product definitions are in Appendix A on page 381.

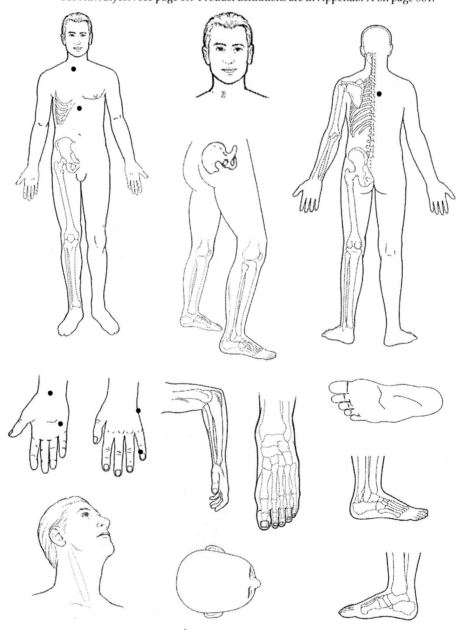

Atrial Flutter

Daily Nutritional Crisis Program	Daily Nutritional Wellness Program
GlycoN*: 5 ¼ tsp & GlycoAO: 4 caps PhytoN: 1 tsp PreH: 3 tabs Cata: 6 tabs CB: 6 caps	GlycoN*: 1 ½ tsp & GlycoAO: 3 caps PhytoN: 3/4 tsp PreH: 3 tabs Cata: 6 tabs CB: 4 caps

*For Adv.GlycoN see page 10. Product definitions are in Appendix A on page 381.

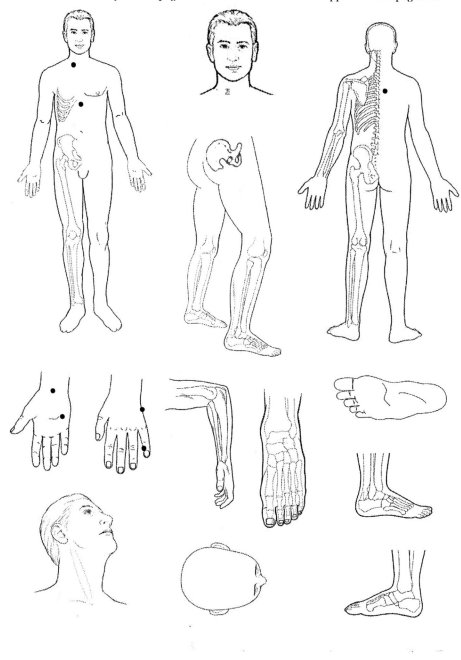

Attention Deficit Disorder (ADD)

Daily Nutritional Crisis Program	Daily Nutritional Wellness Program
GlycoN*: 2 ½ tsp & GlycoAO: 3 caps PhytoN: 1 tsp PreH: 4 tabs Cata: 4 tabs	GlycoN*: 1 ½ tsp & GlycoAO: 3 caps PhytoN: 1 tsp PreH: 3 tabs Cata: 4 tabs

*For Adv.GlycoN see page 10. Product definitions are in Appendix A on page 381.

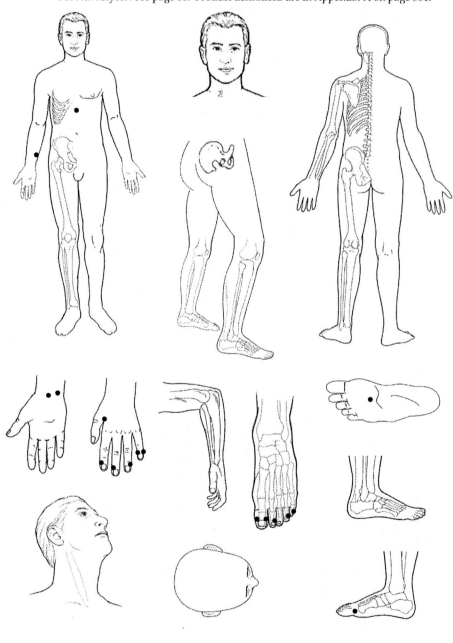

Autism

Daily Nutritional Crisis Program	Daily Nutritional Wellness Program
GlycoN*: 5 ¼ tsp & GlycoAO: 4 caps PhytoN: 1 tsp PreH: 6 tabs Cata: 4 tabs	GlycoN*: 1 ½ tsp & GlycoAO: 3 caps PhytoN: 1 tsp PreH: 3 tabs Cata: 4 tabs

*For Adv.GlycoN see page 10. Product definitions are in Appendix A on page 381.

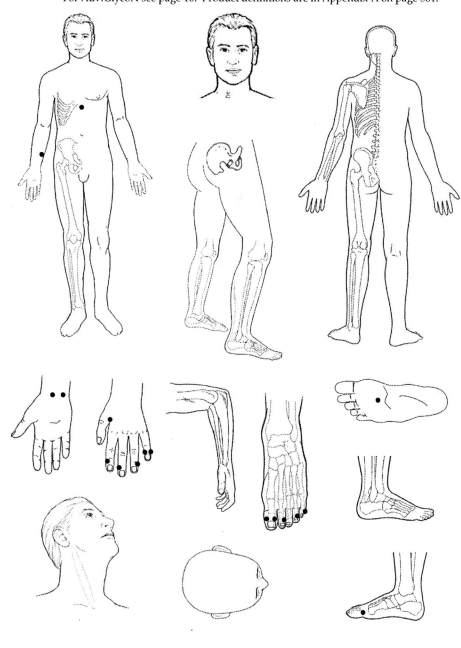

Back Pain w/ Radiation

Daily Nutritional Crisis Program	Daily Nutritional Wellness Program
GlycoN*: 5 ¼ tsp & GlycoAO: 4 caps PhytoN: 1 tsp PreH: 6 tabs Cata: 4 tabs SP: 6 caps	GlycoN*: 1 ½ tsp & GlycoAO: 3 caps PhytoN: 3/4 tsp PreH: 3 tabs Cata: 4 tabs SP: 3 caps

*For Adv.GlycoN see page 10. Product definitions are in Appendix A on page 381.

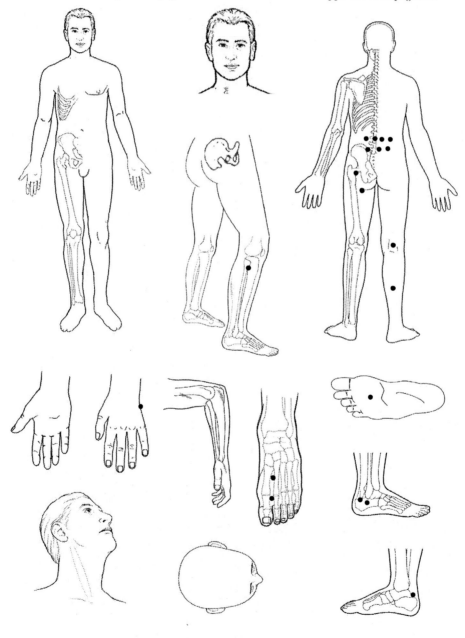

Bacteremia (Not Septicemia)

Daily Nutritional Crisis Program	Daily Nutritional Wellness Program
GlycoN*: 5 ¼ tsp & GlycoAO: 4 caps PhytoN: 1 tsp PreH: 6 tabs Cata: 4 tabs MC: 6 caps ImmS: 8 tabs	GlycoN*: ½ tsp & GlycoAO: 2 caps PhytoN: 1/4 tsp PreH: 3 tabs Cata: 4 tabs MC: 3 caps ImmS: 4 tabs

*For Adv.GlycoN see page 10. Product definitions are in Appendix A on page 381.

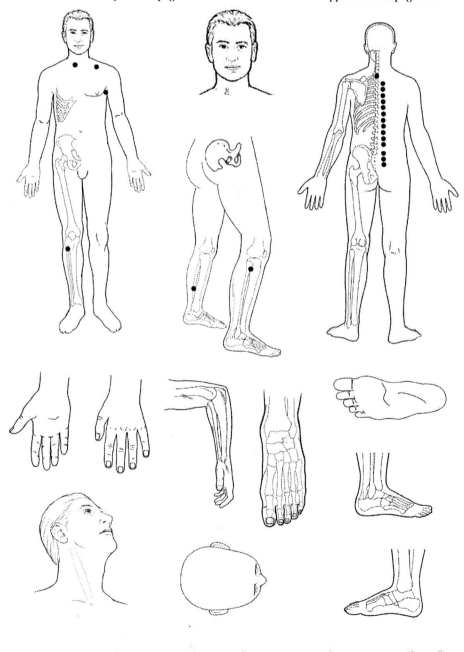

Bacterial Infection

Daily Nutritional Crisis Program	Daily Nutritional Wellness Program
GlycoN*: 5 ¼ tsp & GlycoAO: 4 caps PhytoN: 1 tsp PreH: 6 tabs Cata: 4 tabs MC: 6 caps ImmS: 8 tabs	GlycoN*: ½ tsp & GlycoAO: 2 caps PhytoN: 1/4 tsp PreH: 3 tabs Cata: 4 tabs MC: 3 caps ImmS: 4 tabs

*For Adv.GlycoN see page 10. Product definitions are in Appendix A on page 381.

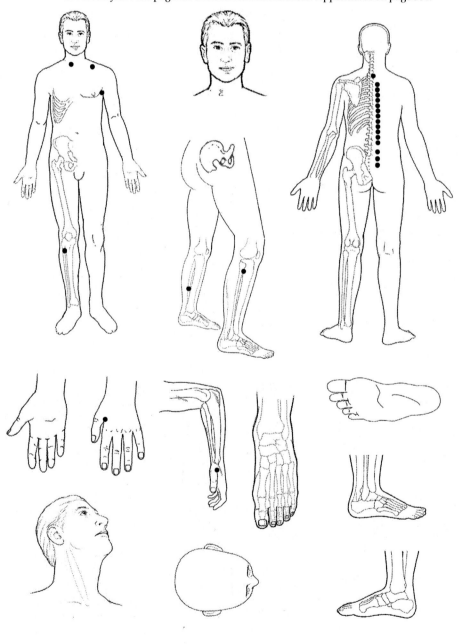

Bed Sores
(apply soft laser to affect areas)

Daily Nutritional Crisis Program	Daily Nutritional Wellness Program
GlycoN*: 5 ¼ tsp & GlycoAO: 4 caps PhytoN: 1 tsp PreH: 4 tabs Cata: 6 tabs MC: 8 caps SkZone: apply to area	GlycoN*: 1 ½ tsp & GlycoAO: 3 caps PhytoN: 1 tsp PreH: 3 tabs Cata: 4 tabs MC: 4 caps SkZone: apply to area

*For Adv.GlycoN see page 10. Product definitions are in Appendix A on page 381.

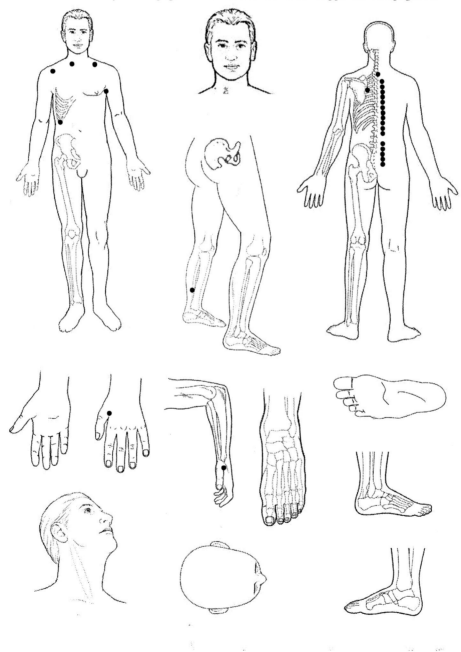

Bell's Palsy

Daily Nutritional Crisis Program	Daily Nutritional Wellness Program
GlycoN*: 2 ½ tsp & GlycoAO: 3 caps PhytoN: 1/2 tsp PreH: 4 tabs Cata: 4 tabs ImmS: 6 tabs MC: 5 caps	GlycoN*: 1 ½ tsp & GlycoAO: 3 caps PhytoN: 1/4 tsp PreH: 3 tabs Cata: 4 tabs ImmS: 4 tabs MC: 3 caps

*For Adv.GlycoN see page 10. Product definitions are in Appendix A on page 381.

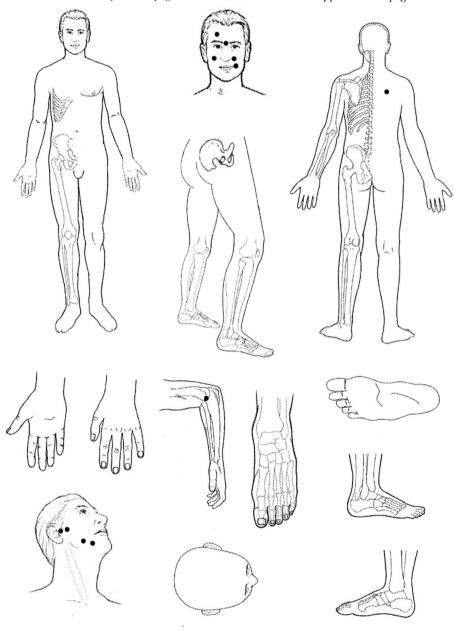

Bipolar Affective Disorder

Daily Nutritional Crisis Program	Daily Nutritional Wellness Program
GlycoN*: 5 ¼ tsp & GlycoAO: 4 caps PhytoN: 1 tsp PreH: 6 tabs Cata: 6 tabs Clean: 3 caps twice a day (2 weeks)	GlycoN*: 1 ½ tsp & GlycoAO: 3 caps PhytoN: 3/4 tsp PreH: 4 tabs Cata: 4 tabs Clean: 1 cap

*For Adv.GlycoN see page 10. Product definitions are in Appendix A on page 381.

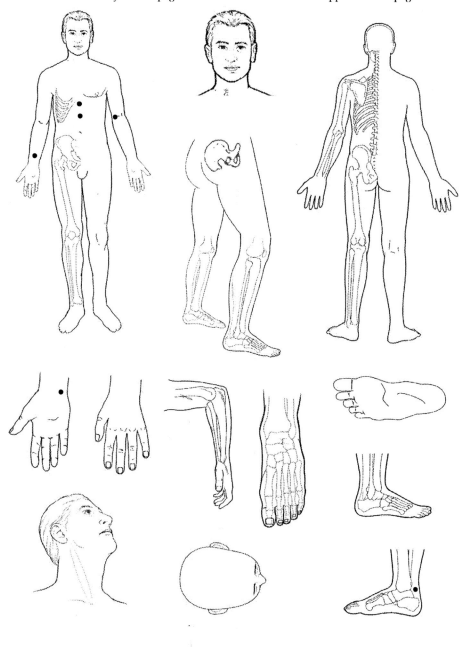

Bladder Problems

Daily Nutritional Crisis Program	Daily Nutritional Wellness Program
GlycoN*: 2 ½ tsp & GlycoAO: 3 caps	GlycoN*: ½ tsp & GlycoAO: 2 caps
PhytoN: 1/2 tsp	PhytoN: 1/4 tsp
PreH: 3 tabs	PreH: 3 tabs
GEssentials: 4 tabs	GEssentials: 4 tabs
ImmS: 6 tabs	ImmS: 4 tabs
MC: 4 caps	MC: 2 caps

*For Adv.GlycoN see page 10. Product definitions are in Appendix A on page 381.

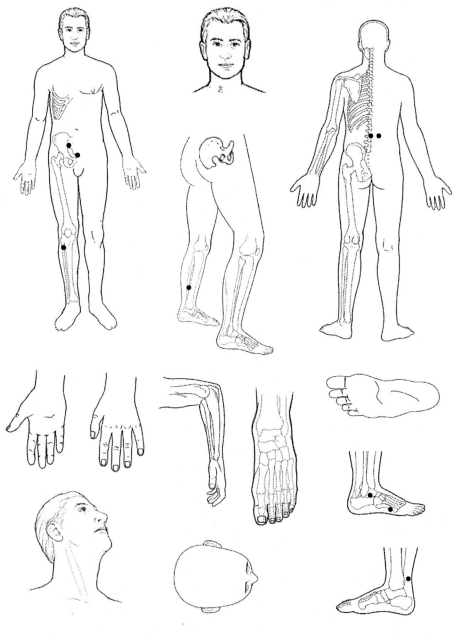

Bloating / Flatulence / Gas

Daily Nutritional Crisis Program	Daily Nutritional Wellness Program
GlycoN*: 2 ½ tsp & GlycoAO: 3 caps	GlycoN*: ½ tsp & GlycoAO: 2 caps
PhytoN: 1/2 tsp	PhytoN: 1/4 tsp
PreH: 4 tabs	PreH: 3 tabs
GEssentials: 4 tabs	GEssentials: 4 tabs
GstroP: 3 caps	GstroP: 2 caps
GstroZ: 2 caps before meals	GstroZ: 1 cap before meals

*For Adv.GlycoN see page 10. Product definitions are in Appendix A on page 381.

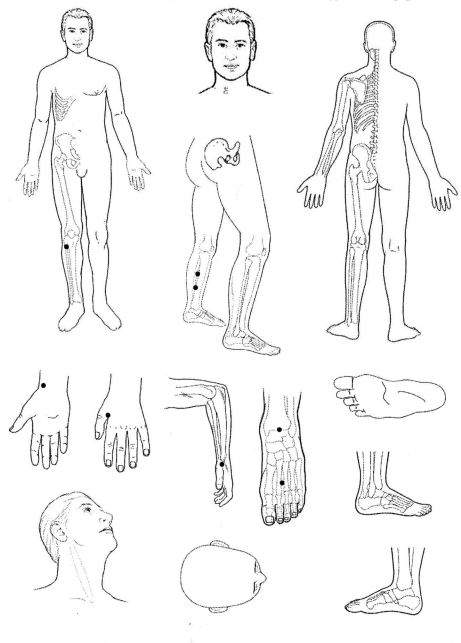

Blocked Tear Duct Lacrimal Duct Obstruction

Daily Nutritional Crisis Program	Daily Nutritional Wellness Program
GlycoN*: ½ tsp & GlycoAO: 2 caps PhytoN: 1/4 tsp PreH: 3 tabs GEssentials: 4 tabs ImmS: 4 tabs	GlycoN*: 1/2 tsp & GlycoAO: 1 caps PhytoN: 1/4 tsp PreH: 3 tabs GEssentials: 4 tabs ImmS: 2 tabs

*For Adv.GlycoN see page 10. Product definitions are in Appendix A on page 381.

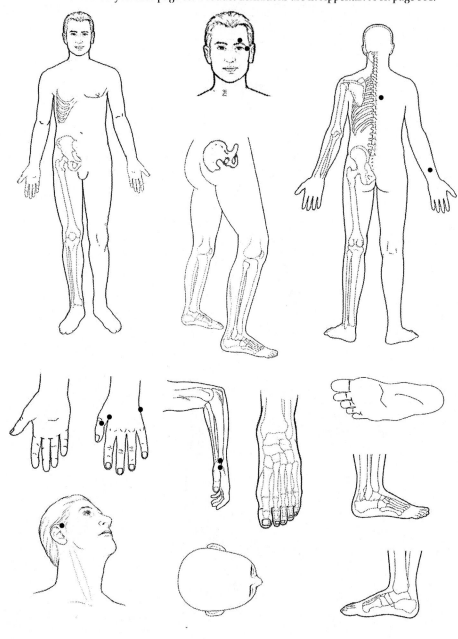

Blood Pressure (Elevated w/o Hypertension)

Daily Nutritional Crisis Program	Daily Nutritional Wellness Program
GlycoN*: 5 ¼ tsp & GlycoAO: 4 caps PhytoN: 1 tsp PreH: 6 tabs Cata: 4 tabs CB: 5 caps	GlycoN*: 1 ½ tsp & GlycoAO: 3 caps PhytoN: 3/4 tsp PreH: 3 tabs Cata: 4 tabs CB: 3 caps

*For Adv.GlycoN see page 10. Product definitions are in Appendix A on page 381.

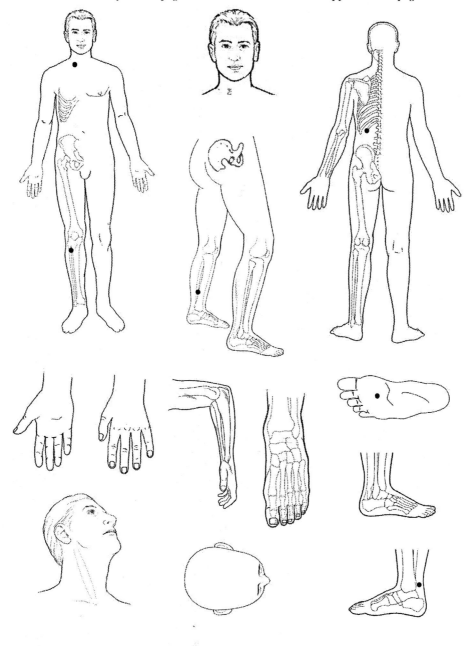

Blood Sugar (Low)

Daily Nutritional Crisis Program	Daily Nutritional Wellness Program
GlycoN*: 2 ½ tsp & GlycoAO: 3 caps PhytoN: 1½ tsp PreH: 6 tabs GEssentials: 6 tabs	GlycoN*: ½ tsp & GlycoAO: 2 caps PhytoN: 3/4 tsp PreH: 3 tabs GEssentials: 4 tabs

*For Adv.GlycoN see page 10. Product definitions are in Appendix A on page 381.

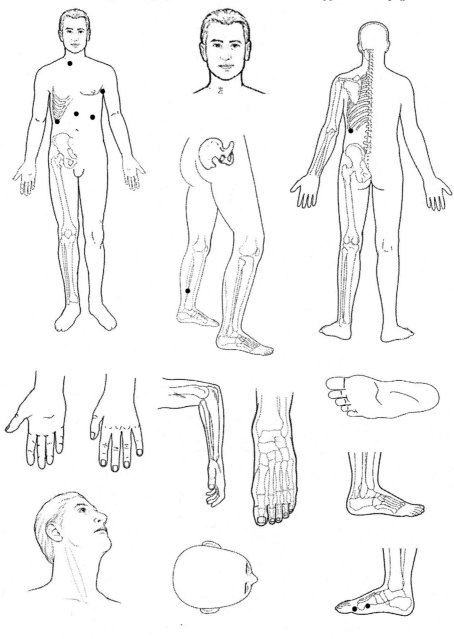

Bowel Detoxification

Daily Nutritional Crisis Program	Daily Nutritional Wellness Program
GlycoN*: 8 tsp & GlycoAO: 5 caps PhytoN: 3/4 tsp PreH: 4 tabs GEssentials: 4 tabs Clean: 3 caps twice a day (2 weeks) GstroP: 3 caps	GlycoN*: ½ tsp & GlycoAO: 2 caps PhytoN: 1/2 tsp PreH: 3 tabs GEssentials: 4 tabs Clean: 2 caps GstroP: 2 caps

*For Adv.GlycoN see page 10. Product definitions are in Appendix A on page 381.

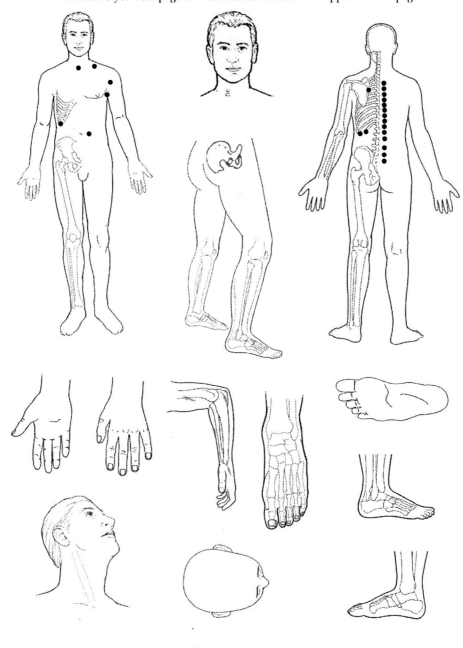

Breast Cyst
(eliminate caffeine from diet)

Daily Nutritional Crisis Program	Daily Nutritional Wellness Program
GlycoN*: 2 ½ tsp & GlycoAO: 3 caps PhytoN: 3/4 tsp PreH: 4 tabs GEssentials: 4 tabs ImmS: 5 tabs MC: 4 caps	GlycoN*: ½ tsp & GlycoAO: 2 caps PhytoN: 1/2 tsp PreH: 4 tabs GEssentials: 4 tabs ImmS: 3 tabs MC: 4 caps

*For Adv.GlycoN see page 10. Product definitions are in Appendix A on page 381.

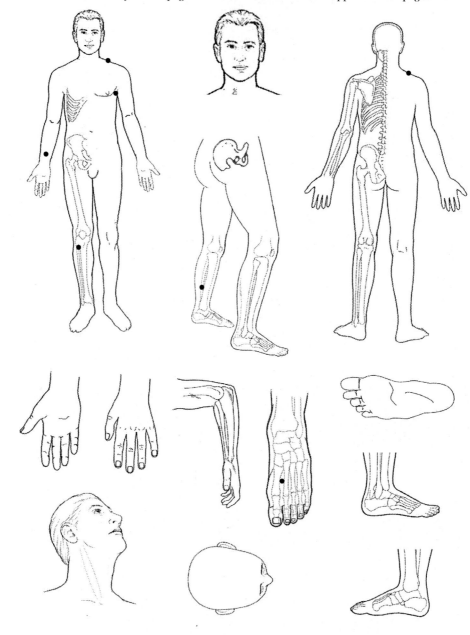

68

Breast Implants (Leaking)

Daily Nutritional Crisis Program	Daily Nutritional Wellness Program
GlycoN*: 5 ¼ tsp & GlycoAO: 4 caps	GlycoN*: 1 ½ tsp & GlycoAO: 3 caps
PhytoN: 1 ½ tsp	PhytoN: 1 tsp
PreH: 4 tabs	PreH: 4 tabs
Cata: 6 tabs	Cata: 4 tabs
ImmS: 6 tabs	ImmS: 4 tabs
MC: 5 caps	MC: 3 caps

*For Adv.GlycoN see page 10. Product definitions are in Appendix A on page 381.

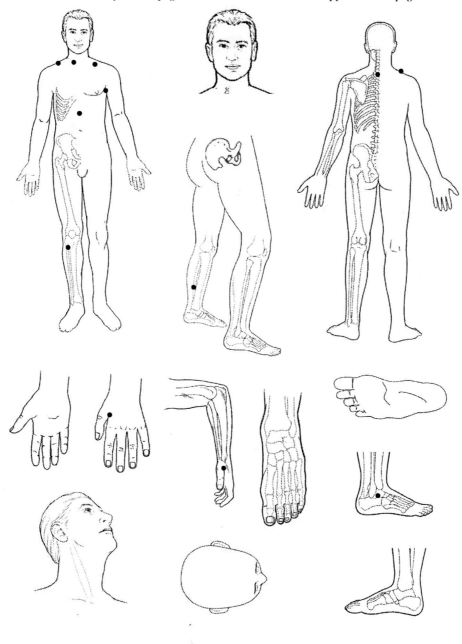

Bronchiectasis

Daily Nutritional Crisis Program	Daily Nutritional Wellness Program
GlycoN*: 2 ½ tsp & GlycoAO: 3 caps PhytoN: 1½ tsp PreH: 4 tabs Cata: 4 tabs ImmS: 6 tabs MC: 6 caps	GlycoN*: 1 ½ tsp & GlycoAO: 3 caps PhytoN: 3/4 tsp PreH: 3 tabs Cata: 4 tabs ImmS: 4 tabs MC: 3 caps

*For Adv.GlycoN see page 10. Product definitions are in Appendix A on page 381.

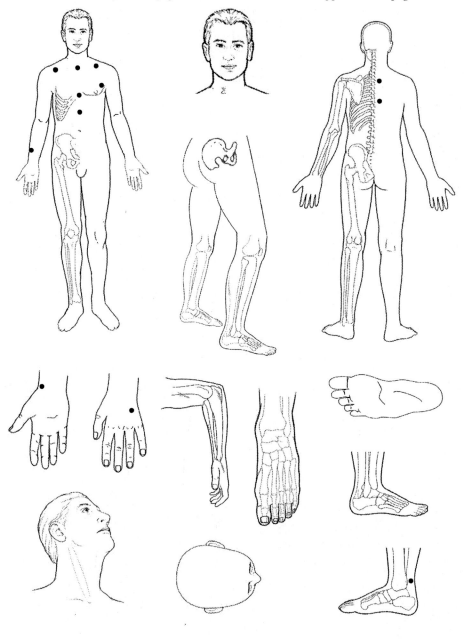

Bronchitis, Chronic

Daily Nutritional Crisis Program	Daily Nutritional Wellness Program
GlycoN*: 2 ½ tsp & GlycoAO: 3 caps PhytoN: 2 tsp PreH: 4 tabs Cata: 4 tabs ImmS: 6 tabs MC: 6 caps	GlycoN*: 1 ½ tsp & GlycoAO: 3 caps PhytoN: 1 tsp PreH: 3 tabs Cata: 4 tabs ImmS: 4 tabs MC: 3 caps

*For Adv.GlycoN see page 10. Product definitions are in Appendix A on page 381.

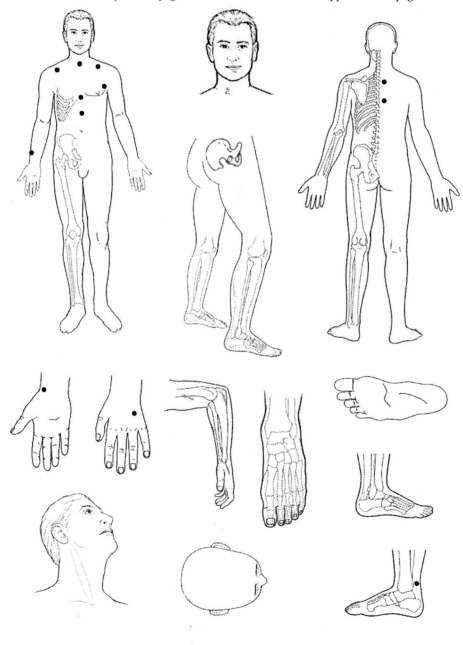

Bruises

Daily Nutritional Crisis Program	Daily Nutritional Wellness Program
GlycoN*: 2 ½ tsp & GlycoAO: 3 caps PhytoN: 1 tsp PreH: 4 tabs Cata: 4 tabs MC: 6 caps	GlycoN*: ½ tsp & GlycoAO: 2 caps PhytoN: 1/4 tsp PreH: 3 tabs Cata: 4 tabs MC: 4 caps

*For Adv.GlycoN see page 10. Product definitions are in Appendix A on page 381.

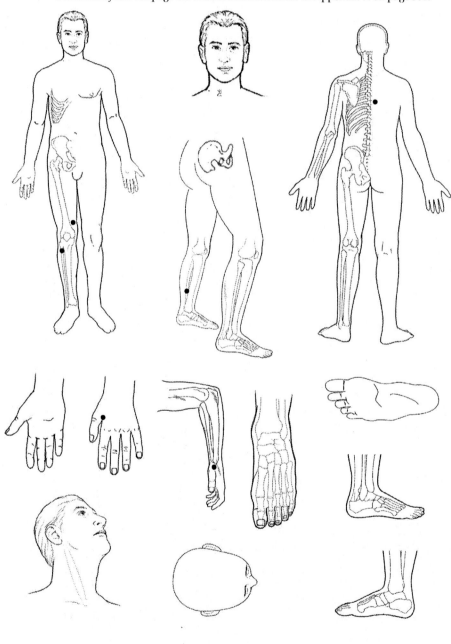

Burns

(soft laser on affected areas)

Daily Nutritional Crisis Program	Daily Nutritional Wellness Program
GlycoN*: 8 tsp & GlycoAO: 5 caps PhytoN: 1 tsp PreH: 6 tabs Cata: 6 tabs MC: 6 caps	GlycoN*: ½ tsp & GlycoAO: 2 caps PhytoN: 1 tsp PreH: 3 tabs Cata: 4 tabs MC: 3 caps

*For Adv.GlycoN see page 10. Product definitions are in Appendix A on page 381.

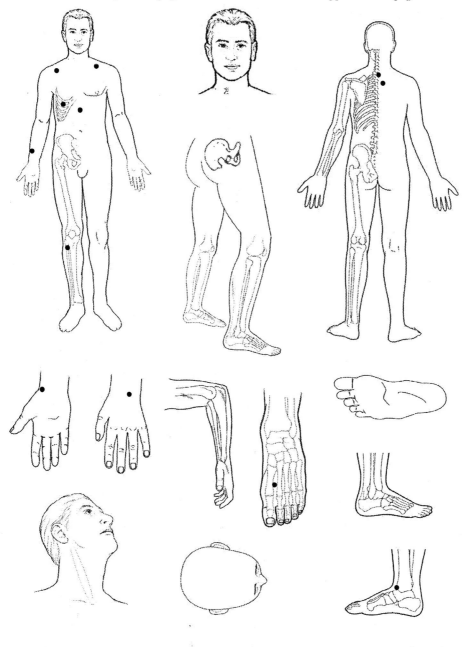

Bursitis

Daily Nutritional Crisis Program	Daily Nutritional Wellness Program
GlycoN*: 2 ½ tsp & GlycoAO: 3 caps PhytoN: 3/4 tsp PreH: 6 tabs Cata: 6 tabs SP: 4 caps	GlycoN*: ½ tsp & GlycoAO: 2 caps PhytoN: 1/2 tsp PreH: 3 tabs Cata: 4 tabs SP: 2 caps

*For Adv.GlycoN see page 10. Product definitions are in Appendix A on page 381.

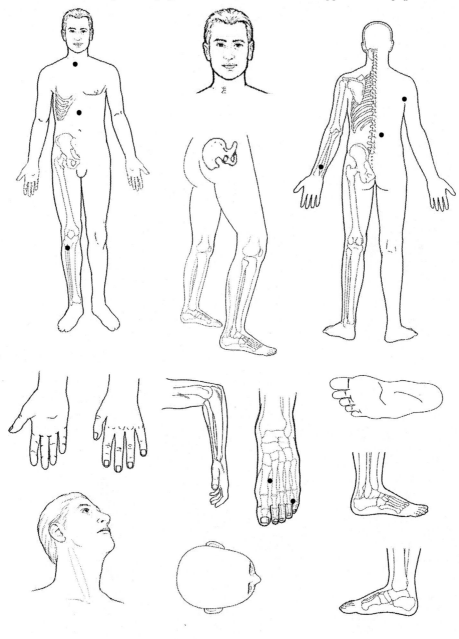

Cancer

Daily Nutritional Crisis Program	Daily Nutritional Wellness Program
GlycoN*: 10 ¾ tsp & GlycoAO: 6 caps PhytoN: 4 tsp PreH: 6 tabs Cata: 6 tabs ImmS: 6 tabs MC: 6 caps	GlycoN*: 2 ½ tsp & GlycoAO: 3 caps PhytoN: 2 tsp PreH: 4 tabs Cata: 6 tabs ImmS: 3 tabs MC: 3 caps

*For Adv.GlycoN see page 10. Product definitions are in Appendix A on page 381.

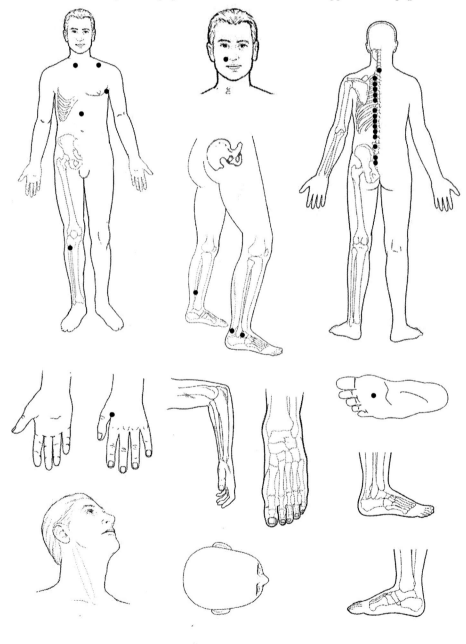

75

Candidiasis

Daily Nutritional Crisis Program	Daily Nutritional Wellness Program
GlycoN*: 5 ¼ tsp & GlycoAO: 4 caps	GlycoN*: 1 ½ tsp & GlycoAO: 3 caps
PhytoN: 1 tsp	PhytoN: 1 tsp
PreH: 4 tabs	PreH: 3 tabs
Cata: 4 tabs	Cata: 4 tabs
ImmS: 4 tabs	ImmS: 3 tabs
GstroP: 3 caps	GastroP: 1 cap

*For Adv.GlycoN see page 10. Product definitions are in Appendix A on page 381.

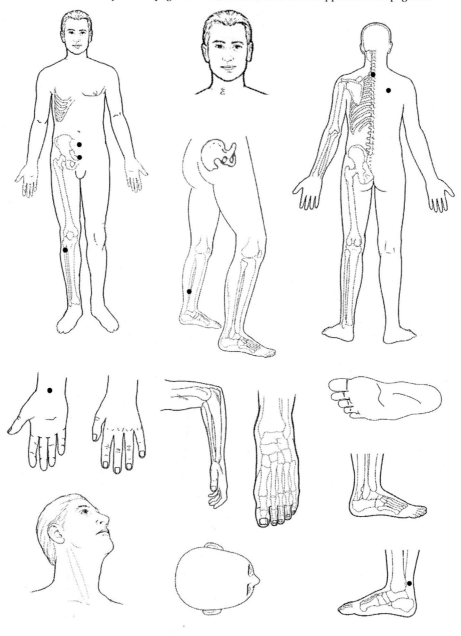

76

Candidiasis (oral)

Daily Nutritional Crisis Program	Daily Nutritional Wellness Program
GlycoN*: 5 ¼ tsp & GlycoAO: 4 caps PhytoN: 1 tsp PreH: 4 tabs Cata: 4 tabs ImmS: 4 tabs GstroP: 3 caps	GlycoN*: 1 ½ tsp & GlycoAO: 3 caps PhytoN: 3/4 tsp PreH: 3 tabs Cata: 4 tabs ImmS: 3 tabs GastroP: 1 cap

*For Adv.GlycoN see page 10. Product definitions are in Appendix A on page 381.

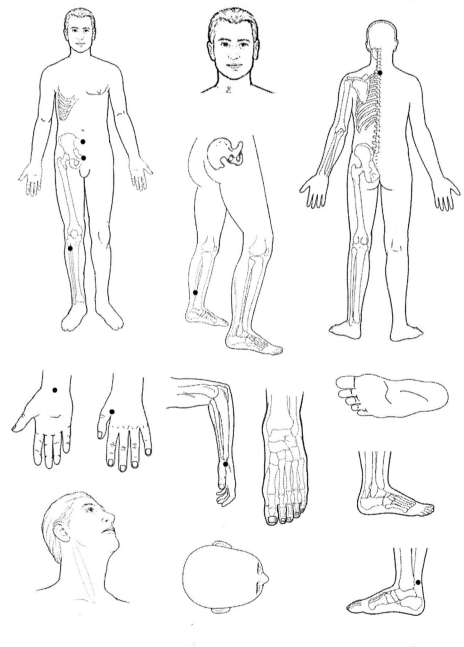

Canker Sores

Daily Nutritional Crisis Program	Daily Nutritional Wellness Program
GlycoN*: 2 ½ tsp & GlycoAO: 3 caps PhytoN: 3/4 tsp PreH: 3 tabs GEssentials: 4 tabs ImmS: 4 tabs	GlycoN*: ½ tsp & GlycoAO: 2 caps PhytoN: 1/2 tsp PreH: 3 tabs GEssentials: 4 tabs ImmS: 2 tabs

*For Adv.GlycoN see page 10. Product definitions are in Appendix A on page 381.

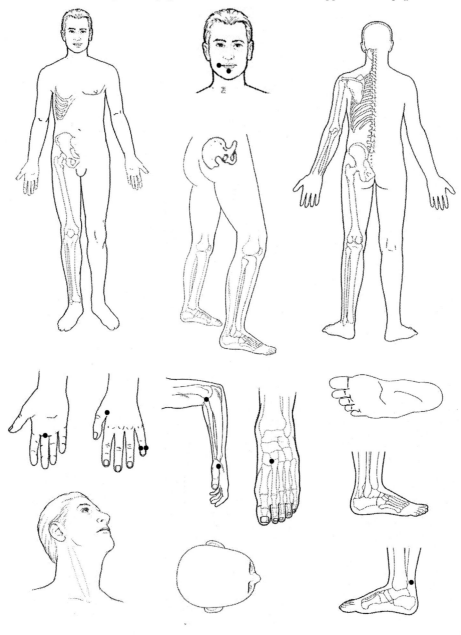

Cardiomyopathy

Daily Nutritional Crisis Program	Daily Nutritional Wellness Program
GlycoN*: 5 ¼ tsp & GlycoAO: 4 caps PhytoN: 1 tsp PreH: 4 tabs Cata: 6 tabs CB: 5 caps	GlycoN*: 1 ½ tsp & GlycoAO: 3 caps PhytoN: 3/4 tsp PreH: 3 tabs Cata: 6 tabs CB: 3 caps

*For Adv.GlycoN see page 10. Product definitions are in Appendix A on page 381.

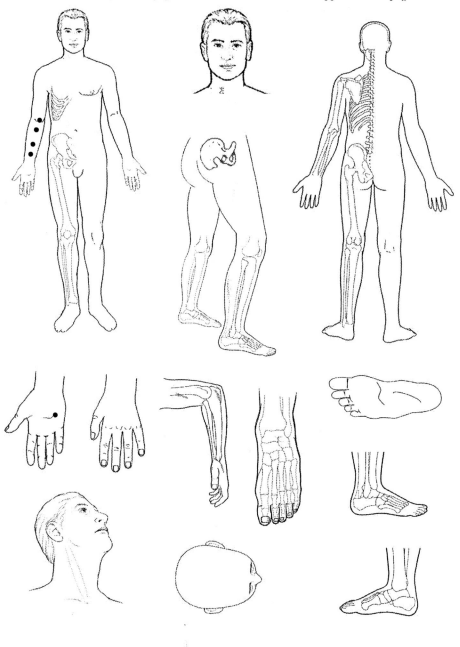

Cellulitis Abscess

Daily Nutritional Crisis Program	Daily Nutritional Wellness Program
GlycoN*: 5 ¼ tsp & GlycoAO: 4 caps	GlycoN*: ½ tsp & GlycoAO: 2 caps
PhytoN: 3/4 tsp	PhytoN: 1/2 tsp
PreH: 4 tabs	PreH: 3 tabs
GEssentials: 4 tabs	GEssentials: 4 tabs
MC: 6 caps	MC: 2 caps

*For Adv.GlycoN see page 10. Product definitions are in Appendix A on page 381.

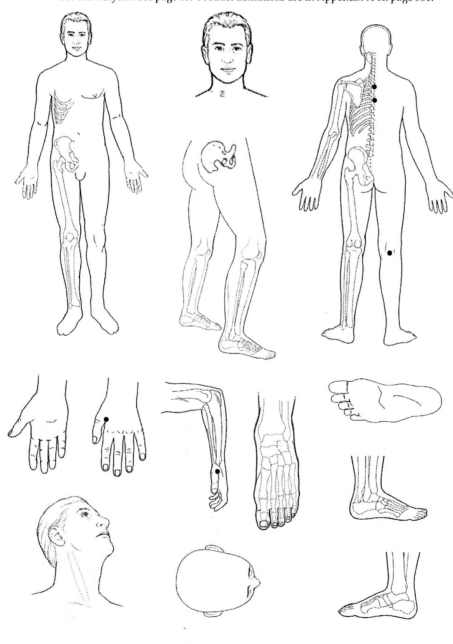

Cerebral Aneurysm (Nonruptured)

Daily Nutritional Crisis Program	Daily Nutritional Wellness Program
GlycoN*: 5 ¼ tsp & GlycoAO: 4 caps PhytoN: 1 tsp PreH: 4 tabs Cata: 4 tabs MC: 5 caps	GlycoN*: 1 ½ tsp & GlycoAO: 3 caps PhytoN: 1/2 tsp PreH: 3 tabs Cata: 4 tabs MC: 3 caps

*For Adv.GlycoN see page 10. Product definitions are in Appendix A on page 381.

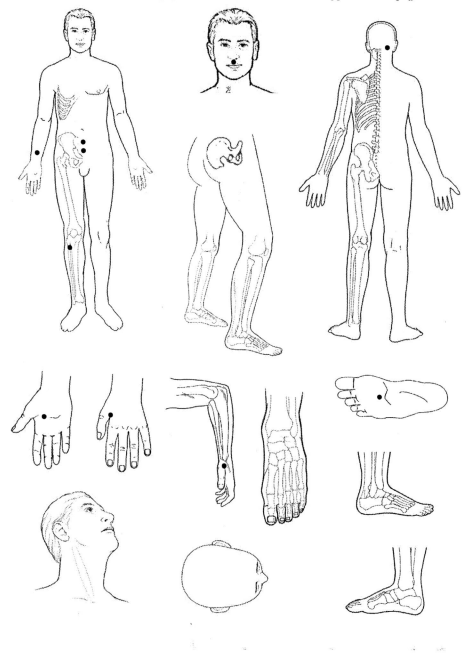

Cerebral Arteriosclerosis

Daily Nutritional Crisis Program	Daily Nutritional Wellness Program
GlycoN*: 5 ¼ tsp & GlycoAO: 4 caps PhytoN: 1 tsp PreH: 4 tabs Cata: 4 tabs MC: 5 caps	GlycoN*: 1 ½ tsp & GlycoAO: 3 caps PhytoN: 3/4 tsp PreH: 3 tabs Cata: 4 tabs MC: 2 caps

*For Adv.GlycoN see page 10. Product definitions are in Appendix A on page 381.

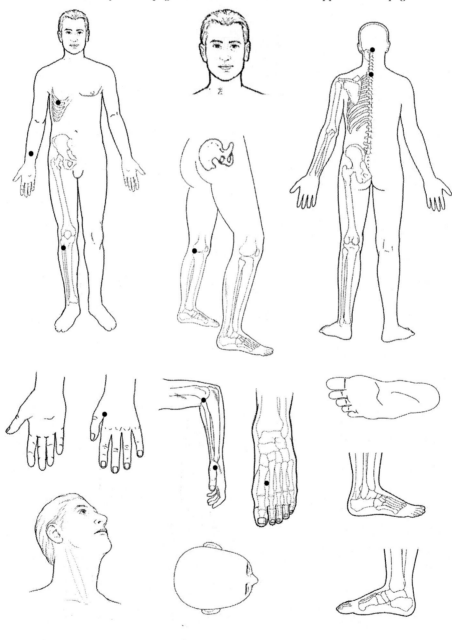

Cerebral Hemorrhage (Intracranial)

Daily Nutritional Crisis Program	Daily Nutritional Wellness Program
GlycoN*: 8 tsp & GlycoAO: 5 caps PhytoN: 1 tsp PreH: 4 tabs Cata: 6 tabs MC: 5 caps	GlycoN*: 1 ½ tsp & GlycoAO: 3 caps PhytoN: 3/4 tsp PreH: 3 tabs Cata: 4 tabs 3 caps

*For Adv.GlycoN see page 10. Product definitions are in Appendix A on page 381.

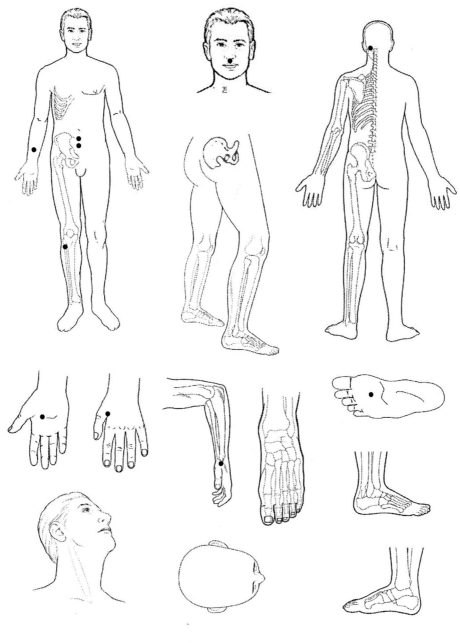

Cerebrovascular Disease

Daily Nutritional Crisis Program	Daily Nutritional Wellness Program
GlycoN*: 8 tsp & GlycoAO: 5 caps PhytoN: 1 tsp PreH: 4 tabs Cata: 6 tabs MC: 5 caps	GlycoN*: 1 ½ tsp & GlycoAO: 3 caps PhytoN: 3/4 tsp PreH: 3 tabs Cata: 4 tabs MC: 3 caps

*For Adv.GlycoN see page 10. Product definitions are in Appendix A on page 381.

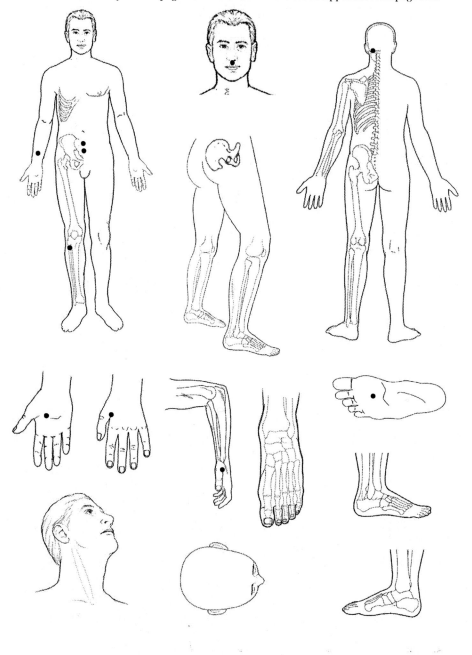

Cervical Dysplasia

Daily Nutritional Crisis Program	Daily Nutritional Wellness Program
GlycoN*: 5 ¼ tsp & GlycoAO: 4 caps PhytoN: 1 tsp PreH: 4 tabs GEssentials: 4 tabs ImmS: 6 tabs MC: 4 caps	GlycoN*: 1 ½ tsp & GlycoAO: 3 caps PhytoN: 3/4 tsp PreH: 3 tabs GEssentials: 4 tabs ImmS: 3 tabs MC: 3 caps

*For Adv.GlycoN see page 10. Product definitions are in Appendix A on page 381.

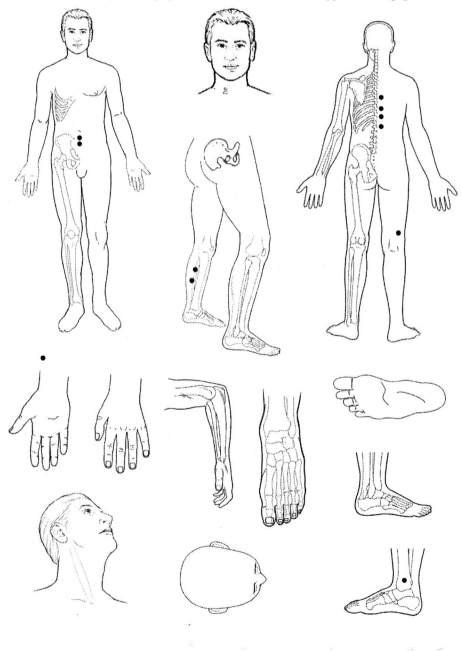

Cervicitis

Daily Nutritional Crisis Program	Daily Nutritional Wellness Program
GlycoN*: 5 ¼ tsp & GlycoAO: 4 caps PhytoN: 1 tsp PreH: 4 tabs GEssentials: 4 tabs ImmS: 6 tabs MC: 4 caps	GlycoN*: 1 ½ tsp & GlycoAO: 3 caps PhytoN: 3/4 tsp PreH: 3 tabs GEssentials: 4 tabs ImmS: 3 tabs MC: 3 caps

*For Adv.GlycoN see page 10. Product definitions are in Appendix A on page 381.

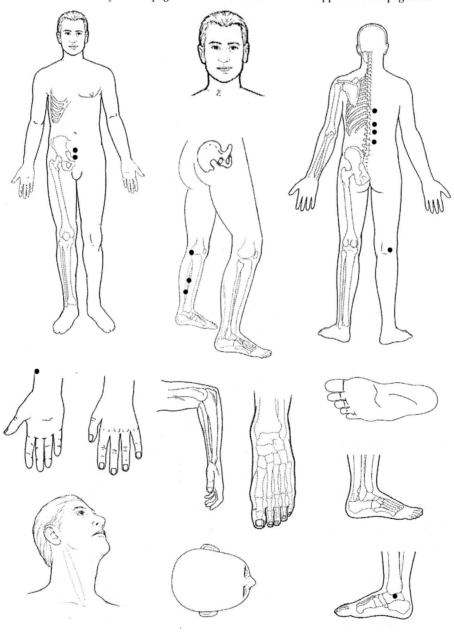

Chest Wall Pain (Costochondritis)

Daily Nutritional Crisis Program	Daily Nutritional Wellness Program
GlycoN*: 2 ½ tsp & GlycoAO: 3 caps PhytoN: 3/4 tsp PreH: 6 tabs GEssentials: 4 tabs MC: 5 caps	GlycoN*: ½ tsp & GlycoAO: 2 caps PhytoN: 1/2 tsp PreH: 3 tabs GEssentials: 4 tabs MC: 3 caps

*For Adv.GlycoN see page 10. Product definitions are in Appendix A on page 381.

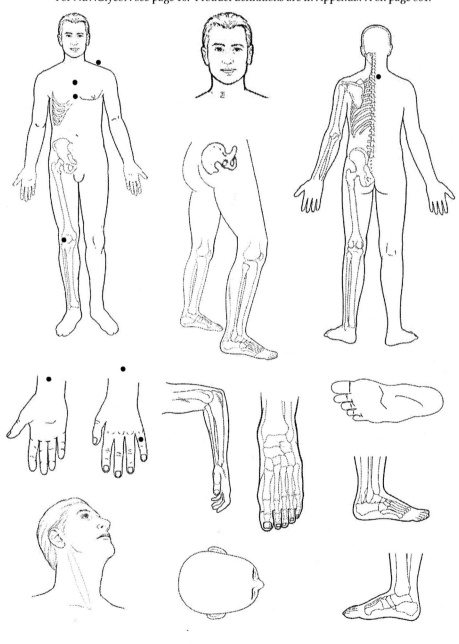

Chickenpox

Daily Nutritional Crisis Program	Daily Nutritional Wellness Program
GlycoN*: 5 ¼ tsp & GlycoAO: 4 caps	GlycoN*: ½ tsp & GlycoAO: 2 caps
PhytoN: 1 tsp	PhytoN: 1/4 tsp
PreH: 4 tabs	PreH: 3 tabs
GEssentials: 4 tabs	GEssentials: 4 tabs
ImmS: 6 tabs	ImmS: 3 tabs
MC: 4 tabs	MC: 4 tabs

*For Adv.GlycoN see page 10. Product definitions are in Appendix A on page 381.

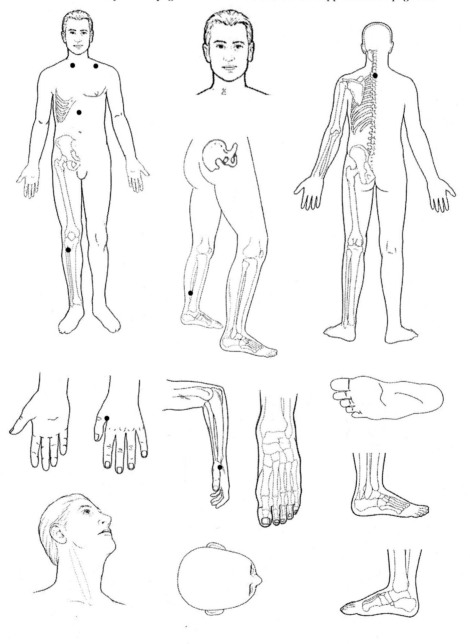

Chlamydia

Daily Nutritional Crisis Program	Daily Nutritional Wellness Program
GlycoN*: 2 ½ tsp & GlycoAO: 3 caps PhytoN: 3/4 tsp PreH: 3 tabs GEssentials: 6 tabs ImmS: 6 tabs MC: 6 caps	GlycoN*: ½ tsp & GlycoAO: 2 caps PhytoN: 1/4 tsp PreH: 3 tabs GEssentials: 4 tabs ImmS: 3 tabs MC: 3 caps

*For Adv.GlycoN see page 10. Product definitions are in Appendix A on page 381.

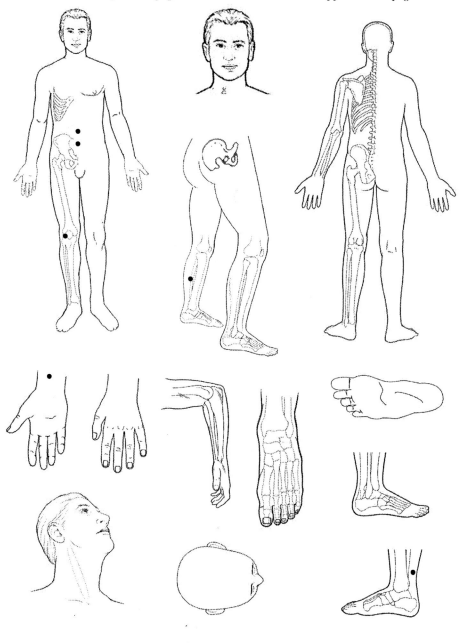

Cholecystitis (Acute)

Daily Nutritional Crisis Program	Daily Nutritional Wellness Program
GlycoN*: 5 ¼ tsp & GlycoAO: 4 caps PhytoN: 1 tsp PreH: 3 tabs GEssentials: 6 tabs GstroZ: 2 caps before meals	GlycoN*: 2 ½ tsp & GlycoAO: 3 caps PhytoN: 3/4 PreH: 3 tabs GEssentials: 4 tabs GastroZ: 1 cap before meals

*For Adv.GlycoN see page 10. Product definitions are in Appendix A on page 381.

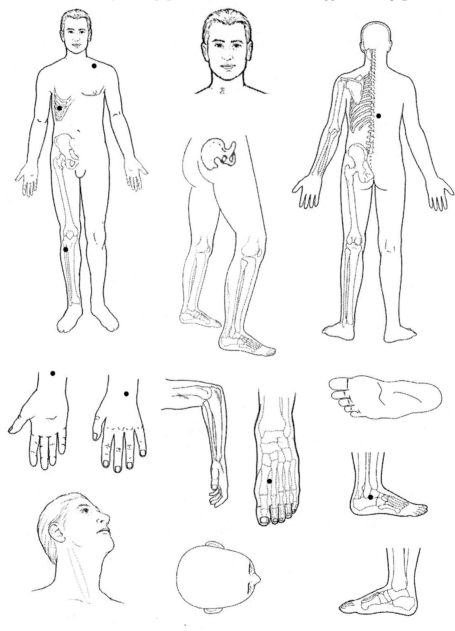

90

Cholecystitis (Chronic)

Daily Nutritional Crisis Program	Daily Nutritional Wellness Program
GlycoN*: 3 ¼ tsp & GlycoAO: 4 caps PhytoN: 1 tsp PreH: 3 tabs GEssentials: 4 tabs GstroZ: 2 caps before meals	GlycoN*: 2 ½ tsp & GlycoAO: 3 caps PhytoN: ¾ tsp PreH: 3 tabs GEssentials: 2 tabs GastroZ: 1 cap before meals

*For Adv.GlycoN see page 10. Product definitions are in Appendix A on page 381.

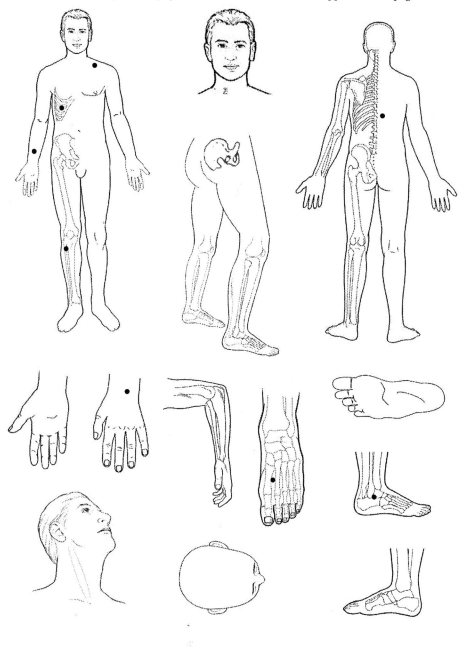

Chronic Fatigue Syndrome

Daily Nutritional Crisis Program	Daily Nutritional Wellness Program
GlycoN*: 5 ¼ tsp & GlycoAO: 4 caps PhytoN: 1 tsp PreH: 6 tabs Cata: 4 tabs ImmS: 4 tabs MC: 4 caps	GlycoN*: 1 ½ tsp & GlycoAO: 3 caps PhytoN: 3/4 tsp PreH: 4 tabs Cata: 4 tabs ImmS: 2 tabs MC: 2 caps

*For Adv.GlycoN see page 10. Product definitions are in Appendix A on page 381.

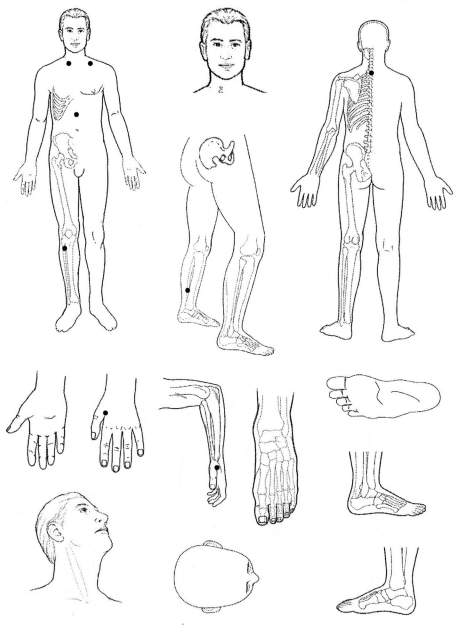

Chronic Ischemic Heart Disease

Daily Nutritional Crisis Program	Daily Nutritional Wellness Program
GlycoN*: 5 ¼ tsp & GlycoAO: 4 caps PhytoN: 1 tsp PreH: 3 tabs Cata: 4 tabs CB: 7 caps MC: 4 caps	GlycoN*: 2 ½ tsp & GlycoAO: 3 caps PhytoN: 3/4 tsp PreH: 3 tabs Cata: 4 tabs CB: 4 caps MC: 2 caps

*For Adv.GlycoN see page 10. Product definitions are in Appendix A on page 381.

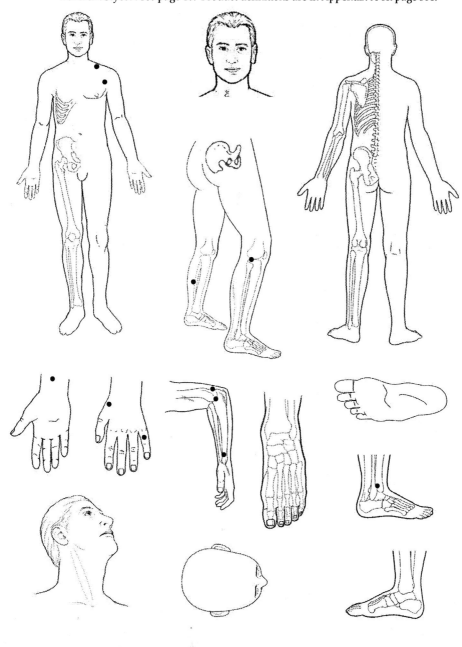

Chronic Liver Disease

Daily Nutritional Crisis Program	Daily Nutritional Wellness Program
GlycoN*: 5 ¼ tsp & GlycoAO: 4 caps PhytoN: 1 tsp PreH: 3 tabs Cata:4 tab ImmS: 6 tabs MC: 5 caps	GlycoN*: 1 ½ tsp & GlycoAO: 3 caps PhytoN: 1/2 tsp PreH: 3 tabs Cata: 4 tabs ImmS: 3 tabs MC: 3 caps

*For Adv.GlycoN see page 10. Product definitions are in Appendix A on page 381.

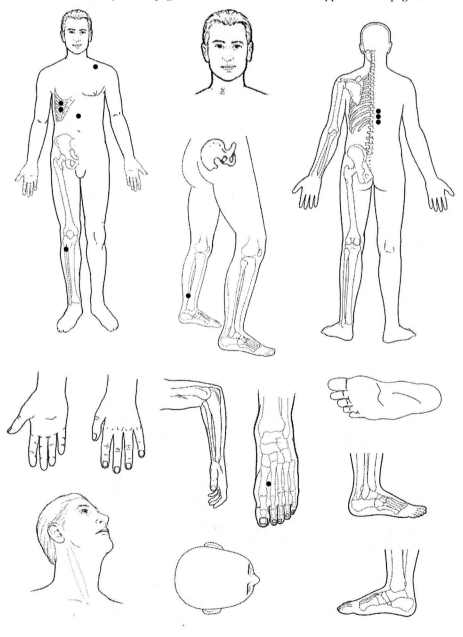

Chronic Skin Ulcer Venous Stasis
(apply soft laser to affect areas)

Daily Nutritional Crisis Program	Daily Nutritional Wellness Program
GlycoN*: 2 ½ tsp & GlycoAO: 3 caps PhytoN: 1 tsp PreH: 3 tabs Cata: 4 tabs MC: 6 caps	GlycoN*: 1 ½ tsp & GlycoAO: 3 caps PhytoN: 3/4 tsp PreH: 3 tabs Cata: 4 tabs MC: 4 caps

*For Adv.GlycoN see page 10. Product definitions are in Appendix A on page 381.

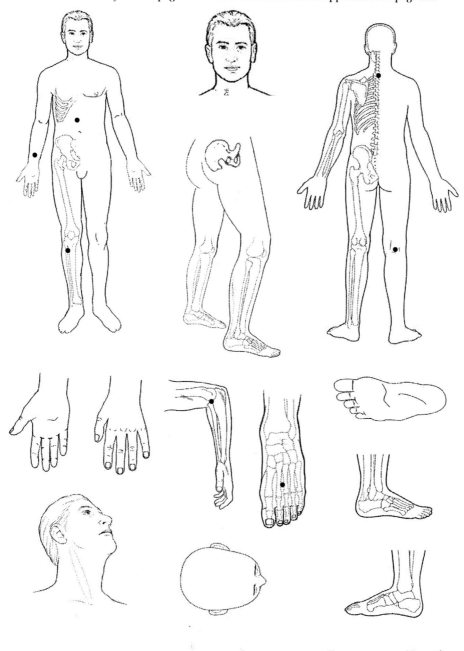

Cirrhosis, Alcoholic Liver

Daily Nutritional Crisis Program	Daily Nutritional Wellness Program
GlycoN*: 5 ¼ tsp GlycoAO: 4 caps PhytoN: 1 tsp PreH: 6 tabs Cata: 4 tabs ImmS: 6 tabs MC: 6 caps	GlycoN*: 1 ½ tsp & GlycoAO: 3 caps PhytoN: 3/4 tsp PreH: 3 tabs Cata: 4 tabs ImmS: 3 tabs MC: 3 caps

*For Adv.GlycoN see page 10. Product definitions are in Appendix A on page 381.

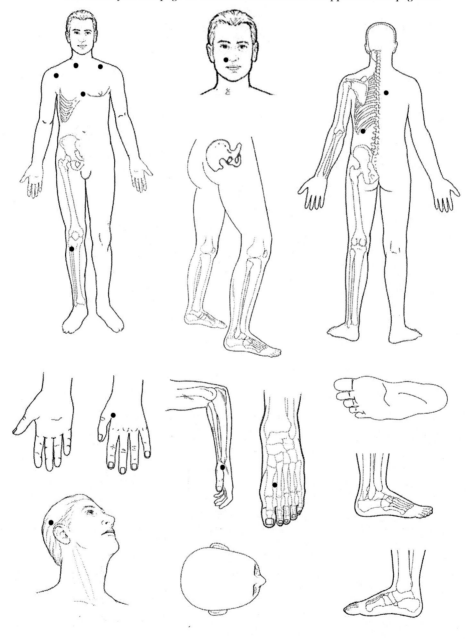

Cirrhosis, Nonalcoholic Liver

Daily Nutritional Crisis Program	Daily Nutritional Wellness Program
GlycoN*: 5 ¼ tsp & GlycoAO: 4 caps PhytoN: 3/4 tsp PreH: 4 tabs Cata: 4 tabs ImmS: 6 tabs MC: 6 caps	GlycoN*: 1 ½ tsp & GlycoAO: 3 caps PhytoN: 1/2 tsp PreH: 3 tabs Cata: 4 tabs ImmS: 3 tabs MC: 3 caps

*For Adv.GlycoN see page 10. Product definitions are in Appendix A on page 381.

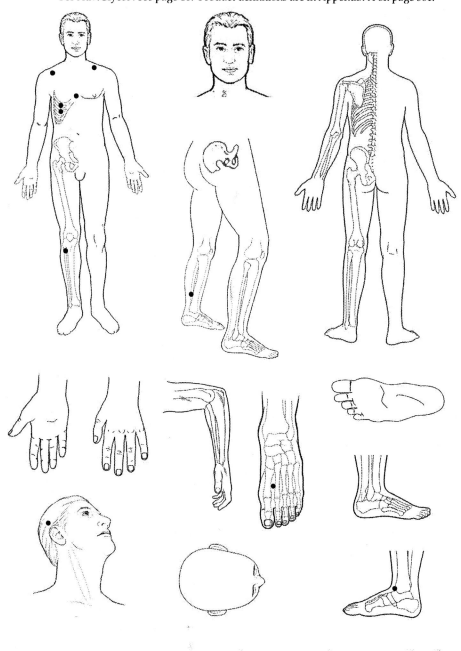

Claudication/Peripheral Vascular Disease

Daily Nutritional Crisis Program	Daily Nutritional Wellness Program
GlycoN*: 5 ¼ tsp & GlycoAO: 4 caps PhytoN: 1 ½ tsp PreH: 6 tabs Cata:6 tabs MC: 6 caps CB: 6 caps	GlycoN*: 1 ½ tsp & GlycoAO: 3 caps PhytoN: 3/4 tsp PreH: 3 tabs Cata: 4 tabs MC: 3 caps CB: 4 caps

*For Adv.GlycoN see page 10. Product definitions are in Appendix A on page 381.

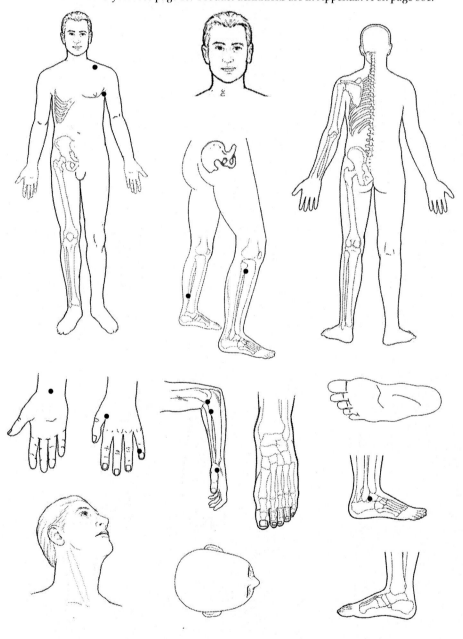

98

Clostridium Difficile

Daily Nutritional Crisis Program	Daily Nutritional Wellness Program
GlycoN*: 2 ½ tsp GlycoAO: 3 caps PhytoN: 3/4 tsp PreH: 3 tabs Cata:6 tabs Clean: 3 caps twice a day (2 weeks) GstroP: 4 caps	GlycoN*: ½ tsp & GlycoAO: 2 caps PhytoN: 1/2 tsp PreH: 3 tabs Cata: 4 tabs Clean: 2 caps GstroP: 2 caps

*For Adv.GlycoN see page 10. Product definitions are in Appendix A on page 381.

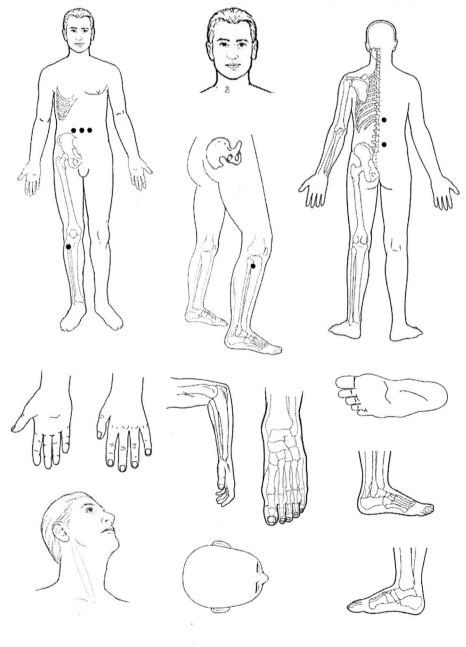

99

Cold Sores
(apply soft laser to affected areas)

Daily Nutritional Crisis Program	Daily Nutritional Wellness Program
GlycoN*: 2 ½ tsp GlycoAO: 3 caps PhytoN: 1/2 tsp PreH: 4 tabs GEssentials: 4 tabs ImmS: 5 tabs MC: 4 caps	GlycoN*: ½ tsp & GlycoAO: 2 caps PhytoN: 1/4 tsp PreH: 3 tabs GEssentials: 4 tabs ImmS: 3 tabs MC: 2 caps

*For Adv.GlycoN see page 10. Product definitions are in Appendix A on page 381.

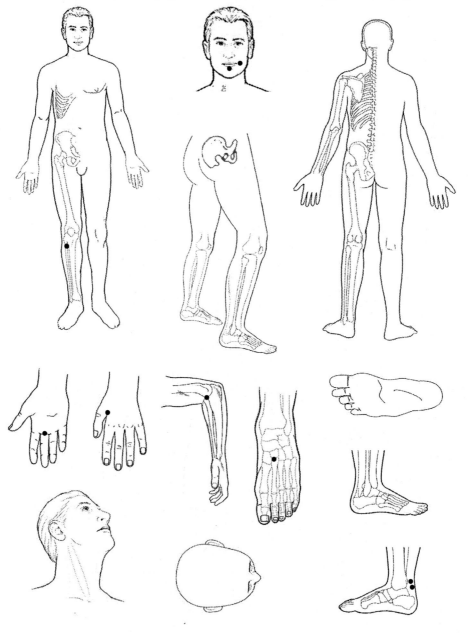

Cold/Flu

Daily Nutritional Crisis Program	Daily Nutritional Wellness Program
GlycoN*: 2 ½ tsp GlycoAO: 3 caps PhytoN: 1 ¾ tsp PreH: 3 tabs GEssentials: 6 tabs ImmS: 6 tabs MC: 6 caps	GlycoN*: ½ tsp & GlycoAO: 2 caps PhytoN: 1/4 tsp PreH: 3 tabs GEssentials: 4 tabs ImmS: 3 tabs MC: 3 caps

*For Adv.GlycoN see page 10. Product definitions are in Appendix A on page 381.

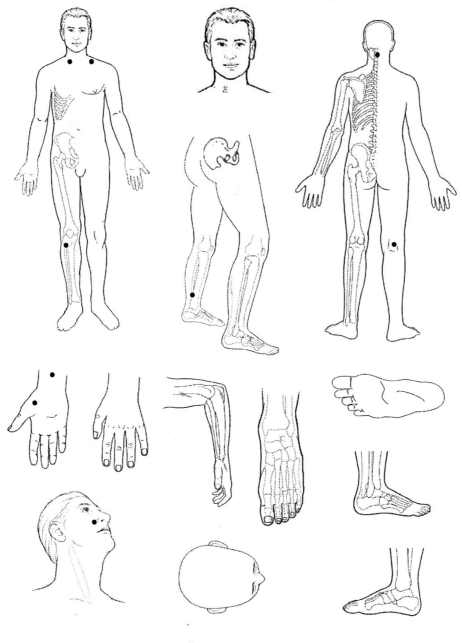

Colitis

Daily Nutritional Crisis Program	Daily Nutritional Wellness Program
GlycoN*: 5 ¼ tsp GlycoAO: 4 caps	GlycoN*: 1 ½ tsp & GlycoAO: 3 caps
PhytoN: 1 ¾ tsp	PhytoN: 3/4 tsp
PreH: 4 tabs	PreH: 3 tabs
Cata: 4 tabs	Cata: 4 tabs
ImmS: 4 tabs	ImmS: 2 tabs
MC: 4 caps & GstroP: 3 caps	MC: 2 caps & GstroP: 1 cap

*For Adv.GlycoN see page 10. Product definitions are in Appendix A on page 381.

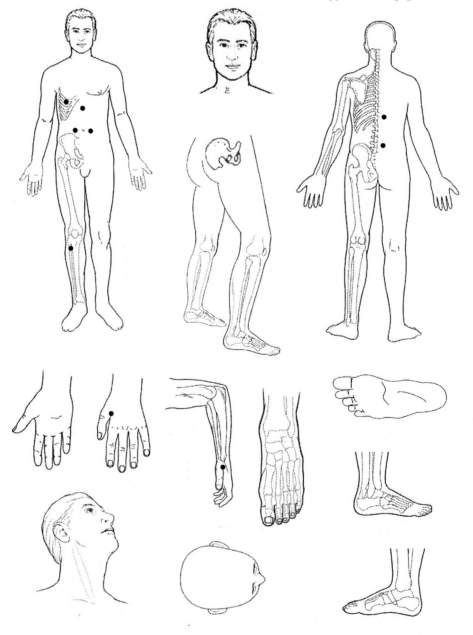

Colon Infection

Daily Nutritional Crisis Program	Daily Nutritional Wellness Program
GlycoN*: 5 ¼ tsp GlycoAO: 4 caps	GlycoN*: 1 ½ tsp & GlycoAO: 3 caps
PhytoN: 1 ¾ tsp	PhytoN: 3/4 tsp
PreH: 4 tabs	PreH: 3 tabs
Cata: 4 tabs	Cata: 4 tabs
ImmS: 4 tabs	ImmS: 2 tabs
MC: 4 caps & GstroP: 3 caps	MC: 2 caps & GstroP: 1 cap

*For Adv.GlycoN see page 10. Product definitions are in Appendix A on page 381.

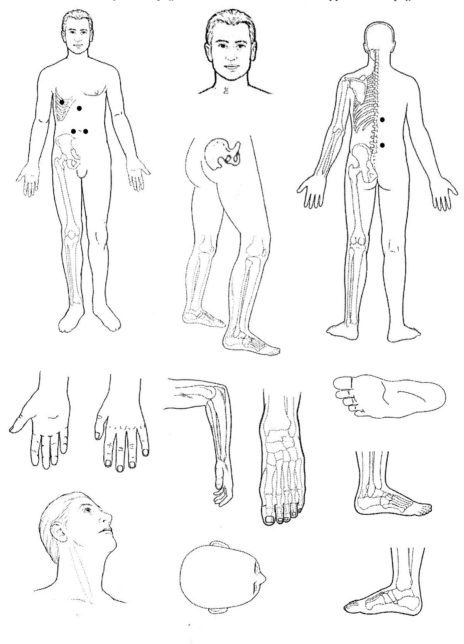

Coma

Daily Nutritional Crisis Program	Daily Nutritional Wellness Program
GlycoN*: 8 tsp & GlycoAO: 5 caps PhytoN: 2 ¾ tsp PreH: 6 tabs Cata:6 tabs CB: 6 caps	GlycoN*: 2 ½ tsp & GlycoAO: 3 caps PhytoN: 3/4 tsp PreH: 3 tabs Cata: 4 tabs CB: 3 caps

*For Adv.GlycoN see page 10. Product definitions are in Appendix A on page 381.

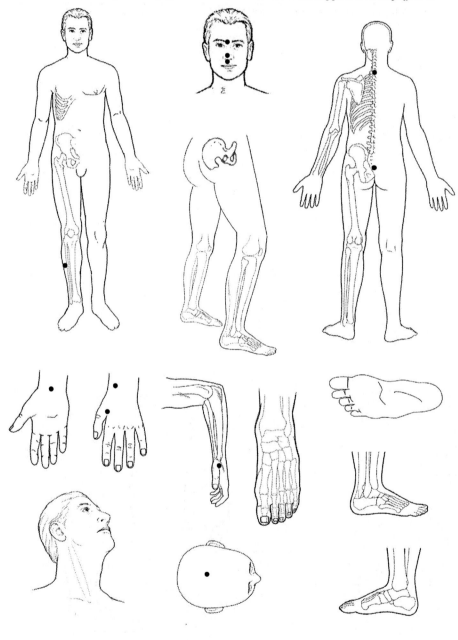

Common Cold

Daily Nutritional Crisis Program	Daily Nutritional Wellness Program
GlycoN*: 2 ½ tsp & GlycoAO: 3 caps PhytoN: 1 ¾ tsp PreH: 3 tabs GEssentials: 6 tabs ImmS: 6 tabs MC: 6 caps	GlycoN*: ½ tsp & GlycoAO: 2 caps PhytoN: 1/4 tsp PreH: 3 tabs GEssentials: 4 tabs ImmS: 3 tabs MC: 3 caps

*For Adv.GlycoN see page 10. Product definitions are in Appendix A on page 381.

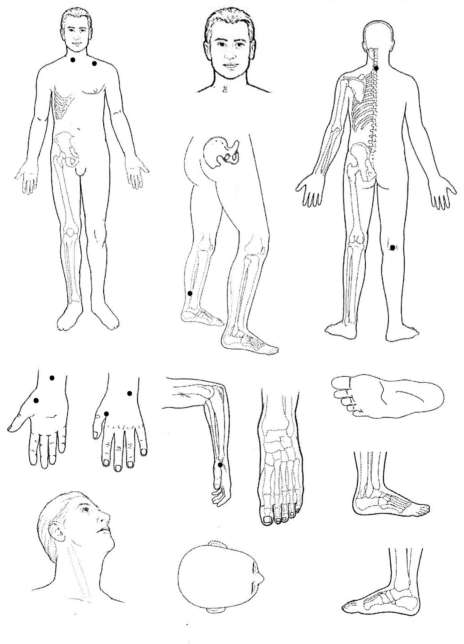

Concussion

Daily Nutritional Crisis Program	Daily Nutritional Wellness Program
GlycoN*: 8 tsp & GlycoAO: 5 caps	GlycoN*: 1 ½ tsp & GlycoAO: 3 caps
PhytoN: 2 ¾ tsp	PhytoN: 3/4 tsp
PreH: 6 tabs	PreH: 3 tabs
Cata:6 tabs	Cata: 4 tabs
SP: 4 caps	SP: 2 caps
MC: 4 caps	MC: 2 caps

*For Adv.GlycoN see page 10. Product definitions are in Appendix A on page 381.

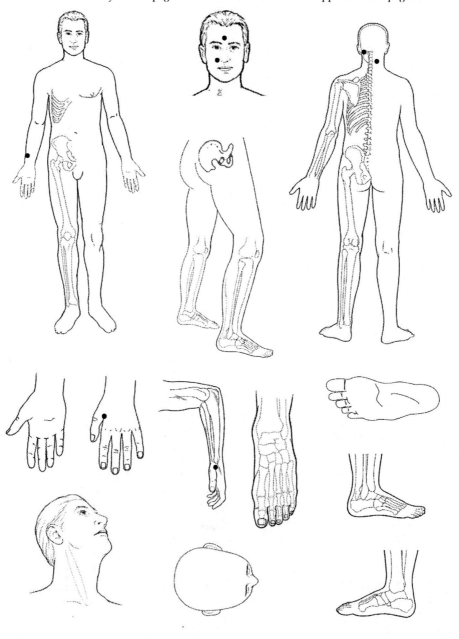

Congenital Heart Defect

Daily Nutritional Crisis Program	Daily Nutritional Wellness Program
GlycoN*: 5 ¼ tsp & GlycoAO: 4 caps PhytoN: 1 ¾ tsp PreH: 3 tabs Cata: 4 tabs CB: 7 caps	GlycoN*: 1 ½ tsp & GlycoAO: 3 caps PhytoN: 3/4 tsp PreH: 3 tabs Cata: 4 tabs CB: 3 caps

*For Adv.GlycoN see page 10. Product definitions are in Appendix A on page 381.

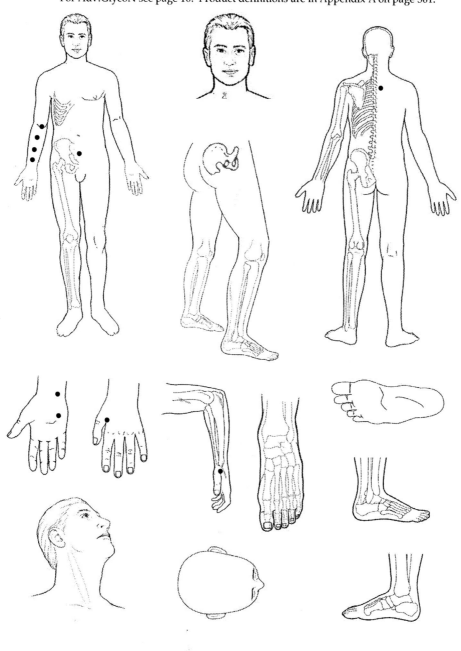

Congestive Heart Failure (CHF)

Daily Nutritional Crisis Program	Daily Nutritional Wellness Program
GlycoN*: 5 ¼ tsp & GlycoAO: 4 caps PhytoN: 1 ¾ tsp PreH: 3 tabs Cata: 4 tabs CB: 7 caps	GlycoN*: 1 ½ tsp & GlycoAO: 3 caps PhytoN: 3/4 tsp PreH: 3 tabs Cata: 4 tabs CB: 3 caps

*For Adv.GlycoN see page 10. Product definitions are in Appendix A on page 381.

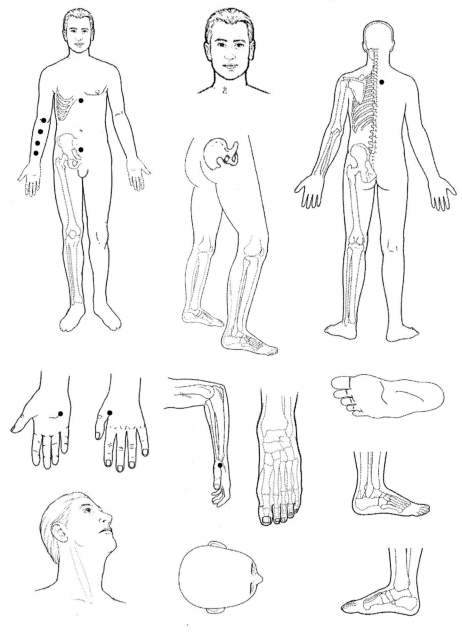

Conjunctivitis

Daily Nutritional Crisis Program	Daily Nutritional Wellness Program
GlycoN*: 1 ½ tsp & GlycoAO: 3 caps PhytoN: 1/2 tsp PreH: 3 tabs GEssentials: 4 tabs ImmS: 6 tabs MC: 6 caps	GlycoN*: ½ tsp & GlycoAO: 2 caps PhytoN: 1/4 tsp PreH: 3 tabs GEssentials: 4 tabs ImmS: 3 tabs MC: 3 caps

*For Adv.GlycoN see page 10. Product definitions are in Appendix A on page 381.

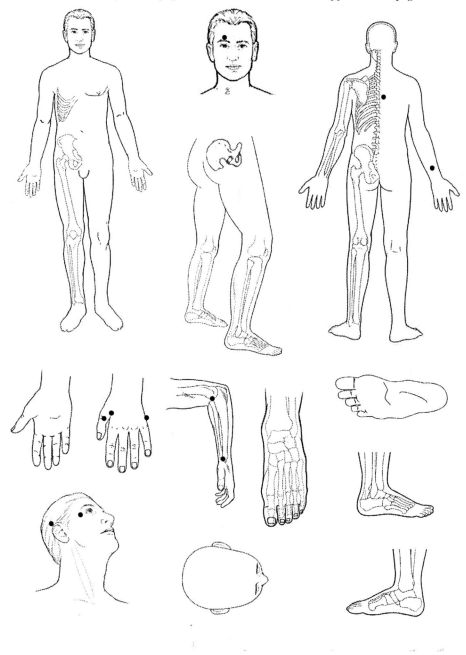

109

Connective Tissue Disease

Daily Nutritional Crisis Program	Daily Nutritional Wellness Program
GlycoN*: 8 tsp & GlycoAO: 5 caps	GlycoN*: 2 ½ tsp & GlycoAO: 3 caps
PhytoN: 1 ¾ tsp	PhytoN: 3/4 tsp
PreH: 6 tabs	PreH: 3 tabs
Cata:6 tabs	Cata:6 tabs
ImmS: 6 tabs	ImmS: 3 tabs
MC: 5 caps	MC: 3 caps

*For Adv.GlycoN see page 10. Product definitions are in Appendix A on page 381.

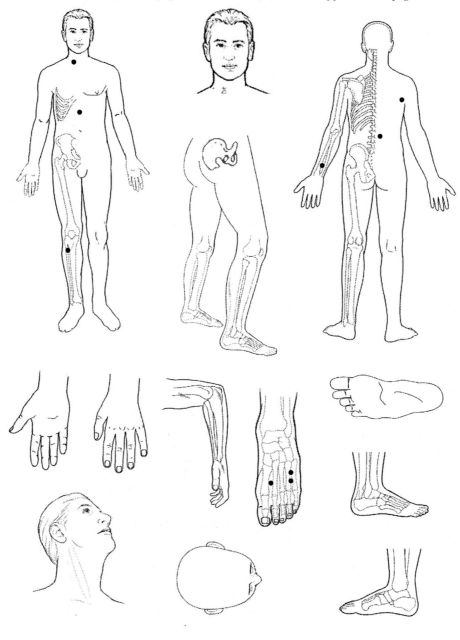

110

Constipation

Daily Nutritional Crisis Program	Daily Nutritional Wellness Program
GlycoN*: 2 ½ tsp & GlycoAO: 3 caps PhytoN: 1 ¾ tsp PreH: 3 tabs GEssentials: 4 tabs Clean: 3 caps twice a day (2 weeks) GstroP: 4 caps	GlycoN*: ½ tsp & GlycoAO: 2 caps PhytoN: 1/4 tsp PreH: 3 tabs GEssentials: 4 tabs Clean: 2 caps GstroP: 3 caps

*For Adv.GlycoN see page 10. Product definitions are in Appendix A on page 381.

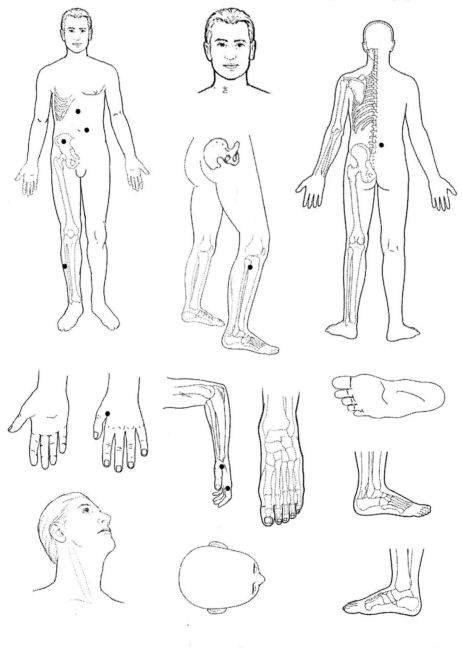

111

Contact Dermatitis

Daily Nutritional Crisis Program	Daily Nutritional Wellness Program
GlycoN*: 2 ½ tsp & GlycoAO: 3 caps	GlycoN*: ½ tsp & GlycoAO: 2 caps
PhytoN: 3/4 tsp	PhytoN: 1/4 tsp
PreH: 3 tabs	PreH: 3 tabs
GEssentials: 4 tabs	GEssentials: 4 tabs
ImmS: 6 tabs	ImmS: 4 tabs
Clean: 3 caps twice a day (2 weeks)	Clean: 2 caps

*For Adv.GlycoN see page 10. Product definitions are in Appendix A on page 381.

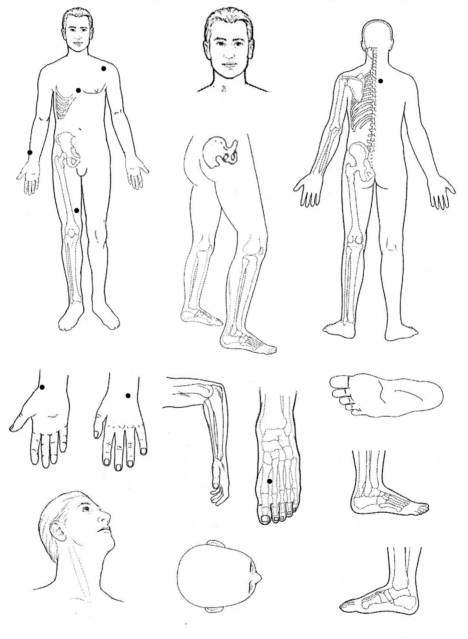

COPD

Daily Nutritional Crisis Program	Daily Nutritional Wellness Program
GlycoN*: 3 ½ tsp & GlycoAO: 3 caps	GlycoN*: 1 ½ tsp & GlycoAO: 3 caps
PhytoN: 1 ¾ tsp	PhytoN: 3/4 tsp
PreH: 3 tabs	PreH: 3 tabs
Cata: 4 tabs	Cata: 4 tabs
ImmS: 5 tabs	ImmS: 3 tabs
Clean: 3 caps twice a day (2 weeks)	Clean: 2 caps

*For Adv.GlycoN see page 10. Product definitions are in Appendix A on page 381.

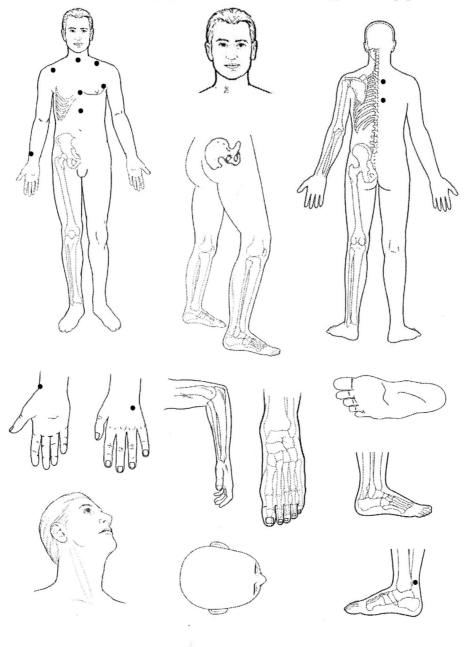

Cor Pulmonale

Daily Nutritional Crisis Program	Daily Nutritional Wellness Program
GlycoN*: 3 ½ tsp & GlycoAO: 3 caps PhytoN: 1 ¾ tsp PreH: 3 tabs Cata: 4 tabs Clean: 3 caps twice a day (2 weeks)	GlycoN*: 1 ½ tsp & GlycoAO: 3 caps PhytoN: 3/4 tsp PreH: 3 tabs Cata: 4 tabs Clean: 3 caps

*For Adv.GlycoN see page 10. Product definitions are in Appendix A on page 381.

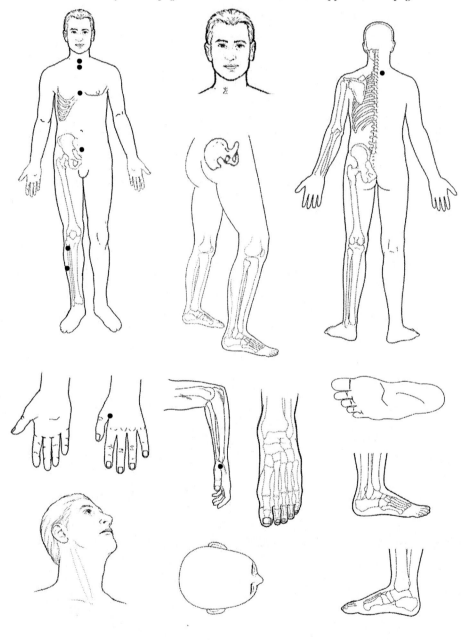

Costochondritis

Daily Nutritional Crisis Program	Daily Nutritional Wellness Program
GlycoN*: 2 ½ tsp & GlycoAO: 3 caps PhytoN: 3/4 tsp PreH: 5 tabs GEssentials: 4 tabs MC: 4 caps	GlycoN*: ½ tsp & GlycoAO: 2 caps PhytoN: 1/4 tsp PreH: 3 tabs GEssentials: 4 tabs MC: 3 caps

*For Adv.GlycoN see page 10. Product definitions are in Appendix A on page 381.

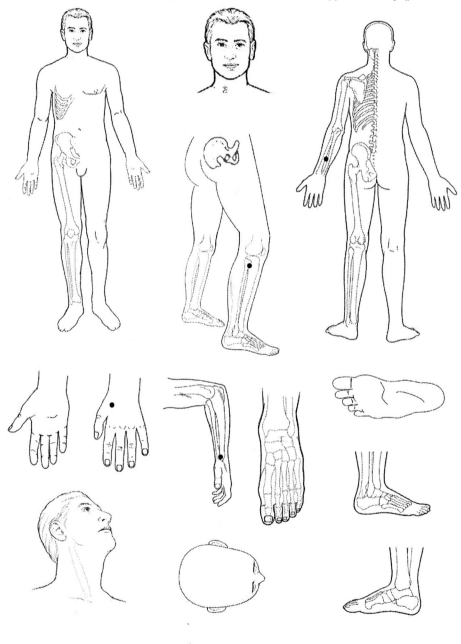

Cough

Daily Nutritional Crisis Program	Daily Nutritional Wellness Program
GlycoN*: 1 ½ tsp & GlycoAO: 3 caps PhytoN: 3/4 tsp PreH: 3 tabs GEssentials: 4 tabs ImmS: 5 tabs MC: 4 caps	GlycoN*: ½ tsp & GlycoAO: 2 caps PhytoN: 1/4 tsp PreH: 3 tabs GEssentials: 4 tabs ImmS: 3 tabs MC: 3 caps

*For Adv.GlycoN see page 10. Product definitions are in Appendix A on page 381.

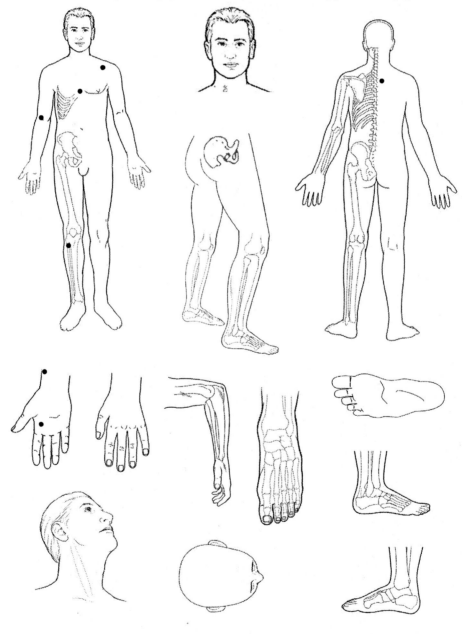

Coumadin Therapy (Long Term)

Daily Nutritional Crisis Program	Daily Nutritional Wellness Program
GlycoN*: ½ tsp & GlycoAO: 2 caps PhytoN: 3/4 tsp PreH: 3 tabs GEssentials: 4 tabs MC: 4 caps CB: 3 caps	GlycoN*: ½ tsp & GlycoAO: 2 caps PhytoN: 1/4 tsp PreH: 3 tabs GEssentials: 4 tabs MC: 2 caps CB: 1 Cap

*For Adv.GlycoN see page 10. Product definitions are in Appendix A on page 381.

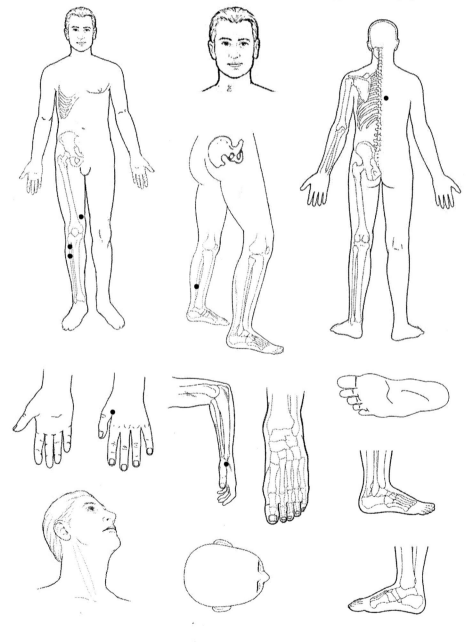

Cramps (Menstrual)

Daily Nutritional Crisis Program	Daily Nutritional Wellness Program
GlycoN*: 1 ½ tsp & GlycoAO: 3 caps PhytoN: 3/4 tsp PreH: 6 tabs GEssentials: 4 tabs MC: 4 caps SP: 4 caps	GlycoN*: ½ tsp & GlycoAO: 2 caps PhytoN: 1/4 tsp PreH: 4 tabs GEssentials: 4 tabs MC: 2 caps SP: 2 caps

*For Adv.GlycoN see page 10. Product definitions are in Appendix A on page 381.

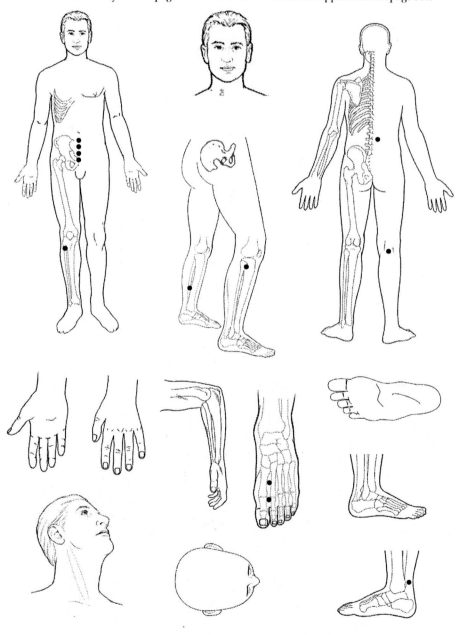

Cravings (Sweets/Alcohol)

Daily Nutritional Crisis Program	Daily Nutritional Wellness Program
GlycoN*: 2 ½ tsp & GlycoAO: 3 caps	GlycoN*: ½ tsp & GlycoAO: 2 caps
PhytoN: 1 ¾ tsp	PhytoN: 3/4 tsp
PreH: 3 tabs	PreH: 4 tabs
Cata: 4 tabs	Cata: 4 tabs
SP: 2 caps	SP: 1 cap
Clean: 3 caps twice a day (2 weeks)	Clean: 2 caps

*For Adv.GlycoN see page 10. Product definitions are in Appendix A on page 381.

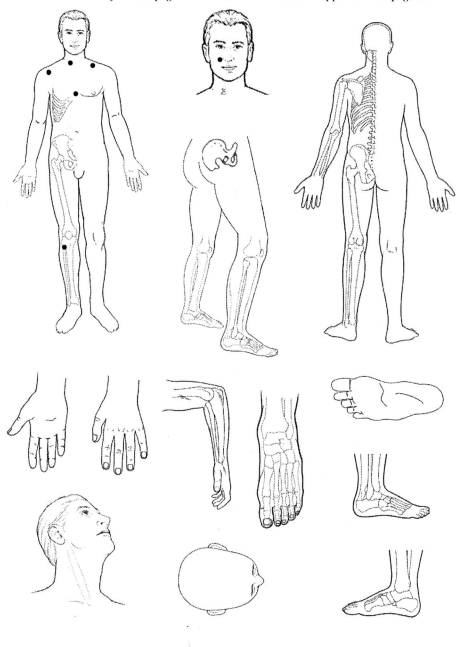

Crohn's Disease

Daily Nutritional Crisis Program	Daily Nutritional Wellness Program
GlycoN*: 5 ¼ tsp & GlycoAO: 4 caps PhytoN: 1 ¾ tsp PreH: 6 tabs Cata: 4 tabs ImmS: 5 tabs GstroP: 3 caps	GlycoN*: 1 ½ tsp & GlycoAO: 3 caps PhytoN: 3/4 tsp PreH: 4 tabs Cata: 4 tabs ImmS: 3 tabs GstroP: 3 caps

*For Adv.GlycoN see page 10. Product definitions are in Appendix A on page 381.

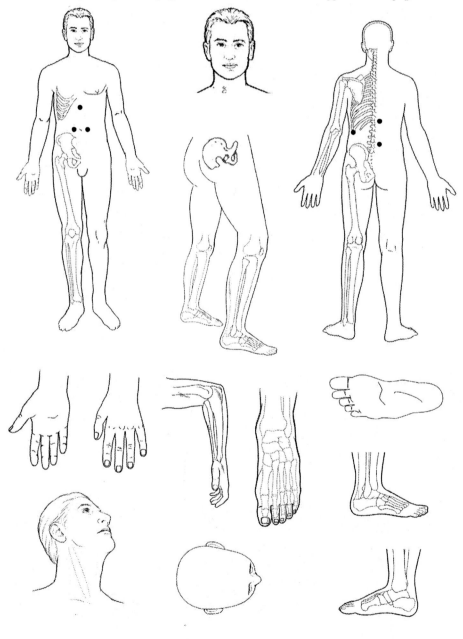

120

Croup

Daily Nutritional Crisis Program	Daily Nutritional Wellness Program
GlycoN*: 2 ½ tsp & GlycoAO: 3 caps PhytoN: 3/4 tsp PreH: 3 tabs GEssentials: 4 tabs ImmS: 4 tabs MC: 5 caps	GlycoN*: ½ tsp & GlycoAO: 2 caps PhytoN: 1/4 tsp PreH: 3 tabs GEssentials: 4 tabs ImmS: 3 tabs MC: 4 caps

*For Adv.GlycoN see page 10. Product definitions are in Appendix A on page 381.

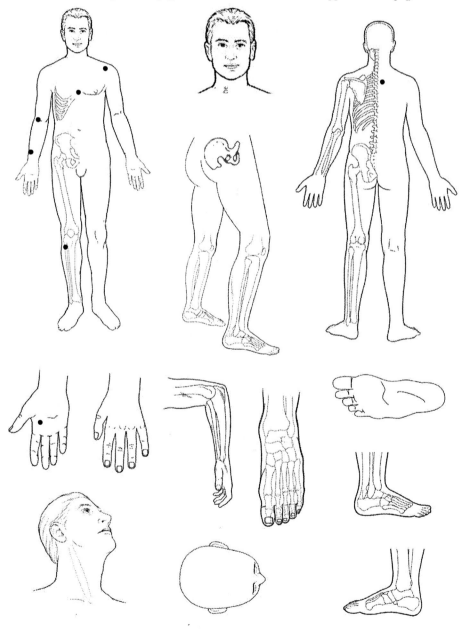

Cushing's Syndrome

Daily Nutritional Crisis Program	Daily Nutritional Wellness Program
GlycoN*: 2 ½ tsp & GlycoAO: 3 caps	GlycoN*: 1 ½ tsp & GlycoAO: 3 caps
PhytoN: 3/4 tsp	PhytoN: 1/2 tsp
PreH: 3 tabs	PreH: 3 tabs
Cata: 4 tabs	Cata: 4 tabs
ImmS: 6 tabs	ImmS: 5 tabs
Clean: 3 caps twice a day (2 weeks)	Clean: 3 caps

*For Adv.GlycoN see page 10. Product definitions are in Appendix A on page 381.

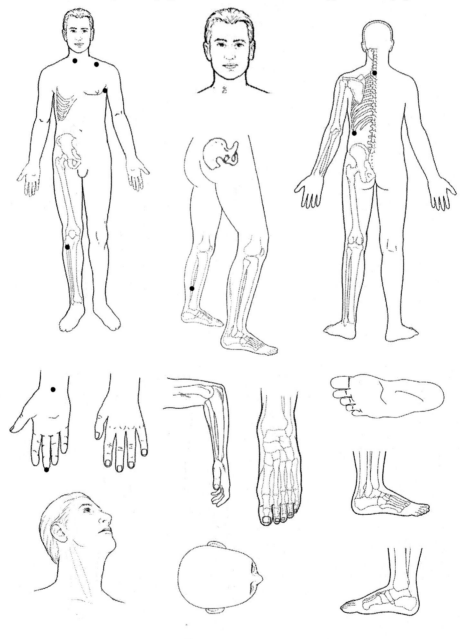

CVA / Stroke

Daily Nutritional Crisis Program	Daily Nutritional Wellness Program
GlycoN*: 5 ¼ tsp & GlycoAO: 4 caps PhytoN: 1 ¾ tsp PreH: 4 tabs Cata:6 tabs CB: 6 caps MC: 5 caps	GlycoN*: 1 ½ tsp & GlycoAO: 3 caps PhytoN: 3/4 tsp PreH: 3 tabs Cata: 4 tabs CB: 4 caps MC: 4 caps

*For Adv.GlycoN see page 10. Product definitions are in Appendix A on page 381.

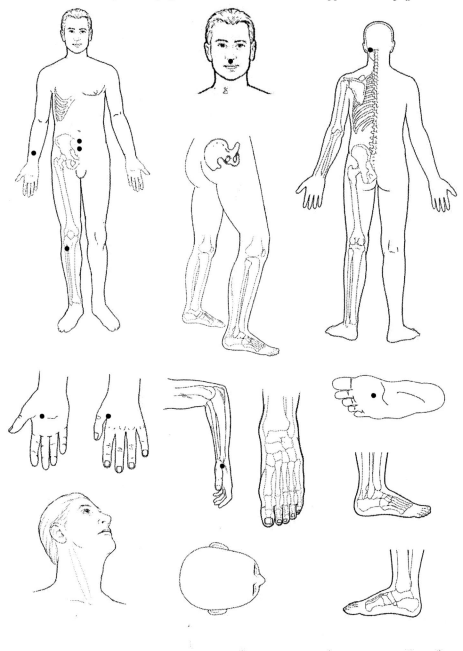

Cystitis (Acute UTI)
(drink only raw unsweetened cranberry juice)

Daily Nutritional Crisis Program	Daily Nutritional Wellness Program
GlycoN*: 2 ½ tsp & GlycoAO: 3 caps PhytoN: 3/4 tsp PreH: 3 tabs GEssentials: 4 tabs ImmS: 7 tabs MC: 6 caps	GlycoN*: ½ tsp & GlycoAO: 2 caps PhytoN: 1/4 tsp PreH: 3 tabs GEssentials: 4 tabs ImmS: 4 tabs MC: 5 caps

*For Adv.GlycoN see page 10. Product definitions are in Appendix A on page 381.

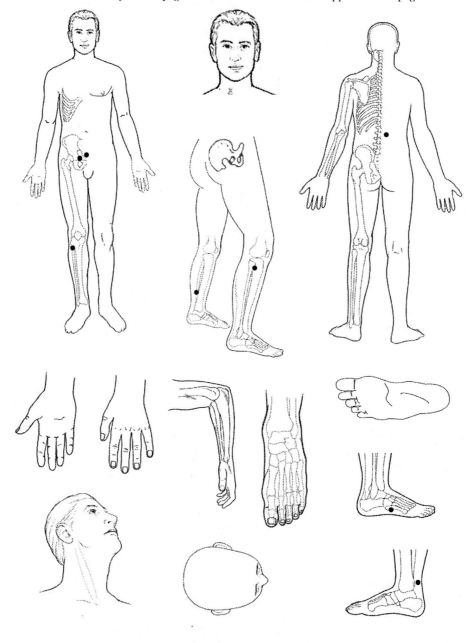

Cystitis (Chronic)
(drink only raw unsweetened cranberry juice)

Daily Nutritional Crisis Program	Daily Nutritional Wellness Program
GlycoN*: 2 ½ tsp & GlycoAO: 3 caps	GlycoN*: ½ tsp & GlycoAO: 2 caps
PhytoN: 3/4 tsp	PhytoN: 1/4 tsp
PreH: 3 tabs	PreH: 3 tabs
GEssentials: 4 tabs	GEssentials: 4 tabs
ImmS: 7 tabs	ImmS: 4 tabs
MC: 6 caps	MC: 5 caps

*For Adv.GlycoN see page 10. Product definitions are in Appendix A on page 381.

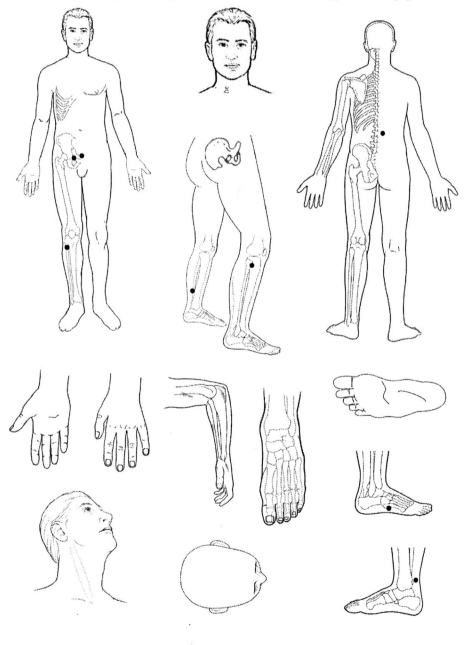

Cysts; Breasts
(eliminate caffeine from diet)

Daily Nutritional Crisis Program	Daily Nutritional Wellness Program
GlycoN*: 2 ½ tsp & GlycoAO: 3 caps	GlycoN*: ½ tsp & GlycoAO: 2 caps
PhytoN: 3/4 tsp	PhytoN: 1/2 tsp
PreH: 4 tabs	PreH: 4 tabs
GEssentials: 4 tabs	GEssentials: 4 tabs
ImmS: 5 tabs	ImmS: 3 tabs
MC: 4 caps	MC: 4 caps

*For Adv.GlycoN see page 10. Product definitions are in Appendix A on page 381.

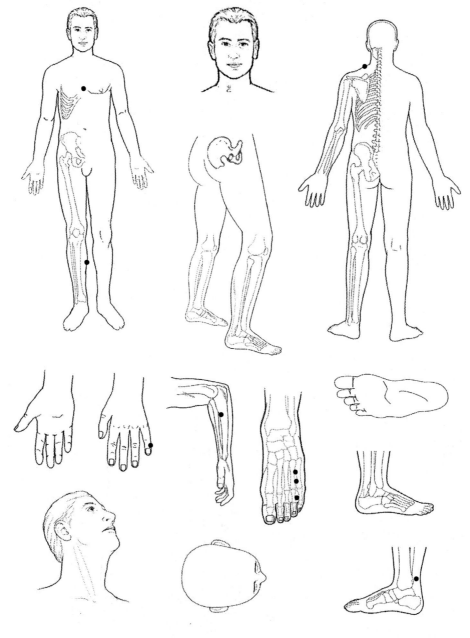

Cytomegalovirus

Daily Nutritional Crisis Program	Daily Nutritional Wellness Program
GlycoN*: 2 ½ tsp & GlycoAO: 3 caps PhytoN: 1 ¾ tsp PreH: 3 tabs Cata:6 tabs ImmS: 7 tabs MC: 5 caps	GlycoN*: 1 ½ tsp & GlycoAO: 3 caps PhytoN: 3/4 tsp PreH: 3 tabs Cata: 4 tabs ImmS: 5 tabs MC: 3 caps

*For Adv.GlycoN see page 10. Product definitions are in Appendix A on page 381.

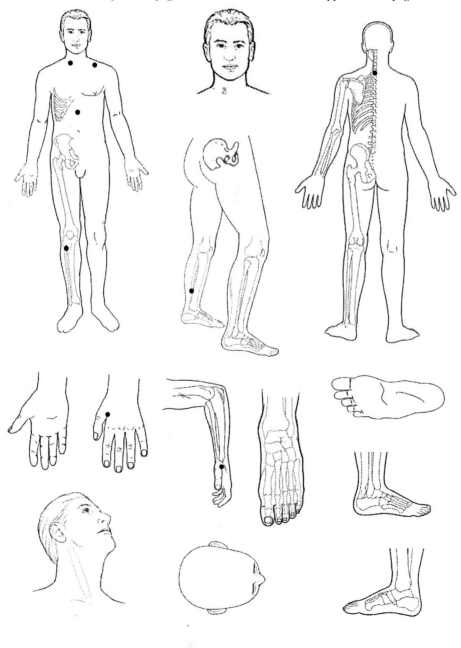

Dandruff

Daily Nutritional Crisis Program	Daily Nutritional Wellness Program
GlycoN*: 1 ½ tsp & GlycoAO: 3 caps	GlycoN*: ½ tsp & GlycoAO: 2 caps
PhytoN: 3/4 tsp	PhytoN: 1/4 tsp
PreH: 3 tabs	PreH: 3 tabs
GEssentials: 4 tabs	GEssentials: 4 tabs
Clean: 3 caps twice a day (2 weeks)	Clean: 2 caps
GstroP: 4 caps	GstroP: 2 caps

*For Adv.GlycoN see page 10. Product definitions are in Appendix A on page 381.

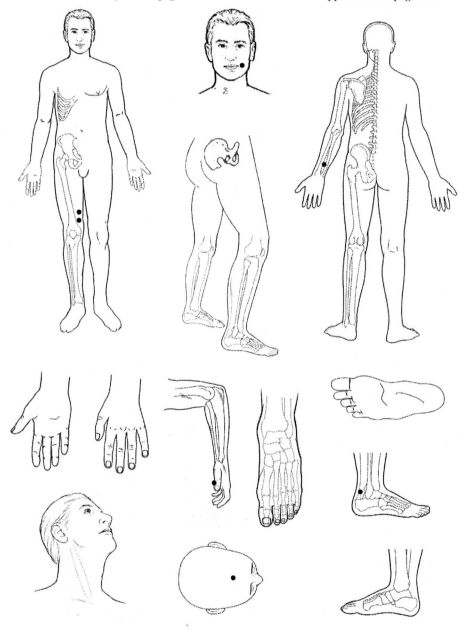

Decubitus Ulcer

(apply soft laser and "SkZone" to affect areas)

Daily Nutritional Crisis Program	Daily Nutritional Wellness Program
GlycoN*: 2 ½ tsp & GlycoAO: 3 caps PhytoN: 1 ¾ tsp PreH: 6 tabs Cata:6 tabs MC: 6 caps ImmS: 5 tabs	GlycoN*: ½ tsp & GlycoAO: 2 caps PhytoN: 3/4 tsp PreH: 3 tabs Cata: 4 tabs MC: 6 caps ImmS: 4 tabs

*For Adv.GlycoN see page 10. Product definitions are in Appendix A on page 381.

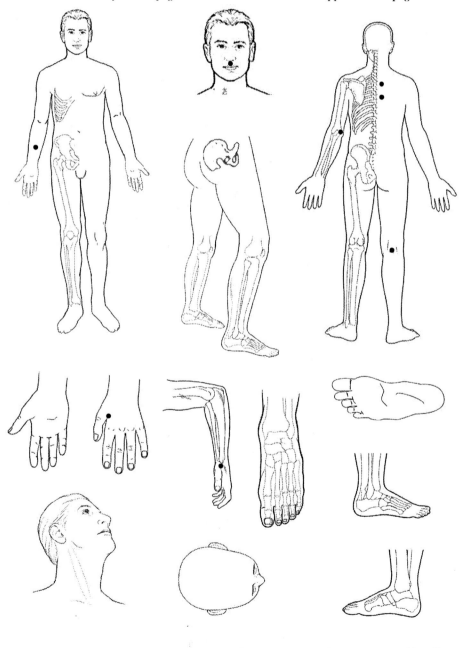

Deep Vein Thrombosis (DVT)

Daily Nutritional Crisis Program	Daily Nutritional Wellness Program
GlycoN*: 1 ½ tsp & GlycoAO: 3 caps	GlycoN*: ½ tsp & GlycoAO: 2 caps
PhytoN: 3/4 tsp	PhytoN: 1/2 tsp
PreH: 3 tabs	PreH: 3 tabs
GEssentials: 4 tabs	GEssentials: 4 tabs
MC: 7 caps	MC: 5 caps
CB: 6 caps	CB: 4 caps

*For Adv.GlycoN see page 10. Product definitions are in Appendix A on page 381.

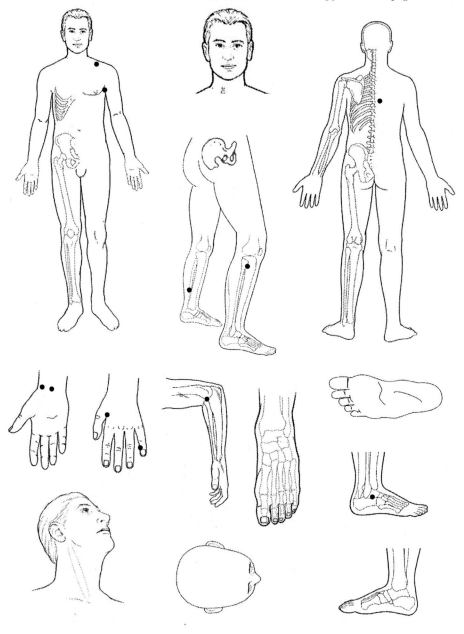

130

Degenerative Disc Disease

Daily Nutritional Crisis Program	Daily Nutritional Wellness Program
GlycoN*: 2 ½ tsp & GlycoAO: 3 caps PhytoN: 3/4 tsp PreH: 3 tabs Cata:6 tabs SP: 6 caps MC: 4 caps	GlycoN*: 1 ½ tsp & GlycoAO: 3 caps PhytoN: 1/2 tsp PreH: 3 tabs Cata: 4 tabs SP: 4 caps MC: 2 caps

*For Adv.GlycoN see page 10. Product definitions are in Appendix A on page 381.

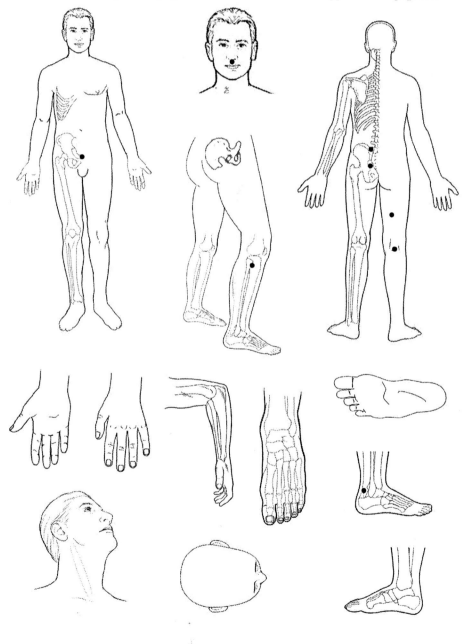

Degenerative Joint Disease (DJD)

Daily Nutritional Crisis Program	Daily Nutritional Wellness Program
GlycoN*: 2 ½ tsp & GlycoAO: 3 caps PhytoN: 3/4 tsp PreH: 3 tabs Cata:6 tabs SP: 6 caps MC: 4 caps	GlycoN*: 1 ½ tsp & GlycoAO: 3 caps PhytoN: 1/2 tsp PreH: 3 tabs Cata: 4 tabs SP: 4 caps MC: 2 caps

*For Adv.GlycoN see page 10. Product definitions are in Appendix A on page 381.

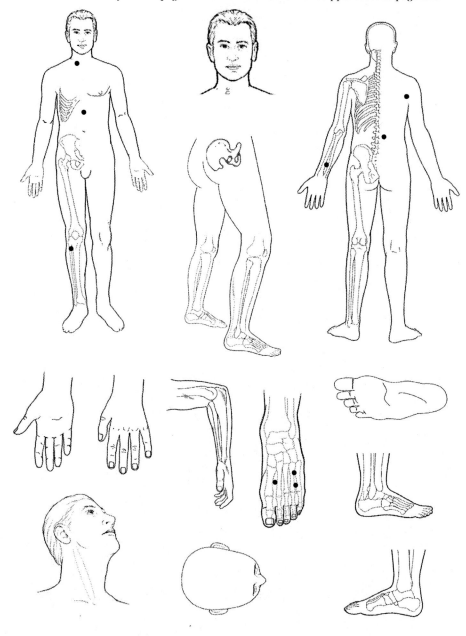

Depression

Daily Nutritional Crisis Program	Daily Nutritional Wellness Program
GlycoN*: 3 ½ tsp & GlycoAO: 3 caps PhytoN: 1 ¾ tsp PreH: 6 tabs Cata: 4 tabs SP: 6 caps	GlycoN*: 1 ½ tsp & GlycoAO: 3 caps PhytoN: 3/4 tsp PreH: 3 tabs Cata:2 tabs SP: 4 caps

*For Adv.GlycoN see page 10. Product definitions are in Appendix A on page 381.

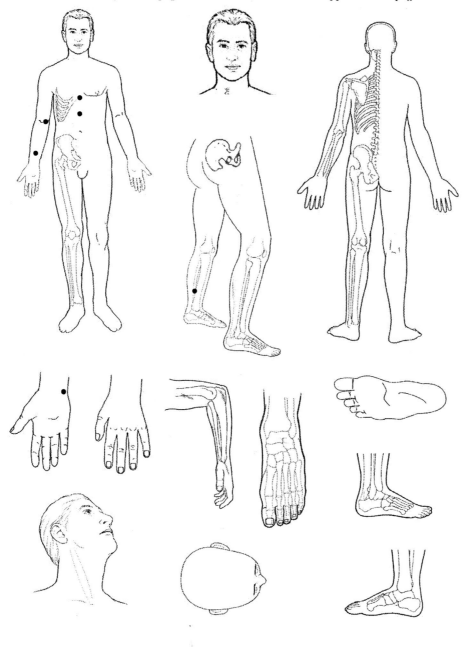

Dermatitis, Atopic Eczema
(apply soft laser to affect areas)

Daily Nutritional Crisis Program	Daily Nutritional Wellness Program
GlycoN*: 2 ½ tsp & GlycoAO: 3 caps PhytoN: 3/4 tsp PreH: 3 tabs GEssentials: 4 tabs Clean: 3 caps twice a day (2 weeks) ImmS: 6 tabs	GlycoN*: ½ tsp & GlycoAO: 2 caps PhytoN: 1/2 tsp PreH: 3 tabs GEssentials: 4 tabs Clean: 2 caps ImmS: 4 tabs

*For Adv.GlycoN see page 10. Product definitions are in Appendix A on page 381.

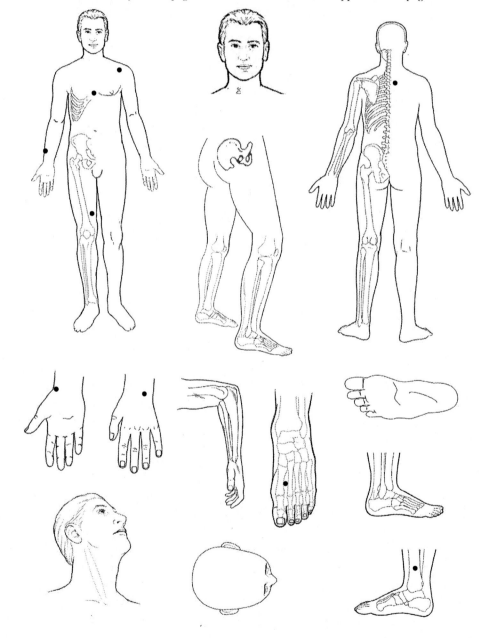

134

Detoxification (Systemic)

Daily Nutritional Crisis Program	Daily Nutritional Wellness Program
GlycoN*: 8 tsp & GlycoAO: 5 caps PhytoN: 1 ¾ tsp PreH: 4 tabs Cata: 4 tabs Clean: 3 caps twice a day (2 weeks) ImmS: 6 tabs & GstroP: 4 caps	GlycoN*: ½ tsp & GlycoAO: 2 caps PhytoN: 1/4 tsp PreH: 3 tabs Cata: 4 tabs Clean: 2 caps ImmS: 4 tabs & Gstro: 2 caps

*For Adv.GlycoN see page 10. Product definitions are in Appendix A on page 381.

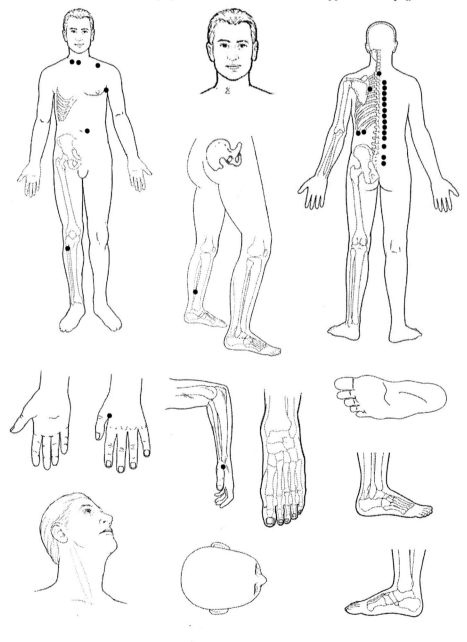

Diabetes

Daily Nutritional Crisis Program	Daily Nutritional Wellness Program
GlycoN*: 3 ½ tsp & GlycoAO: 3 caps PhytoN: 1 ¾ tsp PreH: 6 tabs Cata: 6 tabs ImmS: 4 tabs	GlycoN*: 1 ½ tsp & GlycoAO: 3 caps PhytoN: 1 tsp PreH: 3 tabs Cata: 6 tabs ImmS: 3 tabs

*For Adv.GlycoN see page 10. Product definitions are in Appendix A on page 381.

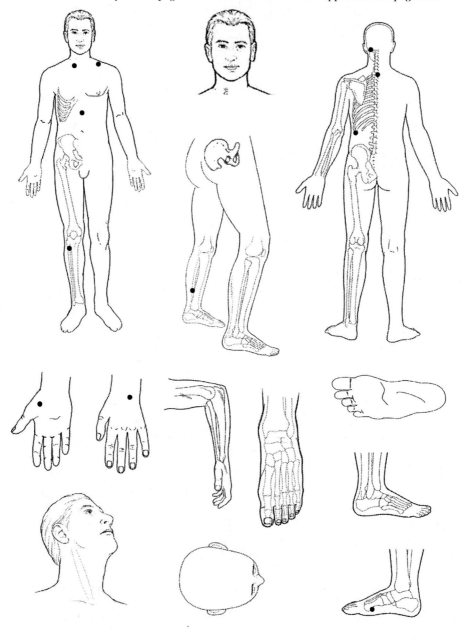

Diabetic Sores
(apply soft laser to affect areas)

Daily Nutritional Crisis Program	Daily Nutritional Wellness Program
GlycoN*: 2 ½ tsp & GlycoAO: 3 caps	GlycoN*: 1 ½ tsp & GlycoAO: 3 caps
PhytoN: 1 ¾ tsp	PhytoN: 3/4 tsp
PreH: 6 tabs	PreH: 3 tabs
Cata:6 tabs	Cata:6 tabs
MC: 6 caps	MC: 5 caps
SkZone: apply to affected areas	SkZone: apply to affected areas

*For Adv.GlycoN see page 10. Product definitions are in Appendix A on page 381.

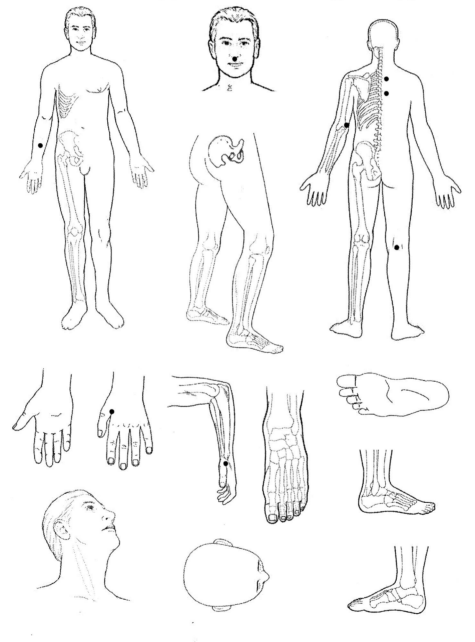

Diarrhea

Daily Nutritional Crisis Program	Daily Nutritional Wellness Program
GlycoN*: 2 ½ tsp & GlycoAO: 3 caps	GlycoN*: ½ tsp & GlycoAO: 2 caps
PhytoN: 3/4 tsp	PhytoN: 1/4 tsp
PreH: 3 tabs	PreH: 1 tabs
GEssentials: 4 tabs	GEssentials: 2 tabs
MC: 2 caps	MC: 1 cap
GstroP: 3 caps	GstroP: 2 caps

*For Adv.GlycoN see page 10. Product definitions are in Appendix A on page 381.

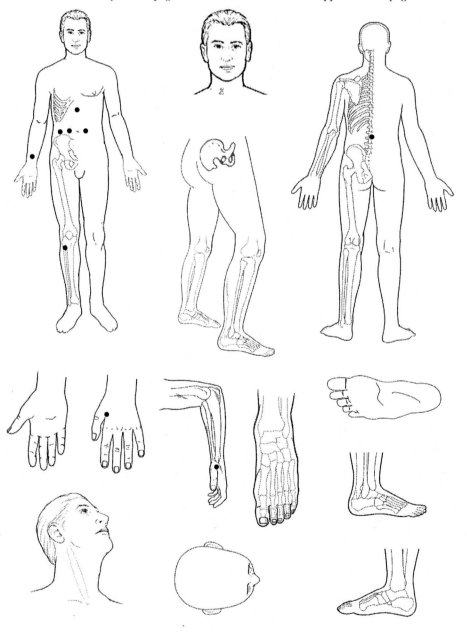

Diverticulitis w/o Hemorrhage

Daily Nutritional Crisis Program	Daily Nutritional Wellness Program
GlycoN*: 2 ½ tsp & GlycoAO: 3 caps PhytoN: 3/4 tsp PreH: 3 tabs GEssentials: 4 tabs MC: 2 caps GstroP: 3 caps	GlycoN*: ½ tsp & GlycoAO: 2 caps PhytoN: 1/4 tsp PreH: 1 tabs GEssentials: 2 tabs MC: 1 cap GstroP: 2 caps

*For Adv.GlycoN see page 10. Product definitions are in Appendix A on page 381.

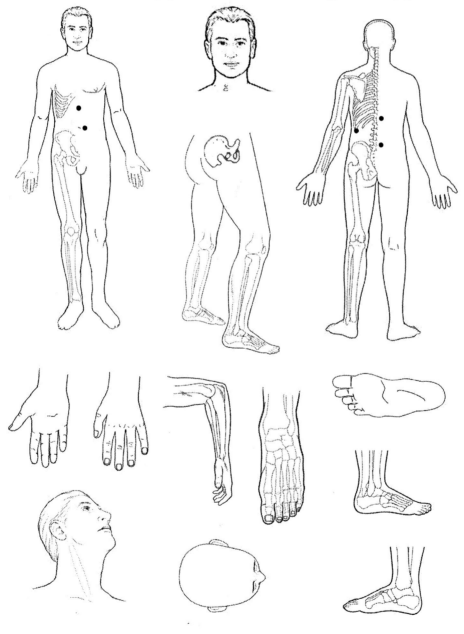

Dizziness (Vertigo)

Daily Nutritional Crisis Program	Daily Nutritional Wellness Program
GlycoN*: 2 ½ tsp & GlycoAO: 3 caps PhytoN: 3/4 tsp PreH: 3 tabs Cata: 4 tabs ImmS: 5 tabs MC: 5 caps	GlycoN*: ½ tsp & GlycoAO: 2 caps PhytoN: 1/4 tsp PreH: 3 tabs Cata: 4 tabs ImmS: 3 tabs MC: 3 caps

*For Adv.GlycoN see page 10. Product definitions are in Appendix A on page 381.

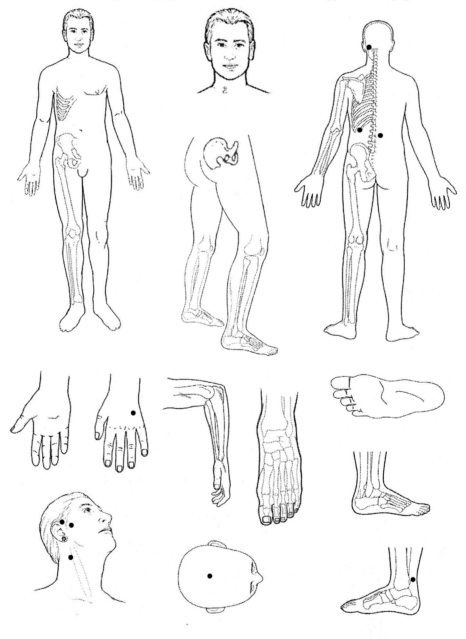

DJD (Degenerative Joint Disease)

Daily Nutritional Crisis Program	Daily Nutritional Wellness Program
GlycoN*: 2 ½ tsp & GlycoAO: 3 caps PhytoN: 3/4 tsp PreH: 3 tabs Cata:6 tabs SP: 6 caps MC: 4 caps	GlycoN*: 1 ½ tsp & GlycoAO: 3 caps PhytoN: 1/2 tsp PreH: 3 tabs Cata: 4 tabs SP: 4 caps MC: 2 caps

*For Adv.GlycoN see page 10. Product definitions are in Appendix A on page 381.

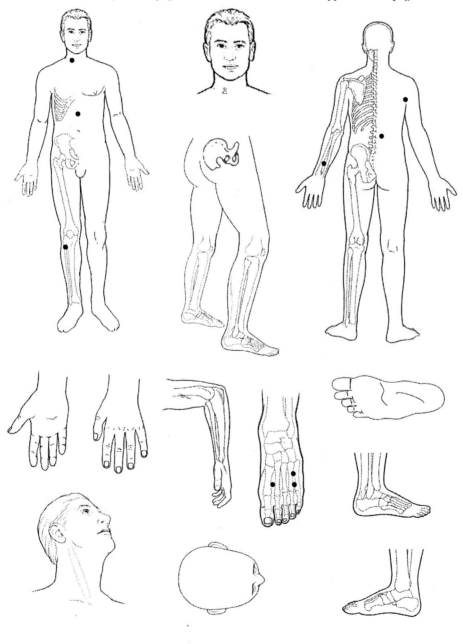

Drug Addiction

Daily Nutritional Crisis Program	Daily Nutritional Wellness Program
GlycoN*: 2½ tsp & GlycoAO: 3 caps PhytoN: 1/2 tsp PreH: 3 tabs Cata: 6 tabs	GlycoN*: 1½ tsp & GlycoAO: 3 caps PhytoN: 1/4 tsp PreH: 3 tabs Cata: 6 tabs

*For Adv.GlycoN see page 10. Product definitions are in Appendix A on page 381.

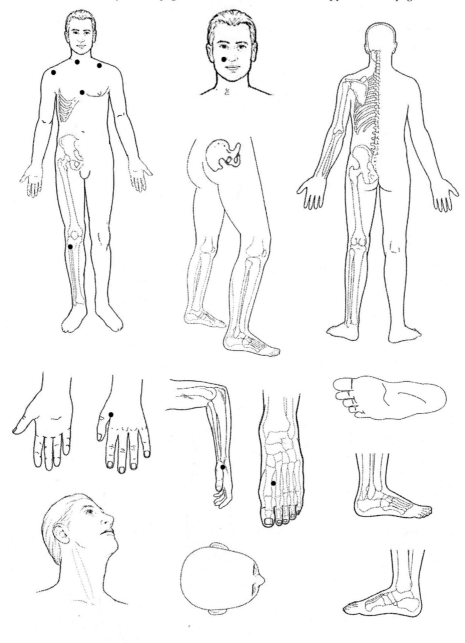

Duodenal Ulcer

Daily Nutritional Crisis Program	Daily Nutritional Wellness Program
GlycoN*: 2 ½ tsp & GlycoAO: 3 caps PhytoN: 3/4 tsp PreH: 3 tabs Cata: 4 tabs ImmS: 5 tabs MC: 4 caps	GlycoN*: ½ tsp & GlycoAO: 2 caps PhytoN: 1/2 tsp PreH: 3 tabs Cata: 4 tabs ImmS: 3 tabs MC: 2 caps

*For Adv.GlycoN see page 10. Product definitions are in Appendix A on page 381.

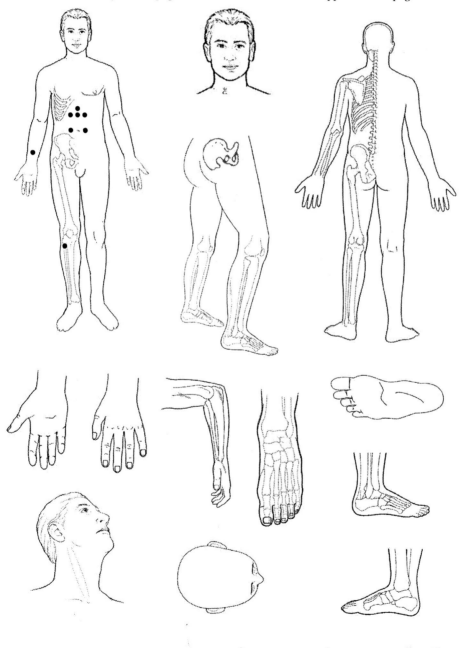

DVT (Deep Vein Thrombosis)

Daily Nutritional Crisis Program	Daily Nutritional Wellness Program
GlycoN*: 1 ½ tsp & GlycoAO: 3 caps	GlycoN*: ½ tsp & GlycoAO: 2 caps
PhytoN: 3/4 tsp	PhytoN: 1/4 tsp
PreH: 3 tabs	PreH: 3 tabs
GEssentials: 4 tabs	GEssentials: 4 tabs
MC: 5 caps	MC: 3 caps
CB: 5 caps	CB: 3 caps

*For Adv.GlycoN see page 10. Product definitions are in Appendix A on page 381.

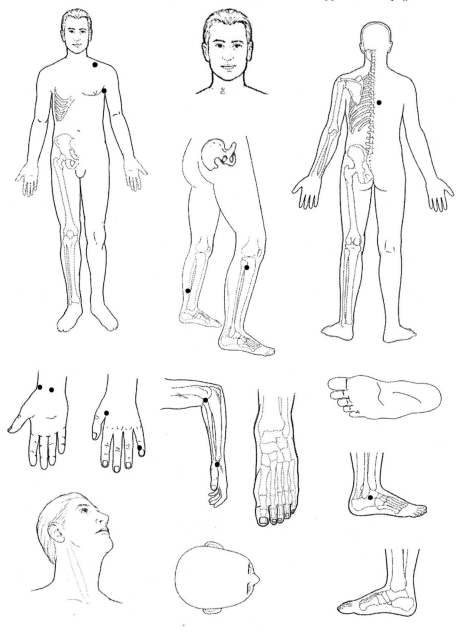

144

Dyslexia

Daily Nutritional Crisis Program	Daily Nutritional Wellness Program
GlycoN*: 5 ¼ tsp & GlycoAO: 4 caps PhytoN: 1 ¾ tsp PreH: 4 tabs Cata: 6 tabs SP: 4 caps	GlycoN*: 1 ½ tsp & GlycoAO: 3 caps PhytoN: 3/4 tsp PreH: 2 tabs Cata: 4 tabs SP: 2 caps

*For Adv.GlycoN see page 10. Product definitions are in Appendix A on page 381.

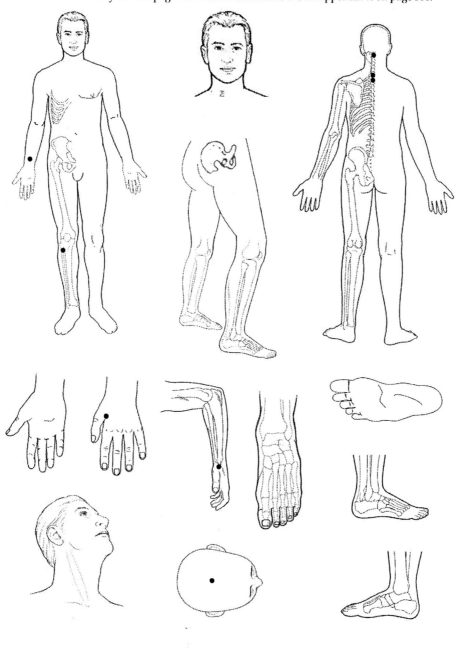

Dyspepsia

Daily Nutritional Crisis Program	Daily Nutritional Wellness Program
GlycoN*: 2 ½ tsp & GlycoAO: 3 caps PhytoN: 3/4 tsp PreH: 3 tabs GEssentials: 5 tabs GstroZ: 2 caps before meals GstroP: 2 caps	GlycoN*: ½ tsp & GlycoAO: 2 caps PhytoN: 1/4 tsp PreH: 2 tabs GEssentials: 3 tabs GstroZ: 2 caps before meals GstroP: 1 cap

*For Adv.GlycoN see page 10. Product definitions are in Appendix A on page 381.

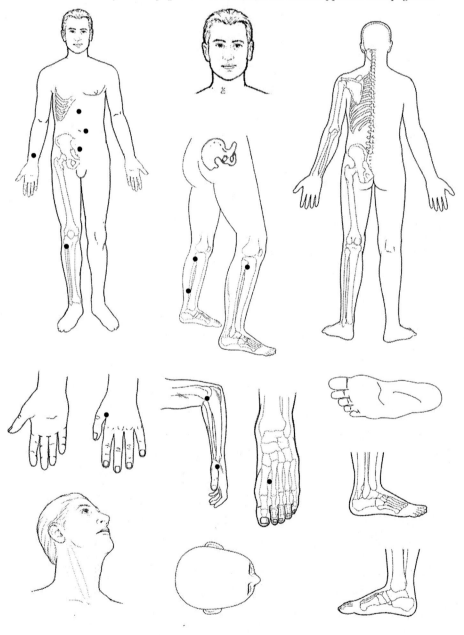

146

Dyspnea

Daily Nutritional Crisis Program	Daily Nutritional Wellness Program
GlycoN*: 2 ½ tsp & GlycoAO: 3 caps PhytoN: 3/4 tsp PreH: 3 tabs GEssentials: 4 tabs Clean: 3 caps twice a day (2 weeks) SP: 4 caps	GlycoN*: ½ tsp & GlycoAO: 2 caps PhytoN: 1/4 tsp PreH: 3 tabs GEssentials: 4 tabs Clean: 2 caps SP: 2 caps

*For Adv.GlycoN see page 10. Product definitions are in Appendix A on page 381.

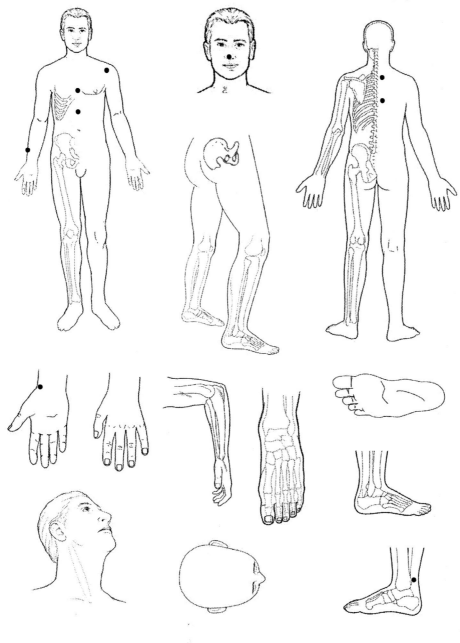

Dysuria

Daily Nutritional Crisis Program	Daily Nutritional Wellness Program
GlycoN*: 2 ½ tsp & GlycoAO: 3 caps PhytoN: 3/4 tsp PreH: 3 tabs GEssentials: 4 tabs ImmS: 5 tabs MC: 4 caps	GlycoN*: ½ tsp & GlycoAO: 2 caps PhytoN: 1/4 tsp PreH: 3 tabs GEssentials: 4 tabs ImmS: 4 tabs MC: 3 caps

*For Adv.GlycoN see page 10. Product definitions are in Appendix A on page 381.

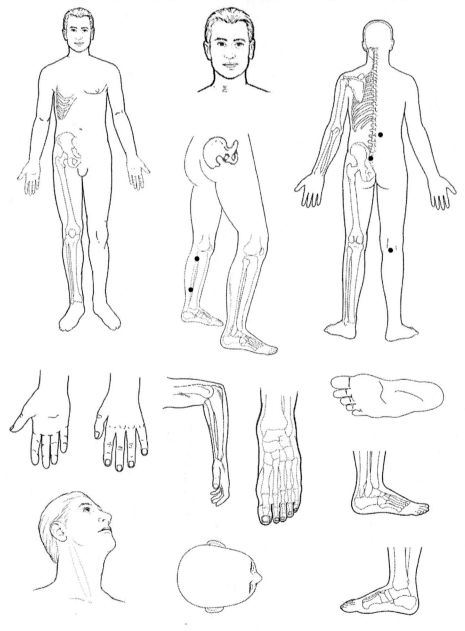

Earache

Daily Nutritional Crisis Program	Daily Nutritional Wellness Program
GlycoN*: 2 tsp & GlycoAO: 3 caps PhytoN: 3/4 tsp PreH: 3 tabs GEssentials: 4 tabs ImmS: 6 tabs MC: 5 caps	GlycoN*: ½ tsp & GlycoAO: 2 caps PhytoN: 1/4 tsp PreH: 3 tabs GEssentials: 4 tabs ImmS: 3 tabs MC: 3 caps

*For Adv.GlycoN see page 10. Product definitions are in Appendix A on page 381.

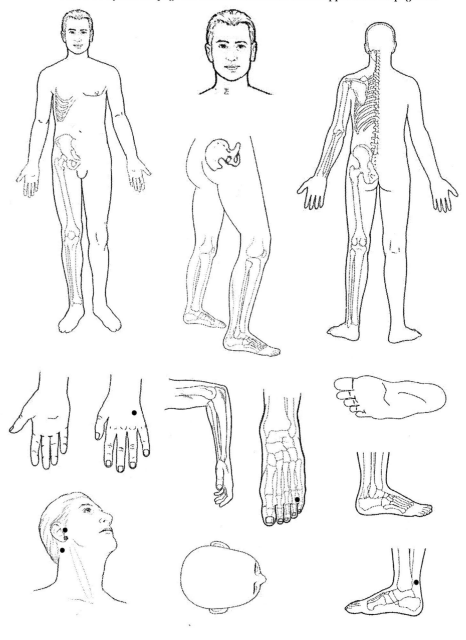

Elevated Blood Pressure w/o Hypertension

Daily Nutritional Crisis Program	Daily Nutritional Wellness Program
GlycoN*: 4 tsp & GlycoAO: 4 caps PhytoN: 1 tsp PreH: 6 tabs Cata: 4 tabs CB: 5 caps	GlycoN*: 1 ½ tsp & GlycoAO: 3 caps PhytoN: 3/4 tsp PreH: 3 tabs Cata: 4 tabs CB: 3 caps

*For Adv.GlycoN see page 10. Product definitions are in Appendix A on page 381.

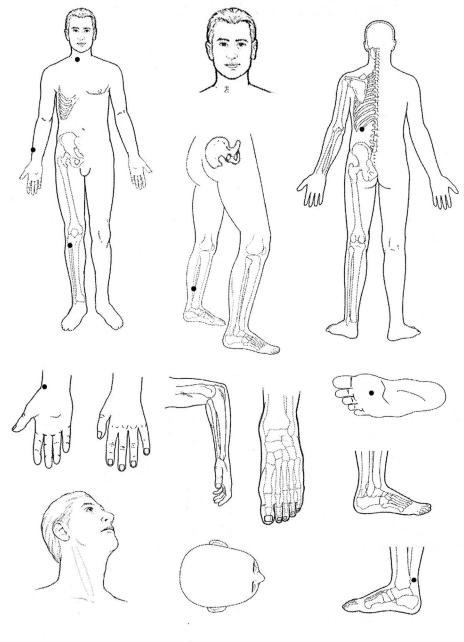

Emphysema

Daily Nutritional Crisis Program	Daily Nutritional Wellness Program
GlycoN*: 4 tsp & GlycoAO: 4 caps PhytoN: 1 tsp PreH: 4 tabs Cata: 4 tabs Clean: 3 caps twice a day (3 weeks) ImmS: 5 tabs	GlycoN*: 1 ½ tsp & GlycoAO: 3 caps PhytoN: 3/4 tsp PreH: 3 tabs Cata: 4 tabs Clean: 2 caps ImmS: 3 tabs

*For Adv.GlycoN see page 10. Product definitions are in Appendix A on page 381.

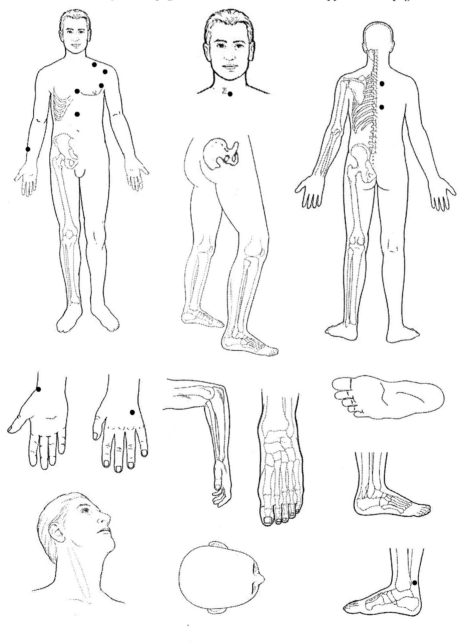

Endocarditis (Acute/Subacute Bacterial)

Daily Nutritional Crisis Program	Daily Nutritional Wellness Program
GlycoN*: 5 tsp & GlycoAO: 4 caps	GlycoN*: 1 ½ tsp & GlycoAO: 3 caps
PhytoN: 1 tsp	PhytoN: 3/4 tsp
PreH: 3 tabs	PreH: 3 tabs
Cata: 6 tabs	Cata: 4 tabs
ImmS: 6 tabs	ImmS: 4 tabs
MC: 6 caps & CB: 6 caps	MC: 3 caps & CB: 3 caps

*For Adv.GlycoN see page 10. Product definitions are in Appendix A on page 381.

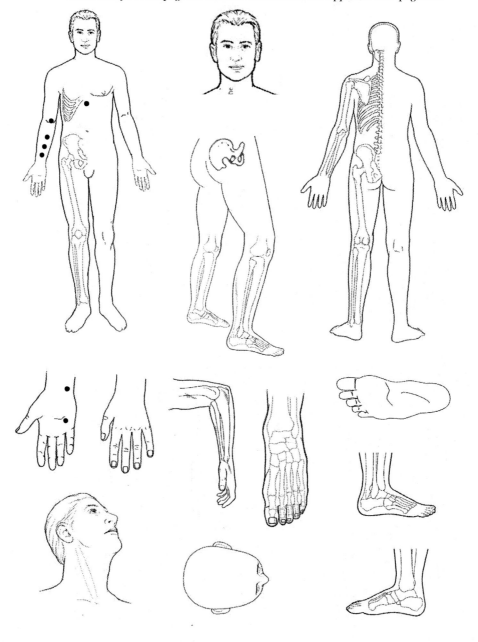

Endocervicitis

Daily Nutritional Crisis Program	Daily Nutritional Wellness Program
GlycoN*: 5 tsp & GlycoAO: 4 caps	GlycoN*: 1 ½ tsp & GlycoAO: 3 caps
PhytoN: 1 tsp	PhytoN: 1/2 tsp
PreH: 4 tabs	PreH: 3 tabs
GEssentials: 4 tabs	GEssentials: 4 tabs
ImmS: 6 tabs	ImmS: 3 tabs
MC: 4 caps	MC: 3 caps

*For Adv.GlycoN see page 10. Product definitions are in Appendix A on page 381.

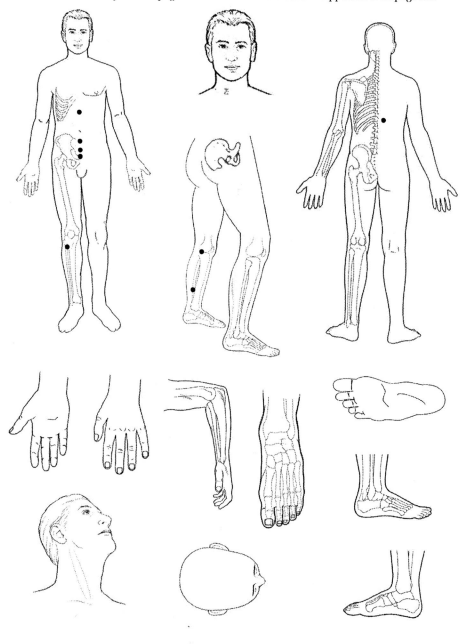

Endometriosis

Daily Nutritional Crisis Program	Daily Nutritional Wellness Program
GlycoN*: 5 tsp & GlycoAO: 4 caps	GlycoN*: 1 ½ tsp & GlycoAO: 3 caps
PhytoN: 1 tsp	PhytoN: 1/2 tsp
PreH: 4 tabs	PreH: 3 tabs
GEssentials: 4 tabs	GEssentials: 4 tabs
ImmS: 6 tabs	ImmS: 3 tabs
MC: 4 caps	MC: 3 caps

*For Adv.GlycoN see page 10. Product definitions are in Appendix A on page 381.

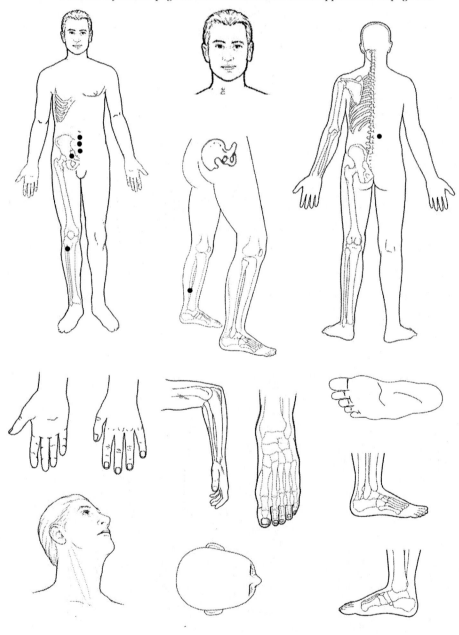

Enteritis (Bacterial)

Daily Nutritional Crisis Program	Daily Nutritional Wellness Program
GlycoN*: 5 tsp & GlycoAO: 4 caps PhytoN: 3/4 tsp PreH: 6 tabs Cata: 4 tabs MC: 6 caps ImmS: 8 tabs	GlycoN*: ½ tsp & GlycoAO: 2 caps PhytoN: 1/4 tsp PreH: 3 tabs Cata: 4 tabs MC: 3 caps ImmS: 4 tabs

*For Adv.GlycoN see page 10. Product definitions are in Appendix A on page 381.

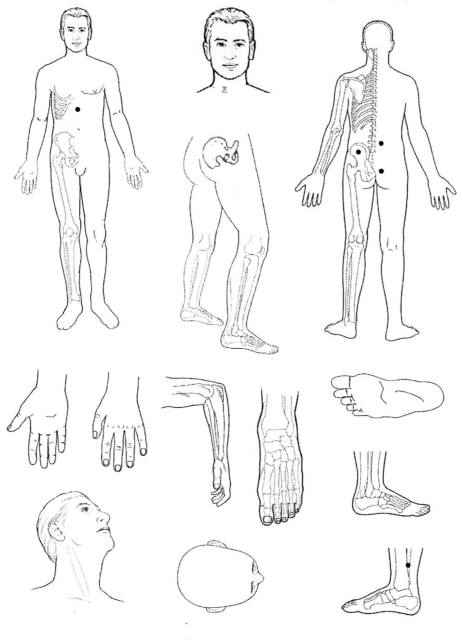

Enterocolitis, Ulcerative, Chronic

Daily Nutritional Crisis Program	Daily Nutritional Wellness Program
GlycoN*: 5 tsp & GlycoAO: 4 caps	GlycoN*: 1 ½ tsp & GlycoAO: 3 caps
PhytoN: 1 tsp	PhytoN: 3/4 tsp
PreH: 4 tabs	PreH: 3 tabs
Cata:4 tabs	Cata:4 tabs
ImmS: 4 tabs	ImmS: 2 tabs
MC: 4 caps & GstroP: 3 caps	MS: 2 caps & GstroP: 1 cap

*For Adv.GlycoN see page 10. Product definitions are in Appendix A on page 381.

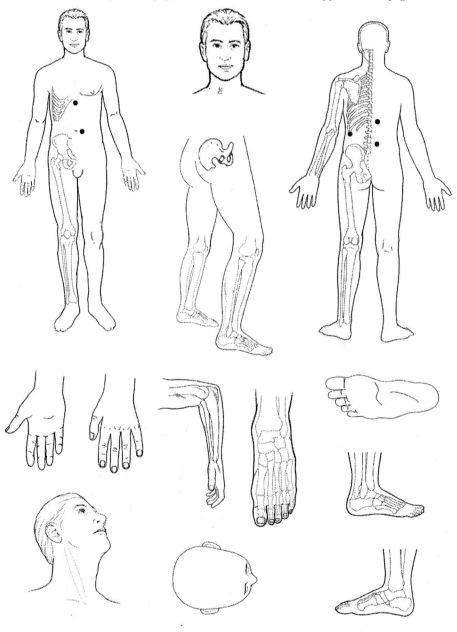

Epstein-Barr Virus

Daily Nutritional Crisis Program	Daily Nutritional Wellness Program
GlycoN*: 4 tsp & GlycoAO: 4 caps PhytoN: 1 tsp PreH: 6 tabs Cata:4 tabs ImmS: 4 tabs MC: 4 caps	GlycoN*: 1 ½ tsp & GlycoAO: 3 caps PhytoN: 3/4 tsp PreH: 4 tabs Cata:4 tabs ImmS: 2 tabs MC: 2 caps

*For Adv.GlycoN see page 10. Product definitions are in Appendix A on page 381.

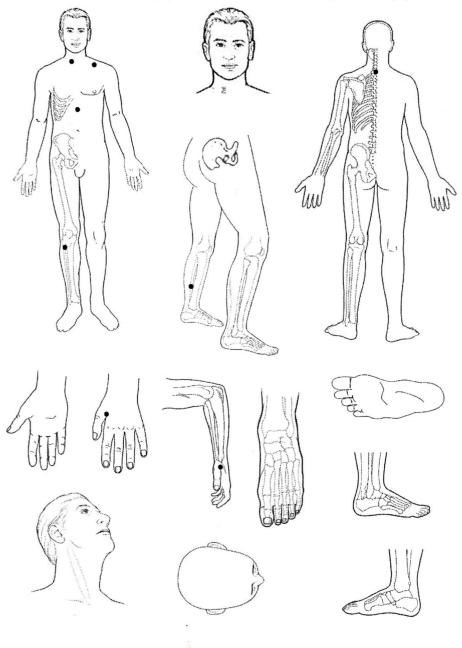

Esophageal Spasm

Daily Nutritional Crisis Program	Daily Nutritional Wellness Program
GlycoN*: 2 tsp & GlycoAO: 3 caps	GlycoN*: ½ tsp & GlycoAO: 2 caps
PhytoN: 3/4 tsp	PhytoN: 1/2 tsp
PreH: 3 tabs	PreH: 3 tabs
GEssentials: 4 tabs	GEssentials: 4 tabs
ImmS: 4 tabs	ImmS: 2 tabs
MC: 6 caps & SP: 4 caps	MC: 3 caps & SP: 2 caps

*For Adv.GlycoN see page 10. Product definitions are in Appendix A on page 381.

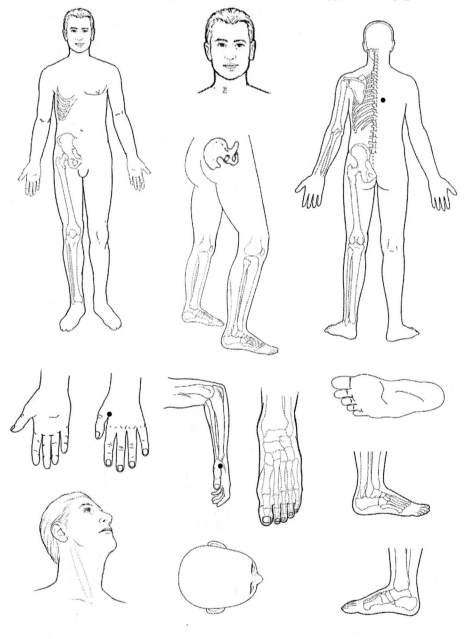

Esophagitis

Daily Nutritional Crisis Program	Daily Nutritional Wellness Program
GlycoN*: 2 tsp & GlycoAO: 3 caps PhytoN: 3/4 tsp PreH: 3 tabs GEssentials: 4 tabs ImmS: 5 tabs MC: 6 caps	GlycoN*: ½ tsp & GlycoAO: 2 caps PhytoN: 1/2 tsp PreH: 3 tabs GEssentials: 4 tabs ImmS: 3 tabs MC: 3 caps

*For Adv.GlycoN see page 10. Product definitions are in Appendix A on page 381.

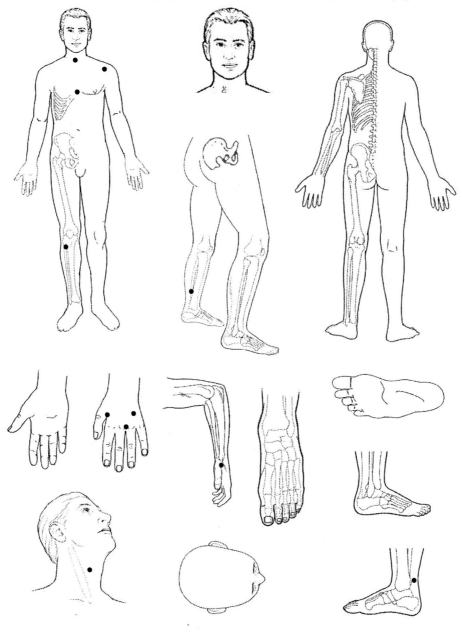

Eustachian Tube Infection

Daily Nutritional Crisis Program	Daily Nutritional Wellness Program
GlycoN*: 2 tsp & GlycoAO: 3 caps	GlycoN*: ½ tsp & GlycoAO: 2 caps
PhytoN: 3/4 tsp	PhytoN: 1/4 tsp
PreH: 3 tabs	PreH: 3 tabs
GEssentials: 4 tabs	GEssentials: 4 tabs
ImmS: 6 tabs	ImmS: 3 tabs
MC: 5 caps	MC: 3 caps

*For Adv.GlycoN see page 10. Product definitions are in Appendix A on page 381.

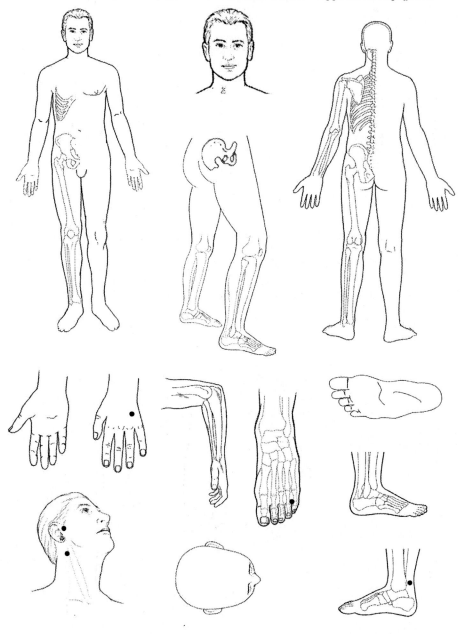

Excessive Sweating (Hyperhidrosis)

Daily Nutritional Crisis Program	Daily Nutritional Wellness Program
GlycoN*: 2 tsp & GlycoAO: 3 caps PhytoN: 1/2 tsp PreH: 4 tabs GEssentials: 4 tabs ImmS: 4 tabs SP: 4 caps & MC: 3 caps	GlycoN*: ½ tsp & GlycoAO: 2 caps PhytoN: 1/4 tsp PreH: 3 tabs GEssentials: 4 tabs ImmS: 3 tabs SP: 2 caps & MC: 2 caps

*For Adv.GlycoN see page 10. Product definitions are in Appendix A on page 381.

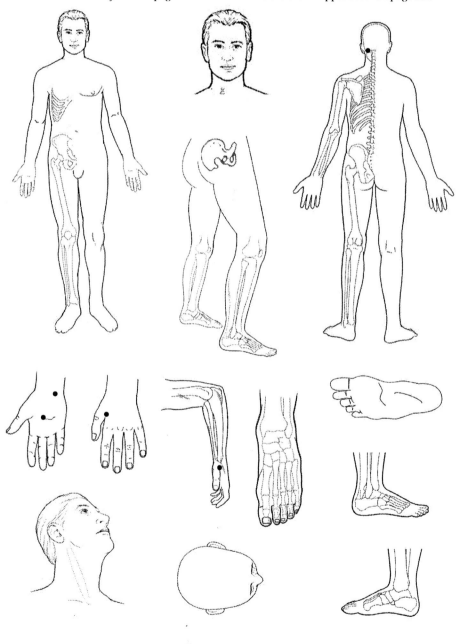

Exercise Intolerance

Daily Nutritional Crisis Program	Daily Nutritional Wellness Program
GlycoN*: 2 tsp & GlycoAO: 3 caps PhytoN: 1/2 tsp PreH: 4 tabs Cata: 4 tabs SP: 5 caps & EM: 1 ½ tblspn CB: 5 caps	GlycoN*: ½ tsp & GlycoAO: 2 caps PhytoN: 1/4 tsp PreH: 4 tabs Cata: 4 tabs SP: 3 caps & EM: 1 ½ tblspn CB: 3 caps

*For Adv.GlycoN see page 10. Product definitions are in Appendix A on page 381.

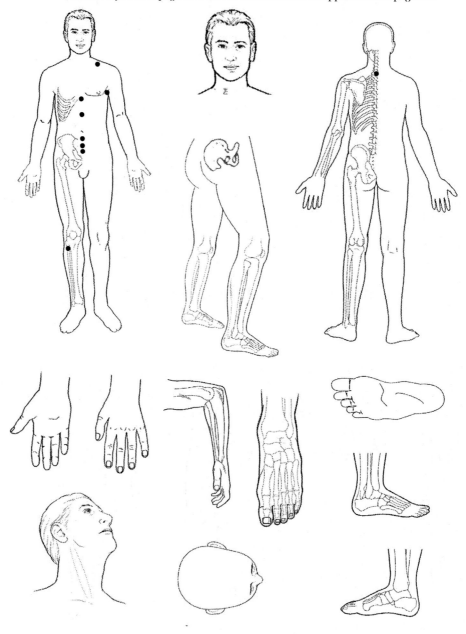

162

Eyes (Swollen)

Daily Nutritional Crisis Program	Daily Nutritional Wellness Program
GlycoN*: 2 tsp & GlycoAO: 3 caps PhytoN: 3/4 tsp PreH: 3 tabs GEssentials: 4 tabs MC: 4 caps SP: 4 caps	GlycoN*: ½ tsp & GlycoAO: 2 caps PhytoN: 1/4 tsp PreH: 3 tabs GEssentials: 4 tabs MC: 2 caps SP: 3 caps

*For Adv.GlycoN see page 10. Product definitions are in Appendix A on page 381.

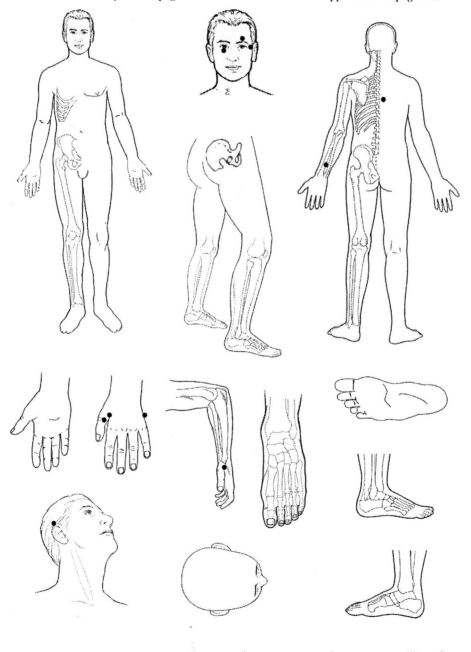

Failure to Thrive

Daily Nutritional Crisis Program	Daily Nutritional Wellness Program
GlycoN*: 5 tsp & GlycoAO: 4 caps	GlycoN*: 1 ½ tsp & GlycoAO: 3 caps
PhytoN: 1/2 tsp	PhytoN: 1/4 tsp
PreH: 3 tabs	PreH: 3 tabs
Cata: 4 tabs	Cata: 4 tabs
ImmS: 4 tabs	ImmS: 2 tabs
MC: 4 caps & SP: 4 caps	MC: 2 caps & SP: 2 caps

*For Adv.GlycoN see page 10. Product definitions are in Appendix A on page 381.

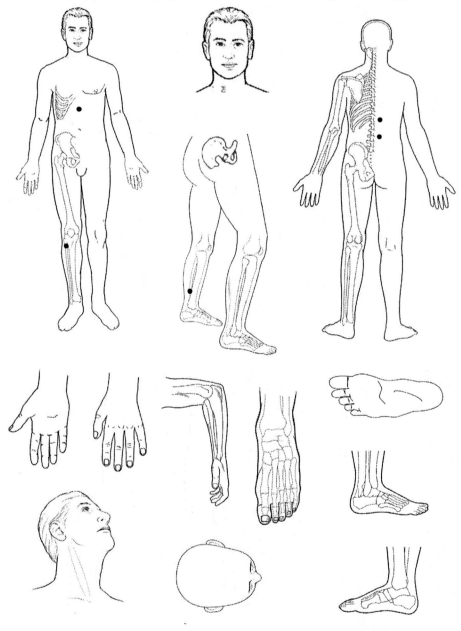

Family History of Breast Cancer

Daily Nutritional Crisis Program	Daily Nutritional Wellness Program
GlycoN*: 10 tsp & GlycoAO: 6 caps PhytoN: 2 tsp PreH: 6 tabs Cata: 6 tabs ImmS: 6 tabs MC: 6 caps	GlycoN*: 2 tsp & GlycoAO: 3 caps PhytoN: 1 tsp PreH: 4 tabs Cata: 6 tabs ImmS: 3 tabs MC: 3 caps

*For Adv.GlycoN see page 10. Product definitions are in Appendix A on page 381.

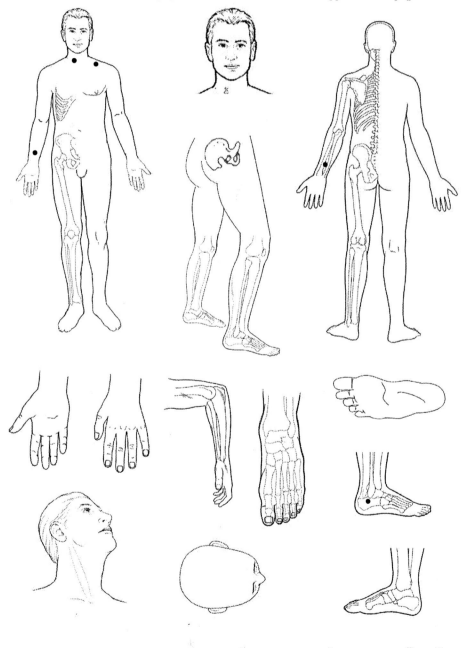

Family History of Coronary Disease

Daily Nutritional Crisis Program	Daily Nutritional Wellness Program
GlycoN*: 5 tsp & GlycoAO: 4 caps PhytoN: 1 ¾ tsp PreH: 3 tabs Cata: 4 tabs CB: 7 caps	GlycoN*: 1 ½ tsp & GlycoAO: 3 caps PhytoN: 3/4 tsp PreH: 3 tabs Cata: 4 tabs CB: 3 caps

*For Adv.GlycoN see page 10. Product definitions are in Appendix A on page 381.

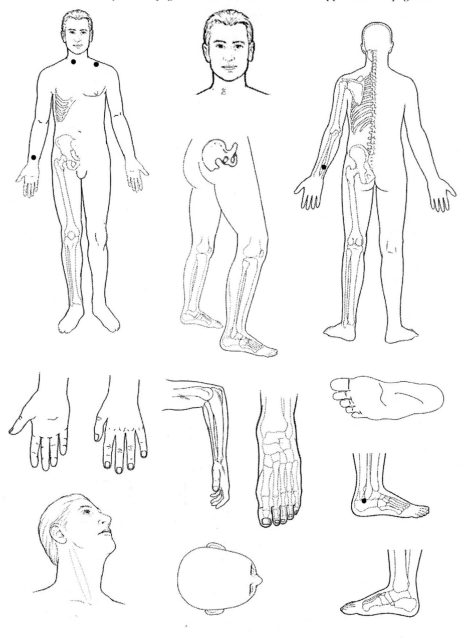

Family History of Diabetes

Daily Nutritional Crisis Program	Daily Nutritional Wellness Program
GlycoN*: 3 tsp & GlycoAO: 3 caps PhytoN: 1 tsp PreH: 6 tabs Cata: 6 tabs ImmS: 4 tabs	GlycoN*: 1 ½ tsp & GlycoAO: 3 caps PhytoN: 1/2 tsp PreH: 3 tabs Cata: 6 tabs ImmS: 3 tabs

*For Adv.GlycoN see page 10. Product definitions are in Appendix A on page 381.

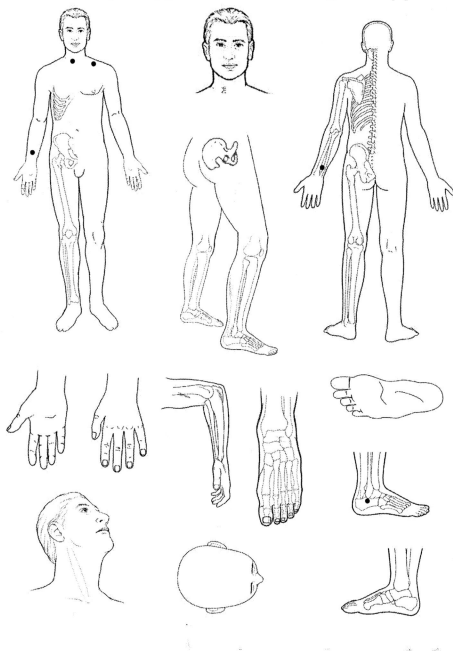

Family History of Gastrointestinal Malignancy

Daily Nutritional Crisis Program	Daily Nutritional Wellness Program
GlycoN*: 10 tsp & GlycoAO: 6 caps PhytoN: 3 tsp PreH: 6 tabs Cata:6 tabs ImmS: 6 tabs MC: 6 caps	GlycoN*: 2 tsp & GlycoAO: 3 caps PhytoN: 1 tsp PreH: 4 tabs Cata:6 tabs ImmS: 3 tabs MC: 3 caps

*For Adv.GlycoN see page 10. Product definitions are in Appendix A on page 381.

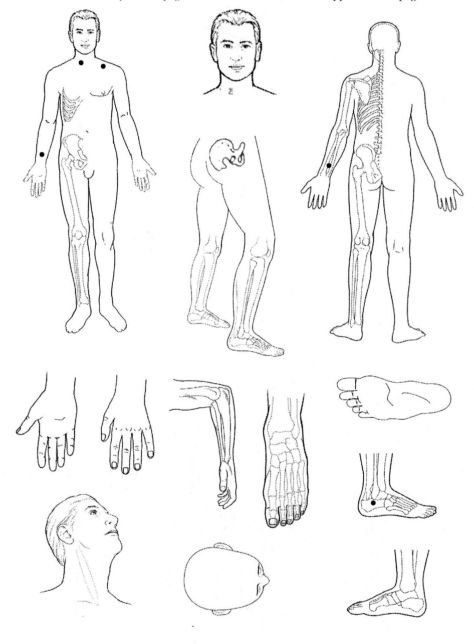

Fasciitis

Daily Nutritional Crisis Program	Daily Nutritional Wellness Program
GlycoN*: 8 tsp & GlycoAO: 5 caps PhytoN: 3/4 tsp PreH: 6 tabs Cata: 6 tabs ImmS: 5 tabs MC: 5 caps	GlycoN*: 1 ½ tsp & GlycoAO: 3 caps PhytoN: 1/4 tsp PreH: 4 tabs Cata: 4 tabs ImmS: 3 tabs MC: 3 caps

*For Adv.GlycoN see page 10. Product definitions are in Appendix A on page 381.

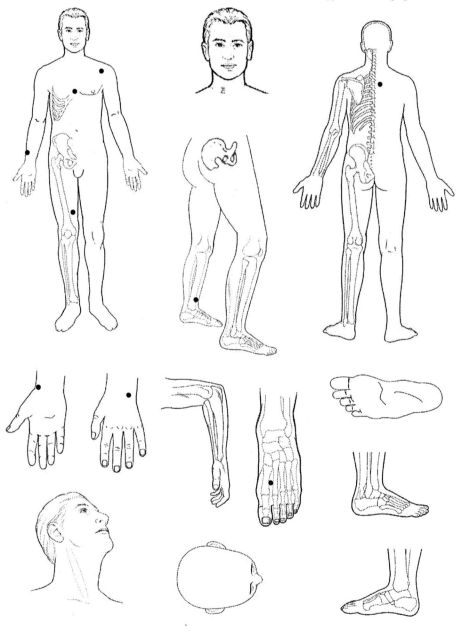

Fatigue/Malaise

Daily Nutritional Crisis Program	Daily Nutritional Wellness Program
GlycoN*: 5 tsp & GlycoAO: 4 caps PhytoN: 1 tsp PreH: 6 tabs Cata: 4 tabs ImmS: 4 tabs MC: 4 caps	GlycoN*: 1 ½ tsp & GlycoAO: 3 caps PhytoN: 1/4 tsp PreH: 4 tabs Cata: 4 tabs ImmS: 2 tabs MC: 2 caps

*For Adv.GlycoN see page 10. Product definitions are in Appendix A on page 381.

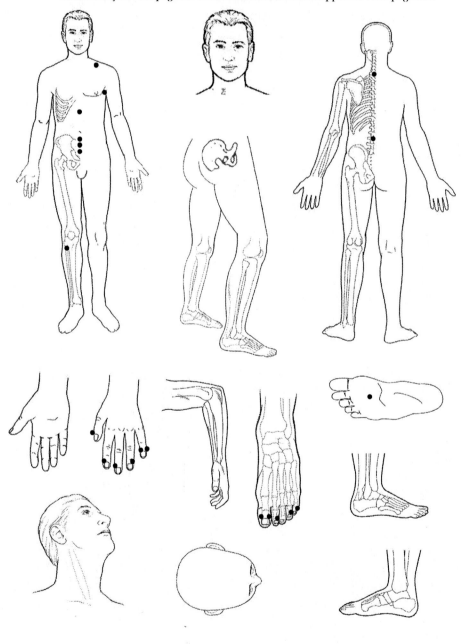

Fever

Daily Nutritional Crisis Program	Daily Nutritional Wellness Program
GlycoN*: 2 tsp & GlycoAO: 3 caps PhytoN: 1 tsp PreH: 3 tabs GEssentials: 6 tabs ImmS: 6 tabs MC: 6 caps	GlycoN*: ½ tsp & GlycoAO: 2 caps PhytoN: 1/4 tsp PreH: 3 tabs GEssentials: 4 tabs ImmS: 3 tabs MC: 3 caps

*For Adv.GlycoN see page 10. Product definitions are in Appendix A on page 381.

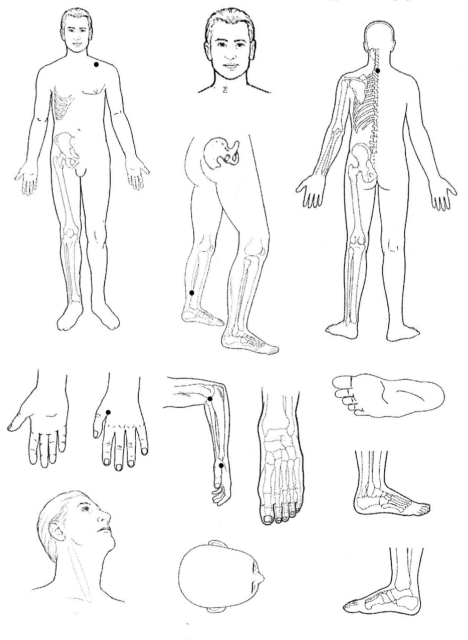

Fibrocystic Breast Disease
(eliminate caffiene from diet)

Daily Nutritional Crisis Program	Daily Nutritional Wellness Program
GlycoN*: 2 tsp & GlycoAO: 3 caps PhytoN: 3/4 tsp PreH: 4 tabs GEssentials: 4 tabs ImmS: 5 tabs MC: 4 caps	GlycoN*: ½ tsp & GlycoAO: 2 caps PhytoN: 1/4 tsp PreH: 4 tabs GEssentials: 4 tabs ImmS: 3 tabs MC: 4 caps

*For Adv.GlycoN see page 10. Product definitions are in Appendix A on page 381.

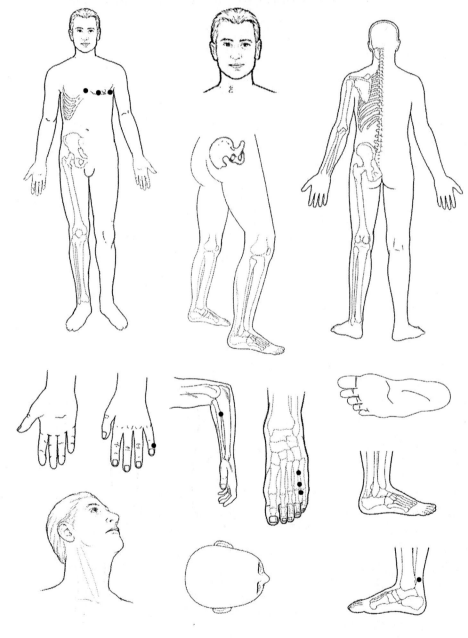

Fibroids (Uterine)

Daily Nutritional Crisis Program	Daily Nutritional Wellness Program
GlycoN*: 2 tsp & GlycoAO: 3 caps	GlycoN*: ½ tsp & GlycoAO: 2 caps
PhytoN: 3/4 tsp	PhytoN: 1/4 tsp
PreH: 4 tabs	PreH: 4 tabs
GEssentials: 4 tabs	GEssentials: 4 tabs
ImmS: 5 tabs	ImmS: 3 tabs
MC: 5 caps	MC: 4 caps

*For Adv.GlycoN see page 10. Product definitions are in Appendix A on page 381.

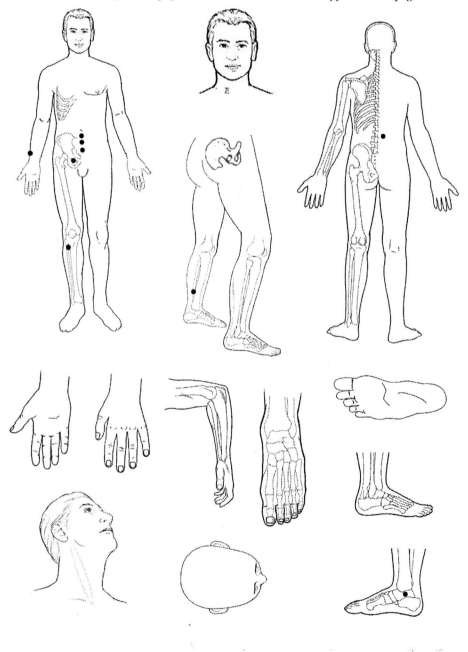

Fibromyalgia

Daily Nutritional Crisis Program	Daily Nutritional Wellness Program
GlycoN*: 5 tsp & GlycoAO: 4 caps PhytoN: 1 tsp PreH: 6 tabs Cata: 6 tabs SP: 6 caps ImmS: 4 tabs & MC: 4 caps	GlycoN*: 1 ½ tsp & GlycoAO: 3 caps PhytoN: 1/2 tsp PreH: 4 tabs Cata: 4 tabs SP: 3 caps ImmS: 3 tabs & MC: 2 caps

*For Adv.GlycoN see page 10. Product definitions are in Appendix A on page 381.

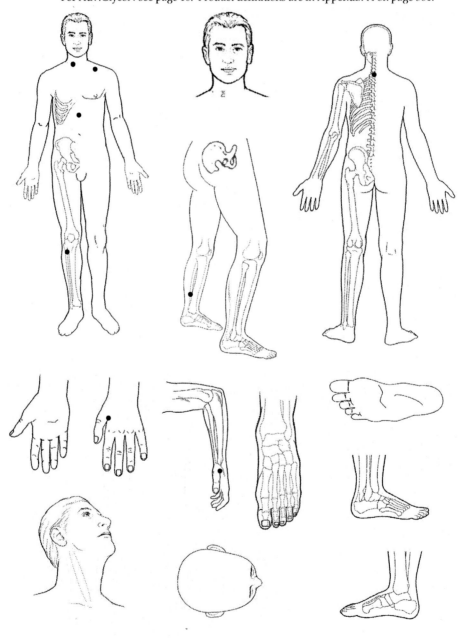

Fibrositis

Daily Nutritional Crisis Program	Daily Nutritional Wellness Program
GlycoN*: 5 tsp & GlycoAO: 4 caps PhytoN: 1 tsp PreH: 6 tabs Cata: 6 tabs ImmS: 6 tabs MC: 5 caps	GlycoN*: 1 ½ tsp & GlycoAO: 3 caps PhytoN: 1/2 tsp PreH: 4 tabs Cata: 4 tabs ImmS: 3 tabs MC: 3 caps

*For Adv.GlycoN see page 10. Product definitions are in Appendix A on page 381.

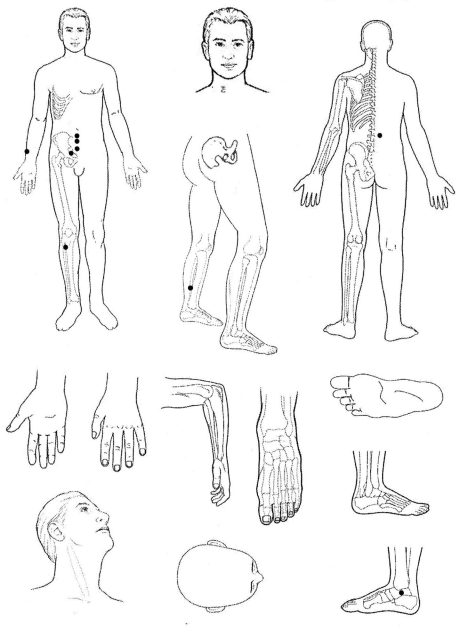

Flatulence

Daily Nutritional Crisis Program	Daily Nutritional Wellness Program
GlycoN*: 2 tsp & GlycoAO: 3 caps PhytoN: 1/2 tsp PreH: 4 tabs GEssentials: 4 tabs GstroP: 3 caps GstroZ: 2 caps before meals	GlycoN*: ½ tsp & GlycoAO: 2 caps PhytoN: 1/4 tsp PreH: 3 tabs GEssentials: 4 tabs GstroP: 2 caps GstroZ: 1 cap before meals

*For Adv.GlycoN see page 10. Product definitions are in Appendix A on page 381.

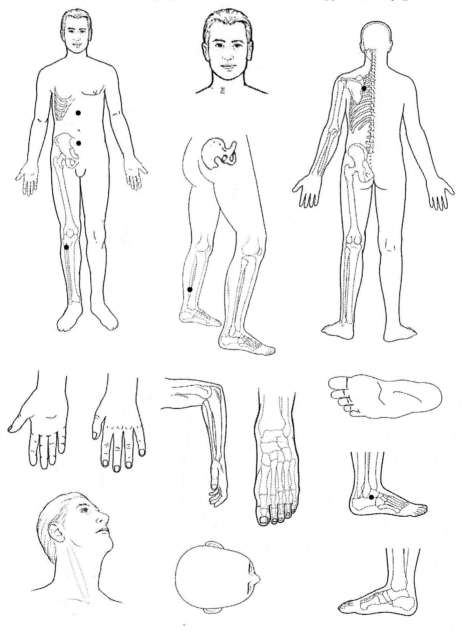

Flora- Restoration Post Antibiotic Therapy

Daily Nutritional Crisis Program	Daily Nutritional Wellness Program
GlycoN*: 2 tsp & GlycoAO: 3 caps PhytoN: 3/4 tsp PreH: 3 tabs Cata: 6 tabs Clean: 3 caps twice a day (2 weeks) GstroP: 4 caps	GlycoN*: ½ tsp & GlycoAO: 2 caps PhytoN: 1/4 tsp PreH: 3 tabs Cata: 4 tabs Clean: 2 caps GstroP: 2 caps

*For Adv.GlycoN see page 10. Product definitions are in Appendix A on page 381.

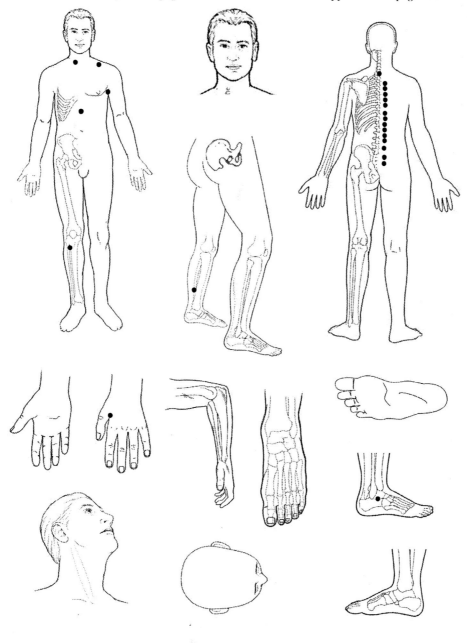

177

Flu Shot Vaccine

Daily Nutritional Crisis Program	Daily Nutritional Wellness Program
GlycoN*: 2 tsp & GlycoAO: 3 caps	GlycoN*: ½ tsp & GlycoAO: 2 caps
PhytoN: 1 tsp	PhytoN: 1/4 tsp
PreH: 3 tabs	PreH: 3 tabs
GEssentials: 6 tabs	GEssentials: 4 tabs
ImmS: 6 tabs	ImmS: 3 tabs
MC: 6 caps	MC: 3 caps

*For Adv.GlycoN see page 10. Product definitions are in Appendix A on page 381.

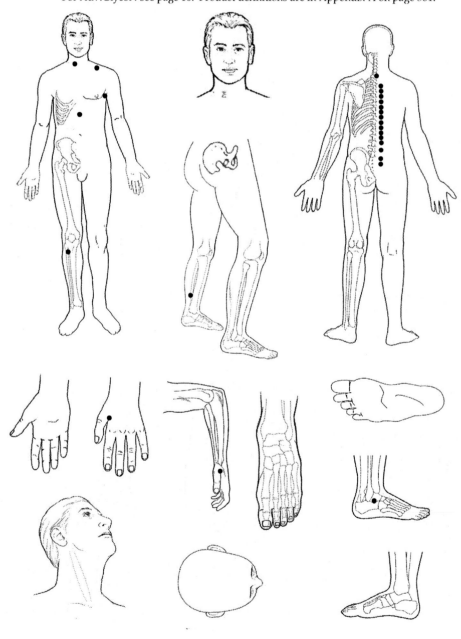

Food Poisoning -Detoxification

Daily Nutritional Crisis Program	Daily Nutritional Wellness Program
GlycoN*: 8 tsp & GlycoAO: 5 caps	GlycoN*: ½ tsp & GlycoAO: 2 caps
PhytoN: 1 tsp	PhytoN: 1/4 tsp
PreH: 4 tabs	PreH: 3 tabs
Cata: 4 tabs	Cata: 4 tabs
Clean: 3 caps twice a day (2 weeks)	Clean: 2 caps
ImmS: 6 tabs & GstroP: 4 caps	ImmS: 4 tabs & GstroP: 2 caps

*For Adv.GlycoN see page 10. Product definitions are in Appendix A on page 381.

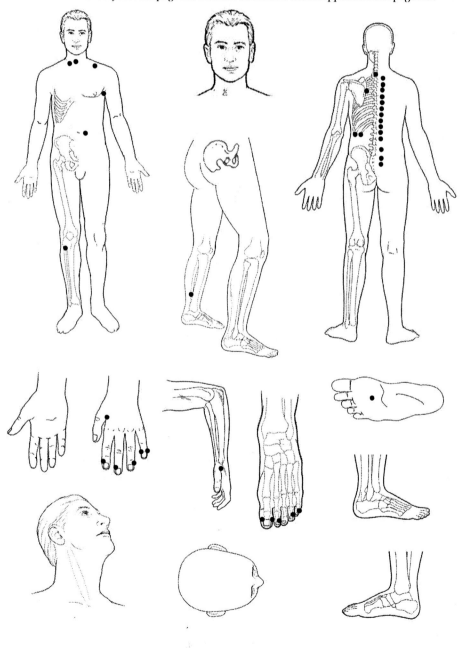

Fracture

Daily Nutritional Crisis Program	Daily Nutritional Wellness Program
GlycoN*: 2 tsp & GlycoAO: 3 caps PhytoN: 3/4 tsp PreH: 6 tabs GEssentials: 4 tabs SP: 6 caps ImmS: 4 tabs & MC: 6 caps	GlycoN*: ½ tsp & GlycoAO: 2 caps PhytoN: 1/4 tsp PreH: 3 tabs GEssentials: 4 tabs SP: 3 caps ImmS: 2 tabs & MC: 4 caps

*For Adv.GlycoN see page 10. Product definitions are in Appendix A on page 381.

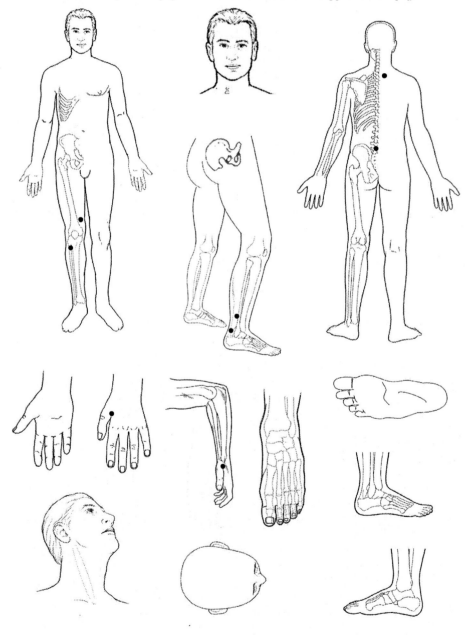

Frostbite
(stimulate meridian points surrounding injured area)

Daily Nutritional Crisis Program	Daily Nutritional Wellness Program
GlycoN*: 5 tsp & GlycoAO: 4 caps PhytoN: 1 tsp PreH: 6 tabs GEssentials: 4 tabs ImmS: 5 tabs MC: 5 caps & CB: 6 caps	GlycoN*: ½ tsp & GlycoAO: 2 caps PhytoN: 1/4 tsp PreH: 3 tabs GEssentials: 4 tabs ImmS: 3 tabs MC: 3 caps & CB: 3 caps

*For Adv.GlycoN see page 10. Product definitions are in Appendix A on page 381.

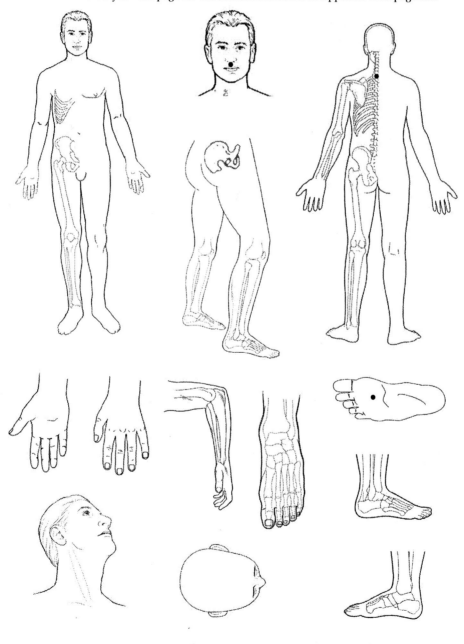

Fungal Infection

Daily Nutritional Crisis Program	Daily Nutritional Wellness Program
GlycoN*: 5 tsp & GlycoAO: 4 caps	GlycoN*: ½ tsp & GlycoAO: 2 caps
PhytoN: 1 tsp	PhytoN: 1/4 tsp
PreH: 6 tabs	PreH: 3 tabs
Cata: 4 tabs	Cata: 4 tabs
Clean: 3 caps twice a day (2 weeks)	Clean: 2 caps
GstroP: 4 caps & ImmS: 4 tabs	GstroP: 2 caps & ImmS: 2 tabs

*For Adv.GlycoN see page 10. Product definitions are in Appendix A on page 381.

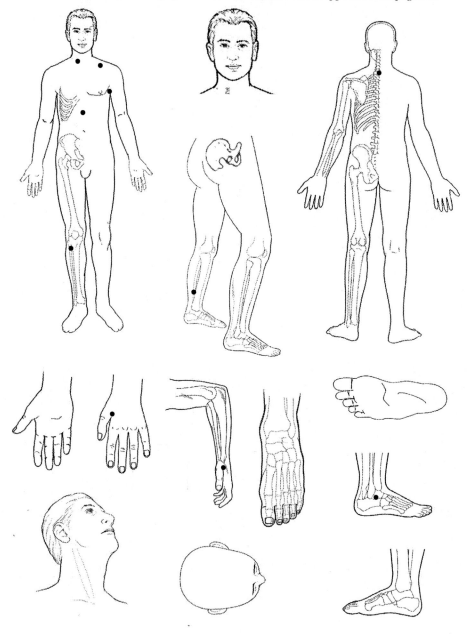

Furuncle/Carbuncle

Daily Nutritional Crisis Program	Daily Nutritional Wellness Program
GlycoN*: 2 tsp & GlycoAO: 3 caps PhytoN: 1 tsp PreH: 6 tabs Cata: 4 tabs ImmS: 4 tabs & MC: 4 caps	GlycoN*: ½ tsp & GlycoAO: 2 caps PhytoN: 1/4 tsp PreH: 3 tabs Cata: 4 tabs ImmS: 2 tabs & MC: 2 caps

*For Adv.GlycoN see page 10. Product definitions are in Appendix A on page 381.

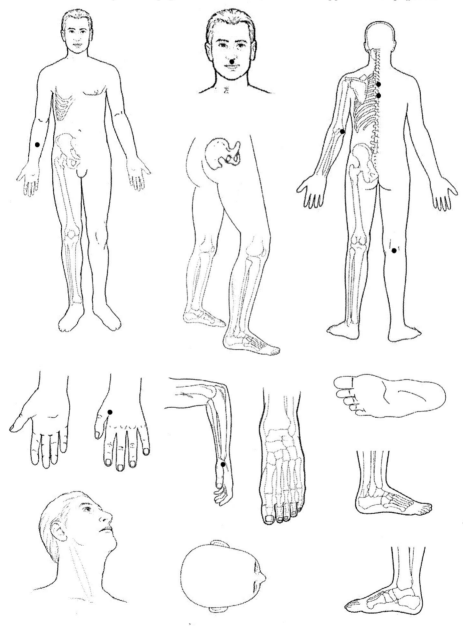

Gallbladder Dysfunction

Daily Nutritional Crisis Program	Daily Nutritional Wellness Program
GlycoN*: 1 ½ tsp & GlycoAO: 3 caps PhytoN: 1/2 tsp PreH: 6 tabs Cata: 4 tabs Clean: 3 caps twice a day (2 weeks) GstroZ: 2 caps before meals	GlycoN*: ½ tsp & GlycoAO: 2 caps PhytoN: 1/4 tsp PreH: 3 tabs Cata: 4 tabs Clean: 1 cap GstroZ: 1 cap before meals

*For Adv.GlycoN see page 10. Product definitions are in Appendix A on page 381.

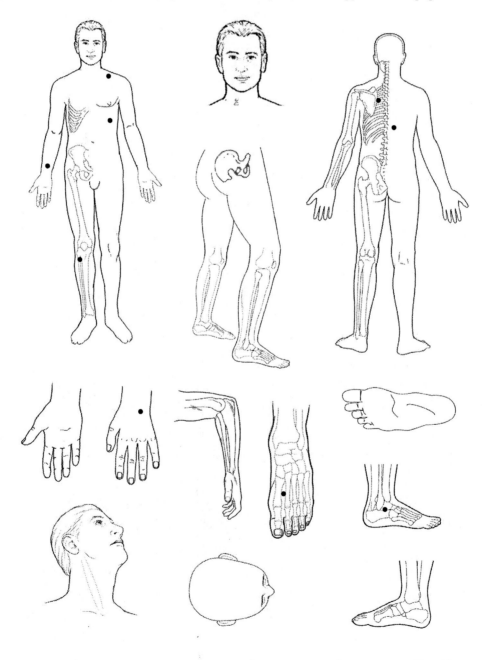

184

Gangrene

Daily Nutritional Crisis Program	Daily Nutritional Wellness Program
GlycoN*: 5 tsp & GlycoAO: 4 caps PhytoN: 1/2 tsp PreH: 6 tabs Cata: 6 tabs CB: 6 tabs MC: 6 caps	GlycoN*: 1 ½ tsp & GlycoAO: 3 caps PhytoN: 1/4 tsp PreH: 3 tabs Cata: 4 tabs CB: 3 tabs MC: 3 caps

*For Adv.GlycoN see page 10. Product definitions are in Appendix A on page 381.

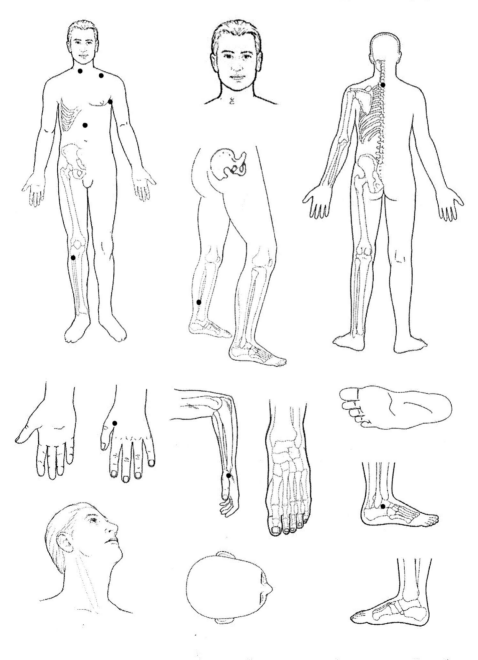

Gas (Intestinal)

Daily Nutritional Crisis Program	Daily Nutritional Wellness Program
GlycoN*: 1 ½ tsp & GlycoAO: 3 caps	GlycoN*: ½ tsp & GlycoAO: 2 caps
PhytoN: 1/2 tsp	PhytoN: 1/4 tsp
PreH: 3 tabs	PreH: 3 tabs
GEssentials: 4 tabs	GEssentials: 4 tabs
GstroP: 4 caps	GstroP: 2 caps
Clean: 3 caps twice a day (2 weeks)	Clean: 2 caps

*For Adv.GlycoN see page 10. Product definitions are in Appendix A on page 381.

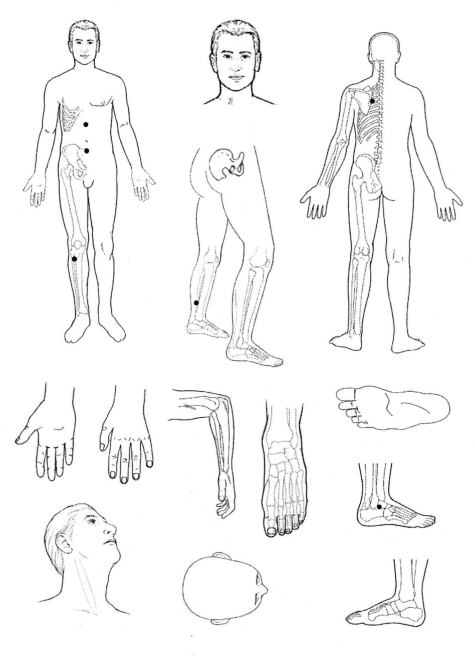

Gastric Ulcer

(drink 3-6 oz of cabbage juice per day)

Daily Nutritional Crisis Program	Daily Nutritional Wellness Program
GlycoN*: 1 ½ tsp & GlycoAO: 3 caps PhytoN: 1/2 tsp PreH: 3 tabs GEssentials: 4 tabs Clean: 3 caps twice a day (2 weeks)	GlycoN*: ½ tsp & GlycoAO: 2 caps PhytoN: 1/4 tsp PreH: 3 tabs GEssentials: 4 tabs Clean: 2 caps

*For Adv.GlycoN see page 10. Product definitions are in Appendix A on page 381.

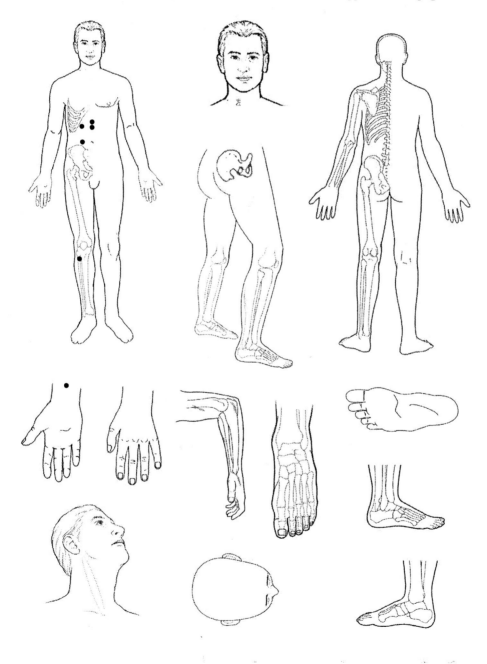

Gastroenteritis

Daily Nutritional Crisis Program	Daily Nutritional Wellness Program
GlycoN*: 1 ½ tsp & GlycoAO: 3 caps PhytoN: 1/2 tsp PreH: 3 tabs GEssentials: 4 tabs Clean: 3 caps twice a day (2 weeks) MC: 4 caps & GstroP: 3 caps	GlycoN*: ½ tsp & GlycoAO: 2 caps PhytoN: 1/4 tsp PreH: 3 tabs GEssentials: 4 tabs Clean: 2 caps MC: 2 caps & GstroP: 1 cap

*For Adv.GlycoN see page 10. Product definitions are in Appendix A on page 381.

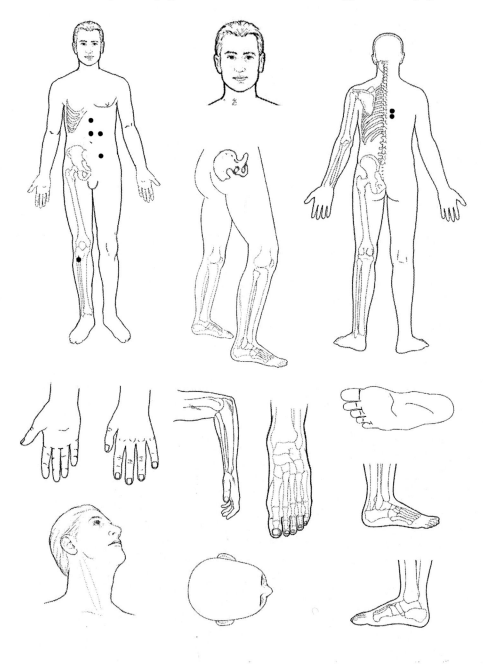

Gastroesophageal Reflux

Daily Nutritional Crisis Program	Daily Nutritional Wellness Program
GlycoN*: 1 ½ tsp & GlycoAO: 3 caps PhytoN: 1/2 tsp PreH: 3 tabs Cata: 4 tabs ImmS: 4 tabs GstroP: 3 caps	GlycoN*: ½ tsp & GlycoAO: 2 caps PhytoN: 1/4 tsp PreH: 3 tabs Cata: 4 tabs Imms: 2 tabs GstroP: 1 cap

*For Adv.GlycoN see page 10. Product definitions are in Appendix A on page 381.

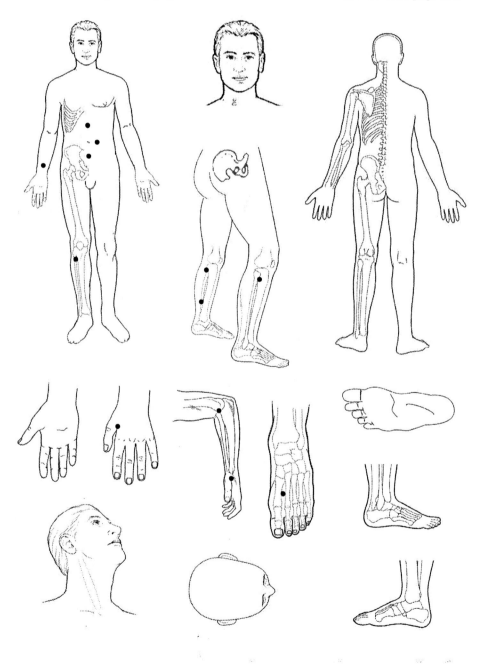

Gastroparesis

Daily Nutritional Crisis Program	Daily Nutritional Wellness Program
GlycoN*: 1 ½ tsp & GlycoAO: 3 caps PhytoN: 1/2 tsp PreH: 3 tabs Cata: 4 tabs GstroZ: 2 caps before meals	GlycoN*: ½ tsp & GlycoAO: 2 caps PhytoN: 1/4 tsp PreH: 3 tabs Cata: 4 tabs GstroP: 1 cap before meals

*For Adv.GlycoN see page 10. Product definitions are in Appendix A on page 381.

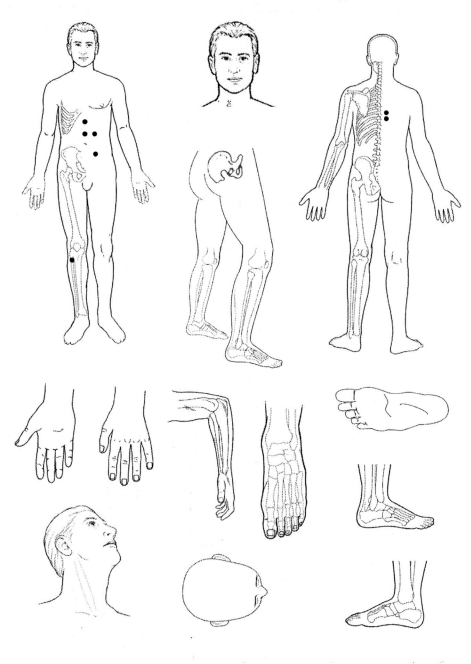

Genital Warts

Daily Nutritional Crisis Program	Daily Nutritional Wellness Program
GlycoN*: 1 ½ tsp & GlycoAO: 3 caps PhytoN: 1/2 tsp PreH: 3 tabs GEssentials: 4 tabs ImmS: 5 tabs MC: 5 caps	GlycoN*: ½ tsp & GlycoAO: 2 caps PhytoN: 1/2 tsp PreH: 3 tabs GEssentials: 4 tabs ImmS: 3 tabs MC: 3 caps

*For Adv.GlycoN see page 10. Product definitions are in Appendix A on page 381.

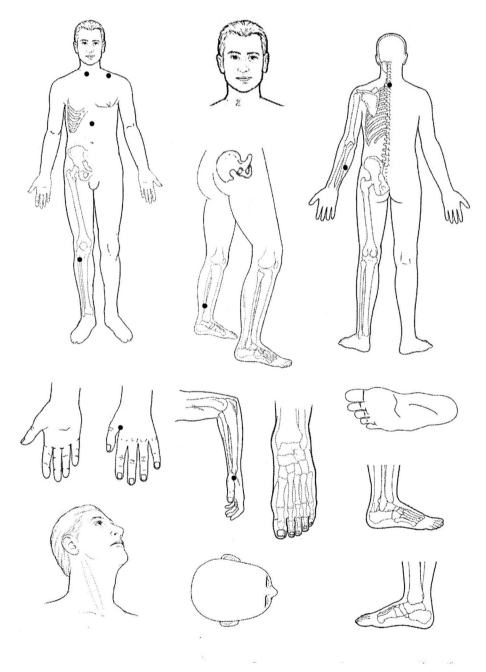

Gingivitis

Daily Nutritional Crisis Program	Daily Nutritional Wellness Program
GlycoN*: 1 ½ tsp & GlycoAO: 3 caps PhytoN: 1/2 tsp PreH: 3 tabs GEssentials: 4 tabs ImmS: 4 tabs MC: 7 caps	GlycoN*: ½ tsp & GlycoAO: 2 caps PhytoN: 1/4 tsp PreH: 3 tabs GEssentials: 4 tabs ImmS: 2 tabs MC: 4 caps

*For Adv.GlycoN see page 10. Product definitions are in Appendix A on page 381.

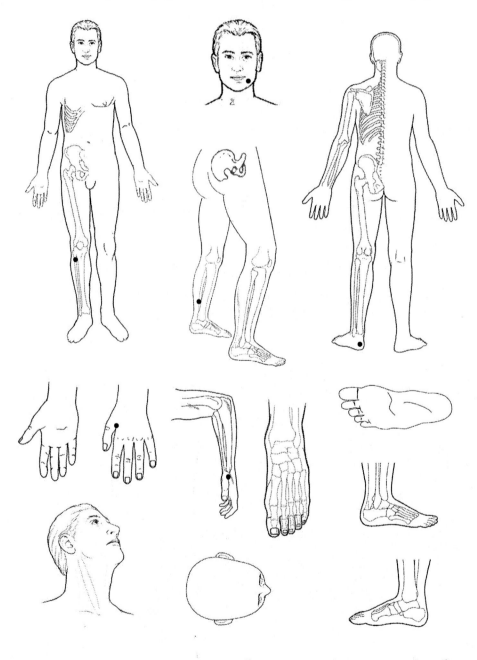

192

Glaucoma

Daily Nutritional Crisis Program	Daily Nutritional Wellness Program
GlycoN*: 1 ½ tsp & GlycoAO: 3 caps PhytoN: 1/2 tsp PreH: 6 tabs Cata: 6 tabs ImmS: 4 tabs MC: 4 caps	GlycoN*: ½ tsp & GlycoAO: 2 caps PhytoN: 1/4 tsp PreH: 3 tabs Cata: 4 tabs ImmS: 2 tabs MC: 2 caps

*For Adv.GlycoN see page 10. Product definitions are in Appendix A on page 381.

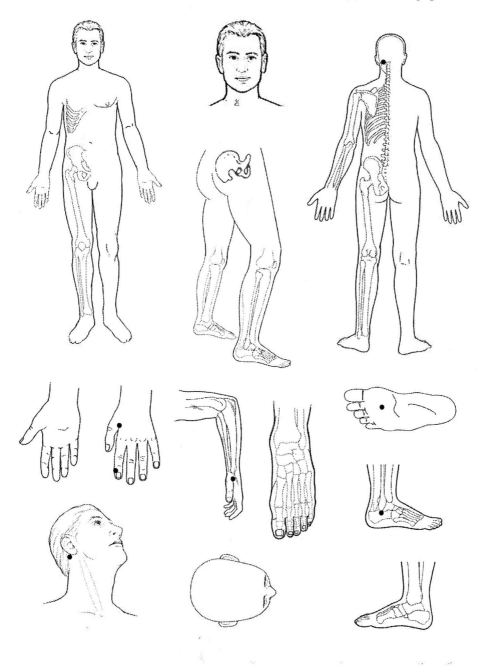

193

Glossitis

Daily Nutritional Crisis Program	Daily Nutritional Wellness Program
GlycoN*: 1 ½ tsp & GlycoAO: 3 caps PhytoN: 1/2 tsp PreH: 3 tabs GEssentials: 4 tabs ImmS: 4 tabs MC: 5 caps	GlycoN*: ½ tsp & GlycoAO: 2 caps PhytoN: 1/4 tsp PreH: 3 tabs GEssentials: 4 tabs ImmS: 2 tabs MC: 3 caps

*For Adv.GlycoN see page 10. Product definitions are in Appendix A on page 381.

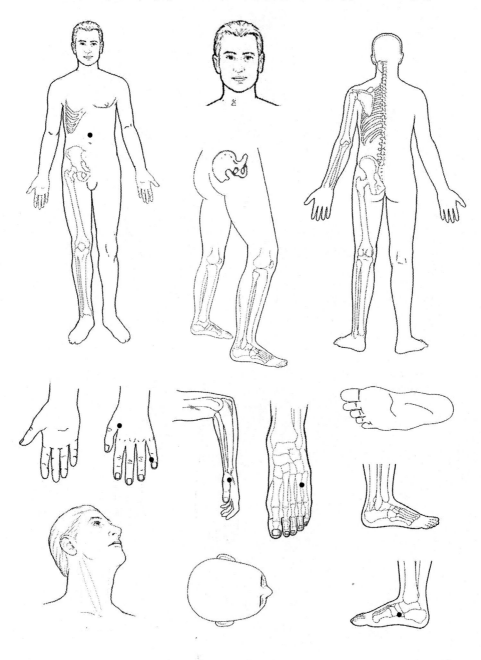

Glucose Intolerance

Daily Nutritional Crisis Program	Daily Nutritional Wellness Program
GlycoN*: 1 ½ tsp & GlycoAO: 3 caps PhytoN: 1/2 tsp PreH: 4 tabs Cata: 4 tabs ImmS: 4 tabs MC: 4 caps	GlycoN*: ½ tsp & GlycoAO: 2 caps PhytoN: 1/4 tsp PreH: 4 tabs Cata: 4 tabs ImmS: 2 tabs MC: 2 caps

*For Adv.GlycoN see page 10. Product definitions are in Appendix A on page 381.

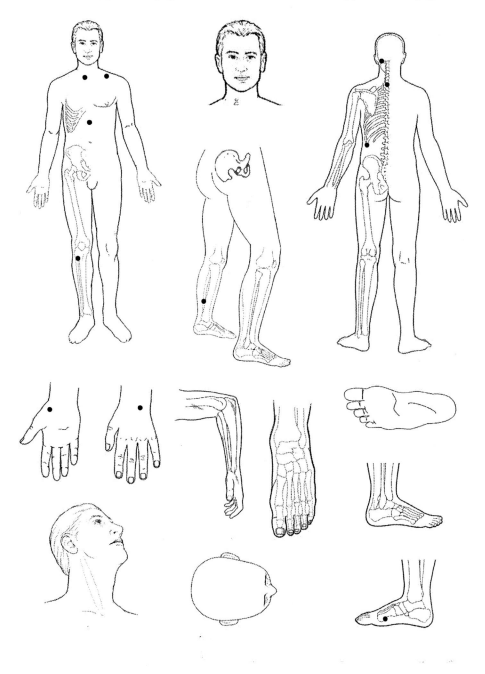

Goiter

Daily Nutritional Crisis Program	Daily Nutritional Wellness Program
GlycoN*: 1 ½ tsp & GlycoAO: 3 caps PhytoN: 1/2 tsp PreH: 4 tabs Cata: 4 tabs ImmS: 5 tabs MC: 5 caps	GlycoN*: ½ tsp & GlycoAO: 2 caps PhytoN: 1/4 tsp PreH: 3 tabs Cata: 4 tabs ImmS: 3 tabs MC: 3 caps

*For Adv.GlycoN see page 10. Product definitions are in Appendix A on page 381.

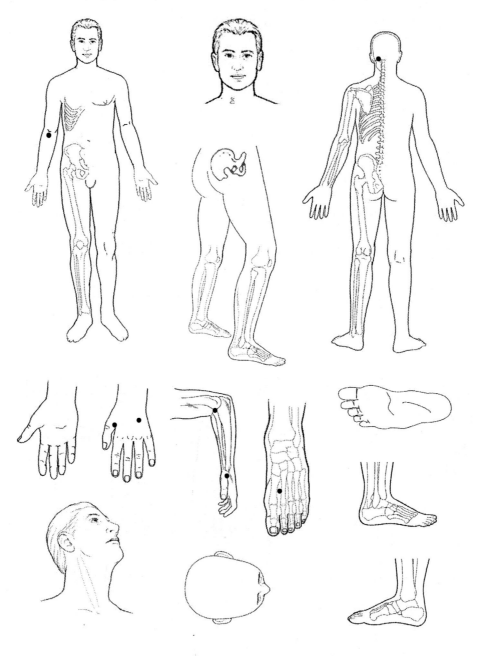

Gonorrhea

Daily Nutritional Crisis Program	Daily Nutritional Wellness Program
GlycoN*: 1 ½ tsp & GlycoAO: 3 caps PhytoN: 1/2 tsp PreH: 3 tabs GEssentials: 4 tabs ImmS: 7 tabs MC: 6 caps	GlycoN*: ½ tsp & GlycoAO: 2 caps PhytoN: 1/4 tsp PreH: 4 tabs GEssentials: 4 tabs ImmS: 4 tabs MC: 3 caps

*For Adv.GlycoN see page 10.   Product definitions are in Appendix A on page 381.

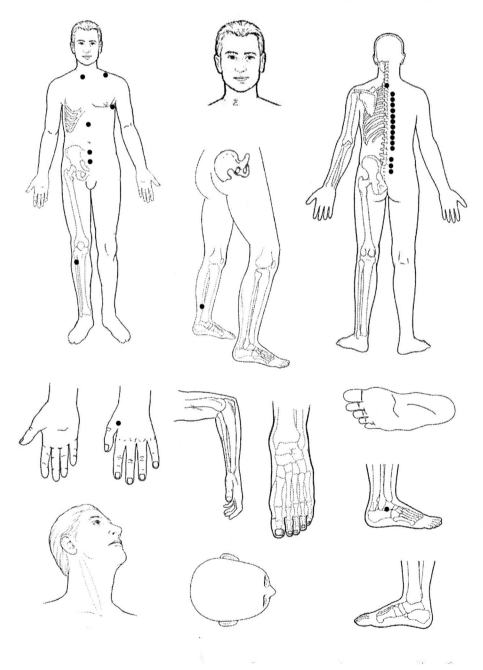

Gout

Daily Nutritional Crisis Program	Daily Nutritional Wellness Program
GlycoN*: 1 ½ tsp & GlycoAO: 3 caps PhytoN: 1/2 tsp PreH: 6 tabs Cata: 5 tabs ImmS: 5 tabs MC: 4 caps	GlycoN*: ½ tsp & GlycoAO: 2 caps PhytoN: 1/4 tsp PreH: 3 tabs Cata: 4 tabs ImmS: 3 tabs MC: 3 caps

*For Adv.GlycoN see page 10. Product definitions are in Appendix A on page 381.

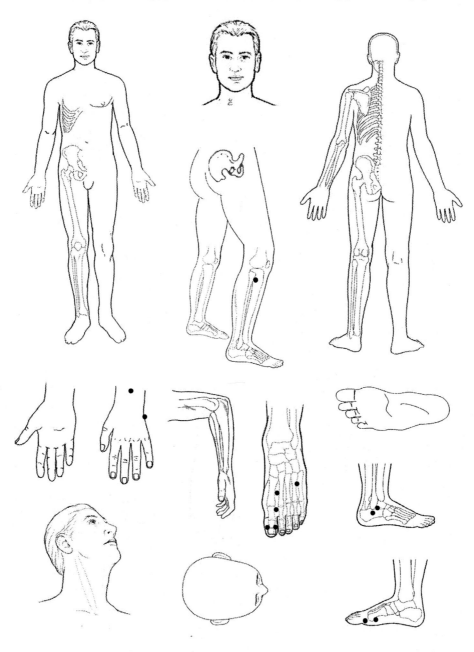

Graves' disease

Daily Nutritional Crisis Program	Daily Nutritional Wellness Program
GlycoN*: 1 ½ tsp & GlycoAO: 3 caps PhytoN: 1/2 tsp PreH: 3 tabs Cata: 4 tabs ImmS: 5 tabs MC: 4 caps	GlycoN*: ½ tsp & GlycoAO: 2 caps PhytoN: 1/4 tsp PreH: 4 tabs Cata: 4 tabs ImmS: 3 tabs MC: 2 caps

*For Adv.GlycoN see page 10. Product definitions are in Appendix A on page 381.

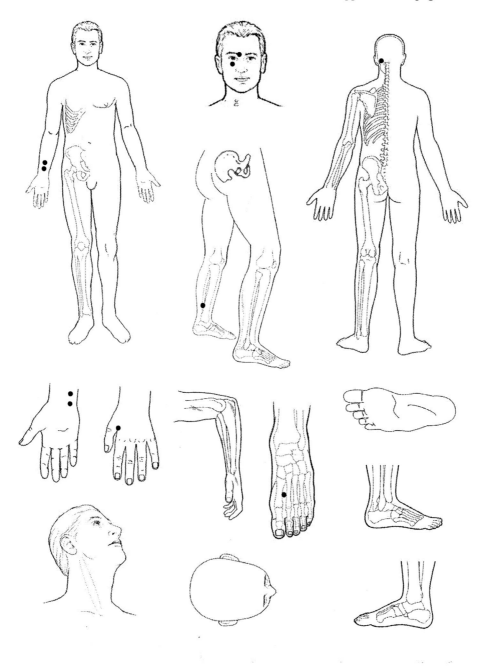

Hair Loss (Non-Genetic)

Daily Nutritional Crisis Program	Daily Nutritional Wellness Program
GlycoN*: 1 ½ tsp & GlycoAO: 3 caps PhytoN: 1/2 tsp PreH: 6 tabs GEssentials: 4 tabs ImmS: 3 tabs SP: 4 caps	GlycoN*: ½ tsp & GlycoAO: 2 caps PhytoN: 1/2 tsp PreH: 3 tabs GEssentials: 4 tabs ImmS: 2 tabs SP: 2 caps

*For Adv.GlycoN see page 10. Product definitions are in Appendix A on page 381.

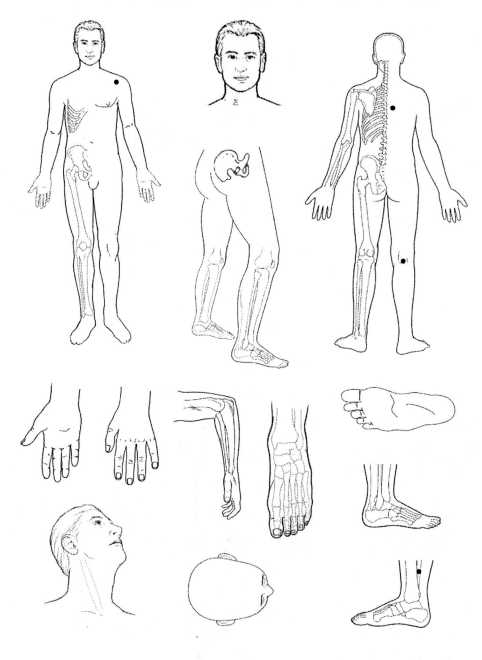

Hangover

Daily Nutritional Crisis Program	Daily Nutritional Wellness Program
GlycoN*: 1 ½ tsp & GlycoAO: 3 caps PhytoN: 1/2 tsp PreH: 6 tabs GEssentials: 4 tabs MC: 5 caps ImmS: 4 tabs	GlycoN*: ½ tsp & GlycoAO: 2 caps PhytoN: 1/2 tsp PreH: 3 tabs GEssentials: 4 tabs MC: 3 caps ImmS: 2 tabs

*For Adv.GlycoN see page 10. Product definitions are in Appendix A on page 381.

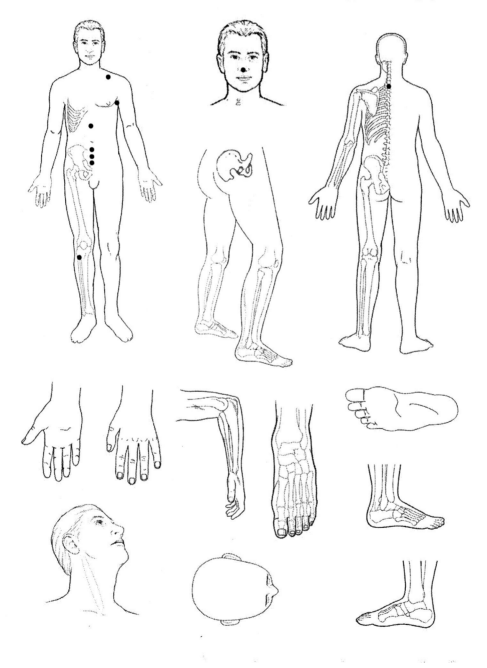

Hay Fever

Daily Nutritional Crisis Program	Daily Nutritional Wellness Program
GlycoN*: 1 ½ tsp & GlycoAO: 3 caps PhytoN: 1/2 tsp PreH: 4 tabs GEssentials: 4 tabs MC: 5 caps ImmS: 5 tabs	GlycoN*: ½ tsp & GlycoAO: 2 caps PhytoN: 1/2 tsp PreH: 3 tabs GEssentials: 4 tabs MC: 3 caps ImmS: 3 tabs

*For Adv.GlycoN see page 10. Product definitions are in Appendix A on page 381.

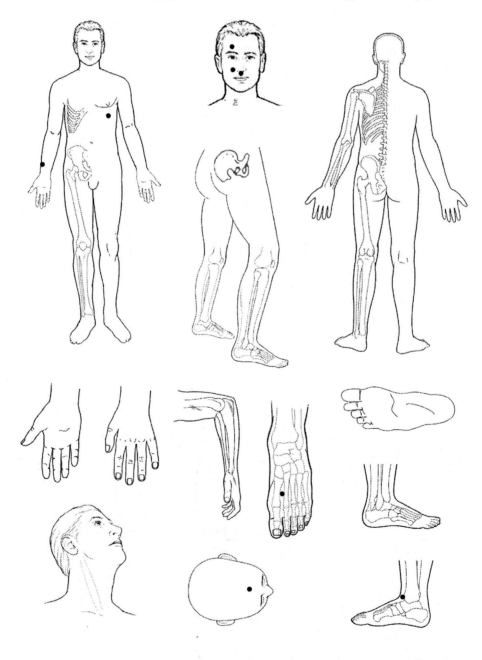

Headache

Daily Nutritional Crisis Program	Daily Nutritional Wellness Program
GlycoN*: 1 ½ tsp & GlycoAO: 3 caps PhytoN: 1/2 tsp PreH: 6 tabs GEssentials: 4 tabs SP: 4 caps ImmS: 4 tabs	GlycoN*: ½ tsp & GlycoAO: 2 caps PhytoN: 1/2 tsp PreH: 3 tabs GEssentials: 4 tabs SP: 3 caps ImmS: 2 tabs

*For Adv.GlycoN see page 10. Product definitions are in Appendix A on page 381.

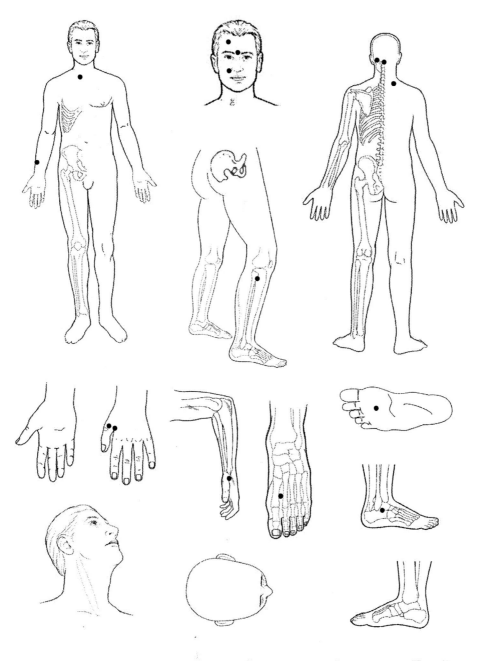

Hearing Loss

Daily Nutritional Crisis Program	Daily Nutritional Wellness Program
GlycoN*: 5 tsp & GlycoAO: 4 caps	GlycoN*: ½ tsp & GlycoAO: 2 caps
PhytoN: 1/2 tsp	PhytoN: 1/4 tsp
PreH: 4 tabs	PreH: 3 tabs
GEssentials: 4 tabs	GEssentials: 4 tabs
ImmS: 5 tabs	ImmS: 3 tabs
MC: 4 caps	MC: 3 caps

*For Adv.GlycoN see page 10. Product definitions are in Appendix A on page 381.

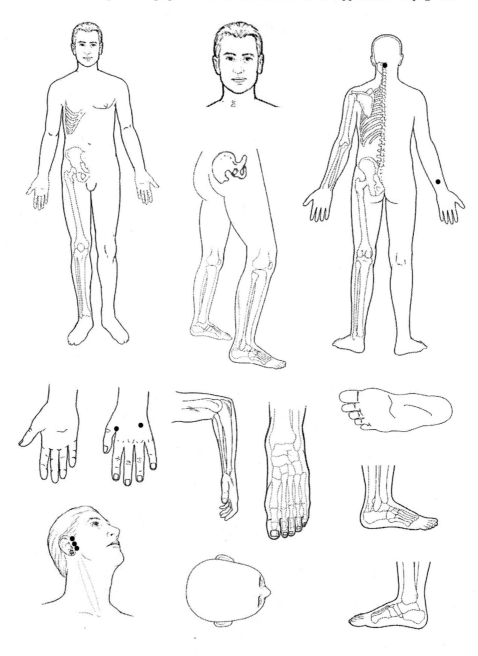

Heavy Metal Toxicity

Daily Nutritional Crisis Program	Daily Nutritional Wellness Program
GlycoN*: 5 ¼ tsp & GlycoAO: 4 caps	GlycoN*: 1 ½ tsp & GlycoAO: 3 caps
PhytoN: 1 tsp	PhytoN: 1/4 tsp
PreH: 3 tabs	PreH: 3 tabs
Cata: 6 tabs	Cata: 6 tabs
Clean: 3 caps twice a day (2 weeks)	Clean: 1 cap
ImmS: 4 tabs	ImmS: 2 tabs

*For Adv.GlycoN see page 10. Product definitions are in Appendix A on page 381.

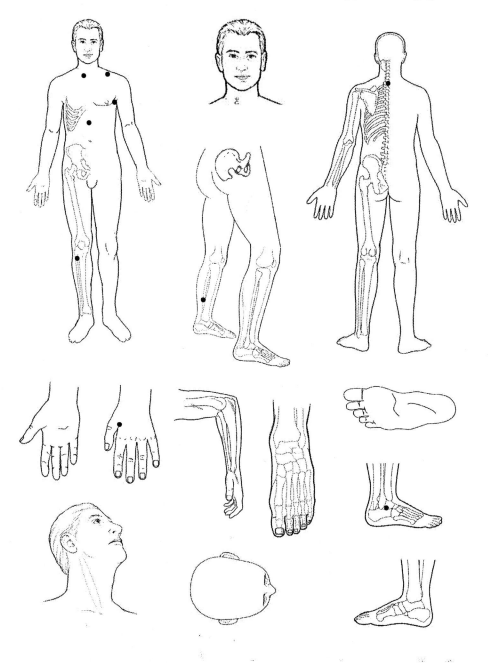

205

Hemiplegia Hemiparesis D/T Stroke

Daily Nutritional Crisis Program	Daily Nutritional Wellness Program
GlycoN*: 8 tsp & GlycoAO: 5 caps PhytoN: 1/2 tsp PreH: 6 tabs Cata: 6 tabs SP: 6 caps ImmS: 6 tabs	GlycoN*: 1 ½ tsp & GlycoAO: 3 caps PhytoN: 1/4 tsp PreH: 4 tabs Cata: 4 tabs SP: 4 caps ImmS: 4 tabs

*For Adv.GlycoN see page 10. Product definitions are in Appendix A on page 381.

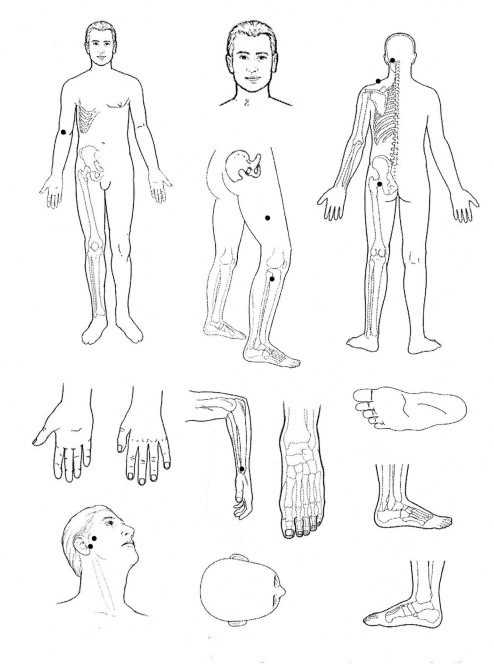

Hepatitis A

Daily Nutritional Crisis Program	Daily Nutritional Wellness Program
GlycoN*: 8 tsp & GlycoAO: 5 caps PhytoN: 1/2 tsp PreH: 4 tabs Cata: 4 tabs Clean: 3 caps twice a day (2 weeks) ImmS: 6 tabs & MC: 6 caps	GlycoN*: ½ tsp & GlycoAO: 2 caps PhytoN: 1/4 tsp PreH: 4 tabs Cata: 4 tabs Clean: 3 caps ImmS: 4 tabs & MC: 4 caps

*For Adv.GlycoN see page 10. Product definitions are in Appendix A on page 381.

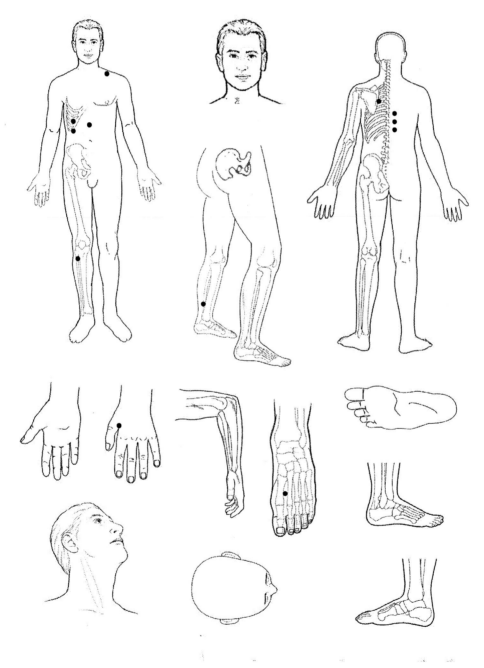

Hepatitis B

Daily Nutritional Crisis Program	Daily Nutritional Wellness Program
GlycoN*: 8 tsp & GlycoAO: 5 caps	GlycoN*: ½ tsp & GlycoAO: 2 caps
PhytoN: 1/2 tsp	PhytoN: 1/4 tsp
PreH: 4 tabs	PreH: 4 tabs
Cata: 4 tabs	Cata: 4 tabs
Clean: 3 caps twice a day (2 weeks)	Clean: 3 caps
ImmS: 6 tabs & MC: 6 caps	ImmS: 4 tabs & MC: 4 caps

*For Adv.GlycoN see page 10. Product definitions are in Appendix A on page 381.

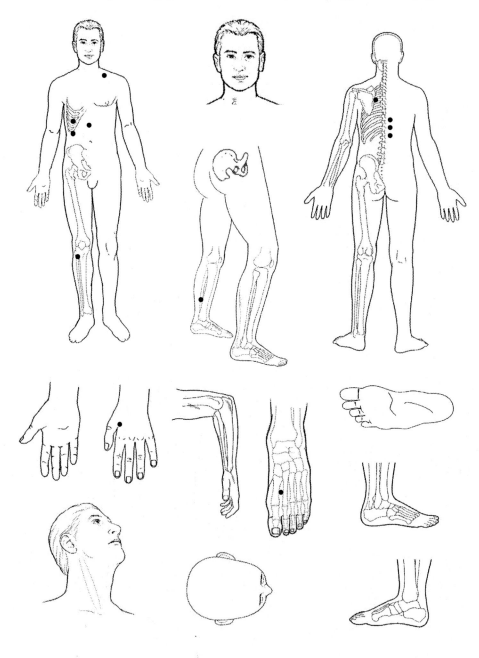

Hepatitis C, Chronic

Daily Nutritional Crisis Program	Daily Nutritional Wellness Program
GlycoN*: 8 tsp & GlycoAO: 5 caps PhytoN: 1/2 tsp PreH: 4 tabs Cata: 4 tabs Clean: 3 caps twice a day (2 weeks) ImmS: 6 tabs & MC: 6 caps	GlycoN*: ½ tsp & GlycoAO: 2 caps PhytoN: 1/4 tsp PreH: 4 tabs Cata: 4 tabs Clean: 3 caps ImmS: 4 tabs & MC: 4 caps

*For Adv.GlycoN see page 10. Product definitions are in Appendix A on page 381.

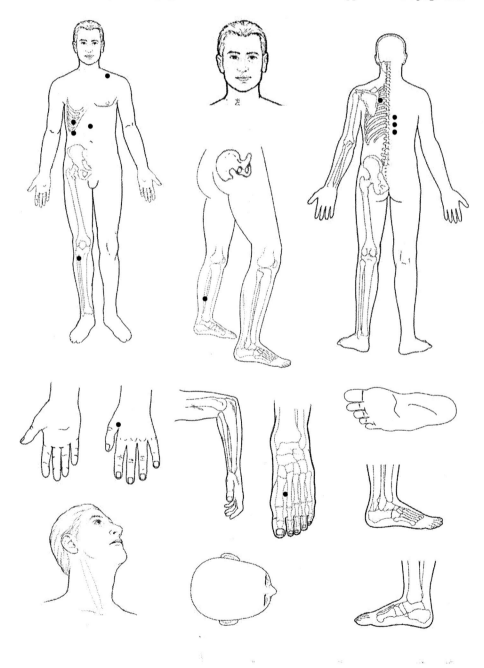

Herniated Intervertebral Disc
(stimulate points surrounding areas of pain)

Daily Nutritional Crisis Program	Daily Nutritional Wellness Program
GlycoN*: 5 tsp & GlycoAO: 4 caps PhytoN: 1/2 tsp PreH: 6 tabs Cata: 4 tabs SP: 6 caps MC: 5 caps	GlycoN*: 1 ½ tsp & GlycoAO: 3 caps PhytoN: 1/4 tsp PreH: 4 tabs Cata: 4 tabs SP: 3 caps MC: 3 caps

*For Adv.GlycoN see page 10. Product definitions are in Appendix A on page 381.

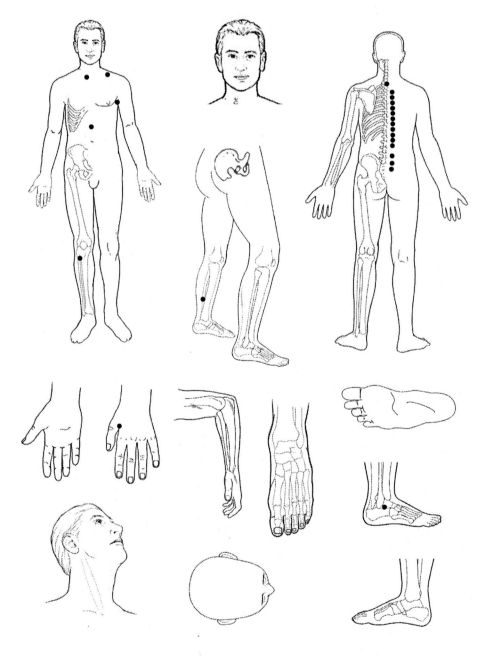

210

Herpes Simplex

(apply soft laser on affected area)

Daily Nutritional Crisis Program	Daily Nutritional Wellness Program
GlycoN*: 1 ½ tsp & GlycoAO: 3 caps PhytoN: 1/2 tsp PreH: 6 tabs Cata: 4 tabs ImmS: 6 tabs MC: 5 caps	GlycoN*: ½ tsp & GlycoAO: 2 caps PhytoN: 1/4 tsp PreH: 3 tabs Cata: 4 tabs ImmS: 4 tabs MC: 4 caps

*For Adv.GlycoN see page 10. Product definitions are in Appendix A on page 381.

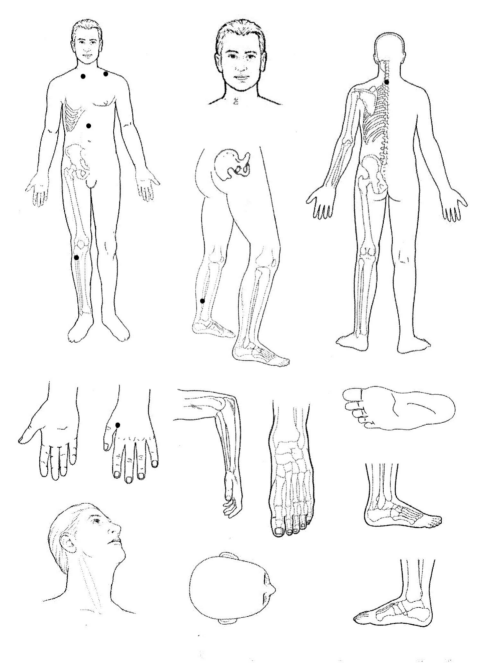

Herpes Zoster

Daily Nutritional Crisis Program	Daily Nutritional Wellness Program
GlycoN*: 1 ½ tsp & GlycoAO: 3 caps	GlycoN*: ½ tsp & GlycoAO: 2 caps
PhytoN: 1/2 tsp	PhytoN: 1/4 tsp
PreH: 6 tabs	PreH: 3 tabs
Cata: 4 tabs	Cata: 4 tabs
ImmS: 6 tabs	ImmS: 4 tabs
MC: 5 caps	MC: 4 caps
SP: 4 caps	SP: 2 caps

*For Adv.GlycoN see page 10. Product definitions are in Appendix A on page 381.

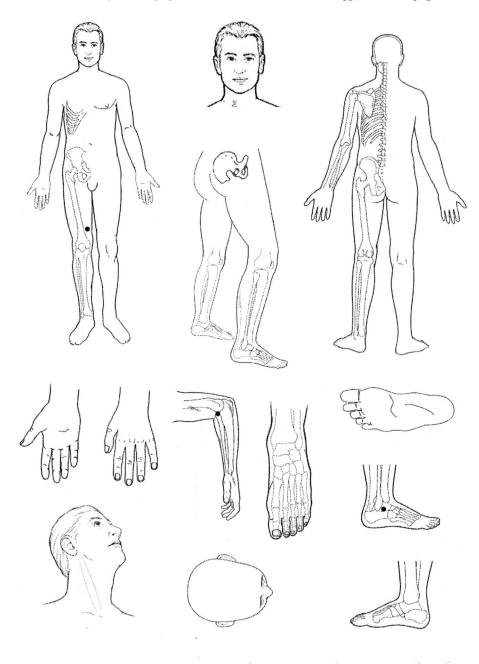

Herpes, Genital
(apply soft laser on affected area)

Daily Nutritional Crisis Program	Daily Nutritional Wellness Program
GlycoN*: 1 ½ tsp & GlycoAO: 3 caps PhytoN: 1/2 tsp PreH: 6 tabs Cata: 4 tabs ImmS: 6 tabs MC: 5 caps	GlycoN*: ½ tsp & GlycoAO: 2 caps PhytoN: 1/4 tsp PreH: 3 tabs Cata: 4 tabs ImmS: 4 tabs MC: 4 caps

*For Adv.GlycoN see page 10. Product definitions are in Appendix A on page 381.

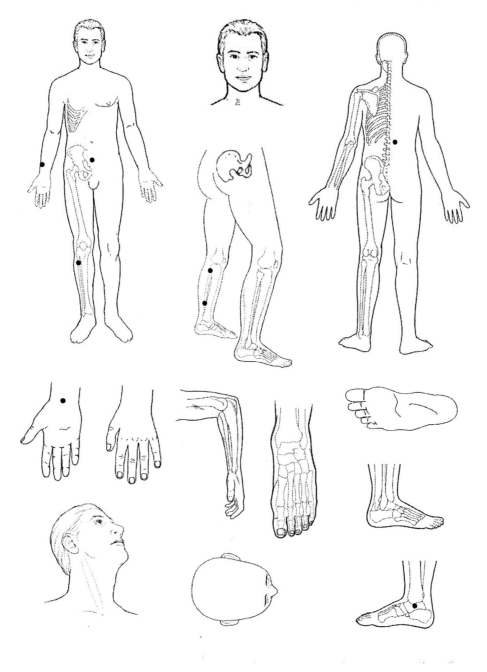

213

HIV Disease

Daily Nutritional Crisis Program	Daily Nutritional Wellness Program
GlycoN*: 10 ¾ tsp & GlycoAO: 6 caps PhytoN: 2 tsp PreH: 6 tabs Cata: 6 tabs ImmS: 7 tabs MC: 7 caps	GlycoN*: 3 ½ tsp & GlycoAO: 3 caps PhytoN: 1/4 tsp PreH: 4 tabs Cata: 4 tabs ImmS: 5 tabs MC: 5 caps

*For Adv.GlycoN see page 10. Product definitions are in Appendix A on page 381.

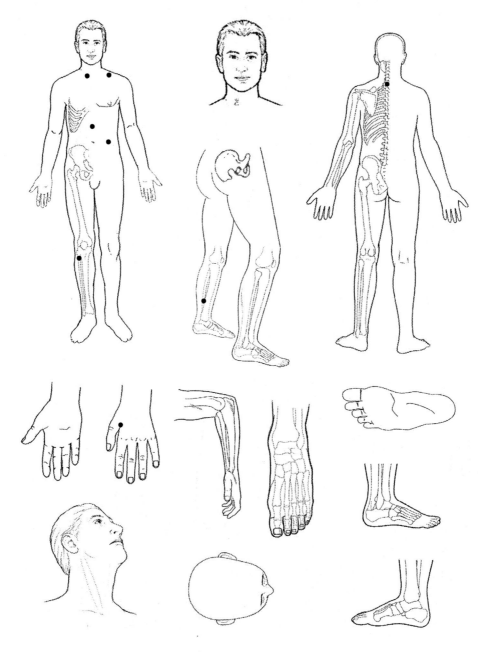

Hives

(apply SkZone to affected area)

Daily Nutritional Crisis Program	Daily Nutritional Wellness Program
GlycoN*: 5 tsp & GlycoAO: 4 caps PhytoN: 1/2 tsp PreH: 4 tabs GEssentials: 4 tabs ImmS: 5 tabs MC: 6 caps	GlycoN*: ½ tsp & GlycoAO: 2 caps PhytoN: 1/4 tsp PreH: 3 tabs GEssentials: 4 tabs ImmS: 2 tabs MC: 3 caps

*For Adv.GlycoN see page 10. Product definitions are in Appendix A on page 381.

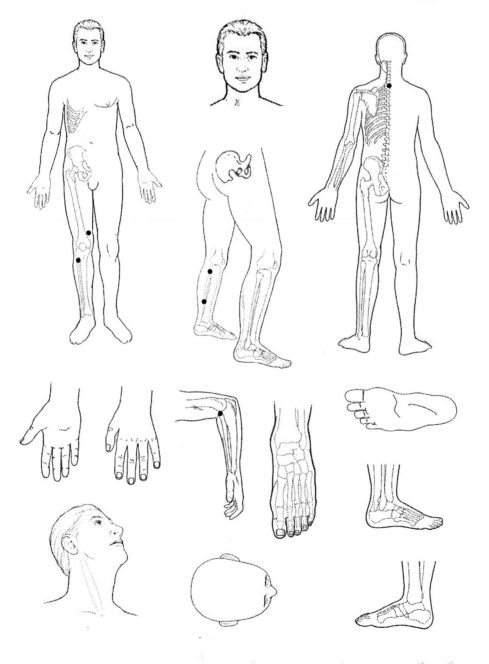

Hodgkins Disease

Daily Nutritional Crisis Program	Daily Nutritional Wellness Program
GlycoN*: 1 ½ tsp & GlycoAO: 3 caps PhytoN: 1/2 tsp PreH: 3 tabs Cata: 4 tabs ImmS: 5 tabs MC: 4 caps	GlycoN*: ½ tsp & GlycoAO: 2 caps PhytoN: 1/4 tsp PreH: 4 tabs Cata: 4 tabs ImmS: 3 tabs MC: 2 caps

*For Adv.GlycoN see page 10. Product definitions are in Appendix A on page 381.

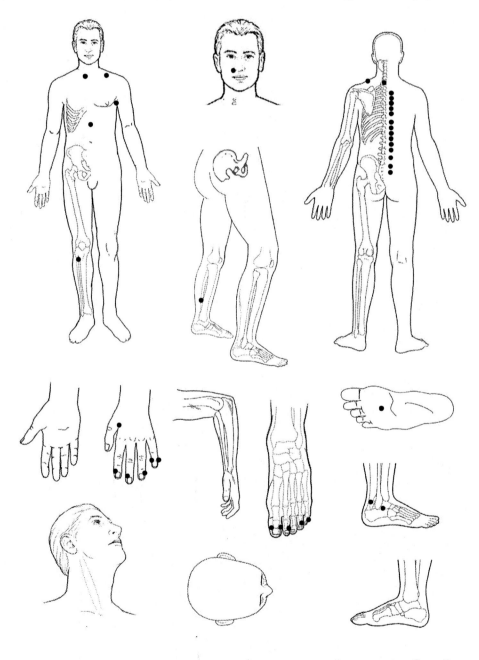

Hyperaldosteronism

Daily Nutritional Crisis Program	Daily Nutritional Wellness Program
GlycoN*: 3½ tsp & GlycoAO: 3 caps PhytoN: 1 tsp PreH: 6 tabs Cata: 6 tabs ImmS: 4 tabs SP: 4 caps	GlycoN*: 1½ tsp & GlycoAO: 3 caps PhytoN: 1/4 tsp PreH: 3 tabs Cata: 4 tabs ImmS: 3 tabs SP: 3 caps

*For Adv.GlycoN see page 10. Product definitions are in Appendix A on page 381.

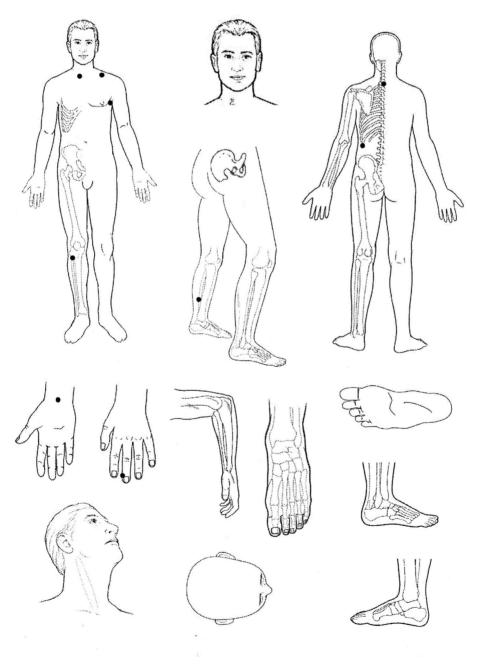

217

Hypercholesterolemia

Daily Nutritional Crisis Program	Daily Nutritional Wellness Program
GlycoN*: 1 ½ tsp & GlycoAO: 3 caps PhytoN: 1/2 tsp PreH: 6 tabs Cata: 4 tabs CB: 7 caps MC: 5 caps	GlycoN*: 1 ½ tsp & GlycoAO: 3 caps PhytoN: 1/4 tsp PreH: 4 tabs Cata: 4 tabs CB: 5 caps MC: 3 caps

*For Adv.GlycoN see page 10. Product definitions are in Appendix A on page 381.

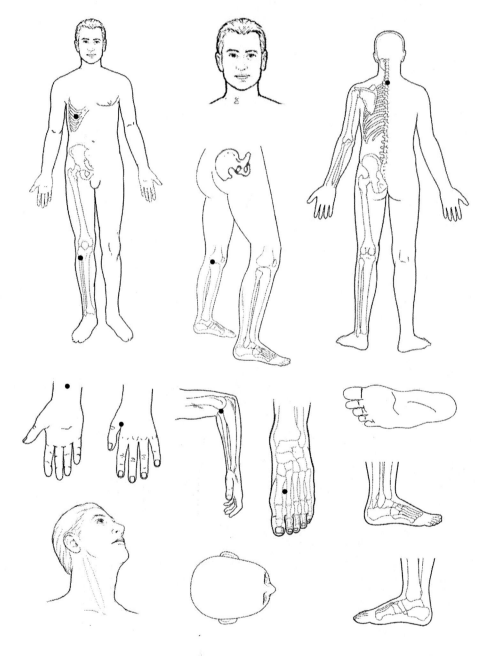

Hyperesthesia

Daily Nutritional Crisis Program	Daily Nutritional Wellness Program
GlycoN*: 8 tsp & GlycoAO: 5 caps PhytoN: 1/2 tsp PreH: 6 tabs Cata: 4 tabs SP: 5 caps ImmS: 5 tabs & MC: 4 caps	GlycoN*: 1 ½ tsp & GlycoAO: 3 caps PhytoN: 1/4 tsp PreH: 3 tabs Cata: 4 tabs SP: 3 caps ImmS & MC: 3 caps

*For Adv.GlycoN see page 10. Product definitions are in Appendix A on page 381.

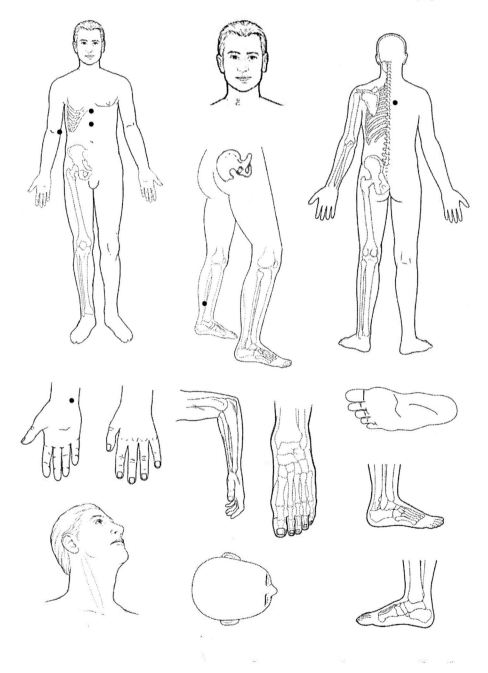

Hyperhidrosos

Daily Nutritional Crisis Program	Daily Nutritional Wellness Program
GlycoN*: 5 tsp & GlycoAO: 4 caps PhytoN: 1/2 tsp PreH: 6 tabs Cata: 4 tabs SP: 4 caps CB: 4 caps	GlycoN*: 1 ½ tsp & GlycoAO: 3 caps PhytoN: 1/4 tsp PreH: 3 tabs Cata: 4 tabs SP: 4 caps CB: 3 caps

*For Adv.GlycoN see page 10. Product definitions are in Appendix A on page 381.

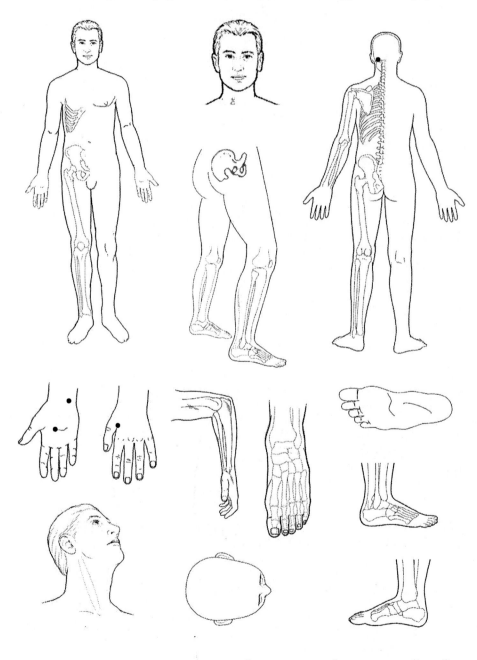

Hyperlipidemia (Triglycerides)

Daily Nutritional Crisis Program	Daily Nutritional Wellness Program
GlycoN*: 1 ½ tsp & GlycoAO: 3 caps PhytoN: 1/2 tsp PreH: 6 tabs Cata: 4 tabs CB: 7 caps MC: 5 caps	GlycoN*: 1 ½ tsp & GlycoAO: 3 caps PhytoN: 1/4 tsp PreH: 4 tabs Cata: 4 tabs CB: 5 caps MC: 3 caps

*For Adv.GlycoN see page 10. Product definitions are in Appendix A on page 381.

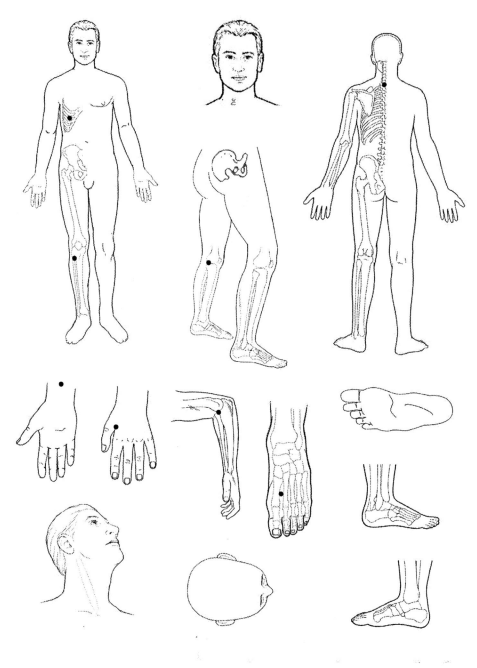

Hypertension

Daily Nutritional Crisis Program	Daily Nutritional Wellness Program
GlycoN*: 5 ¼ tsp & GlycoAO: 4 caps PhytoN: 1 tsp PreH: 6 tabs Cata: 4 tabs CB: 4 caps	GlycoN*: 1 ½ tsp & GlycoAO: 3 caps PhytoN: 3/4 tsp PreH: 3 tabs Cata: 4 tabs CB: 3 caps

*For Adv.GlycoN see page 10. Product definitions are in Appendix A on page 381.

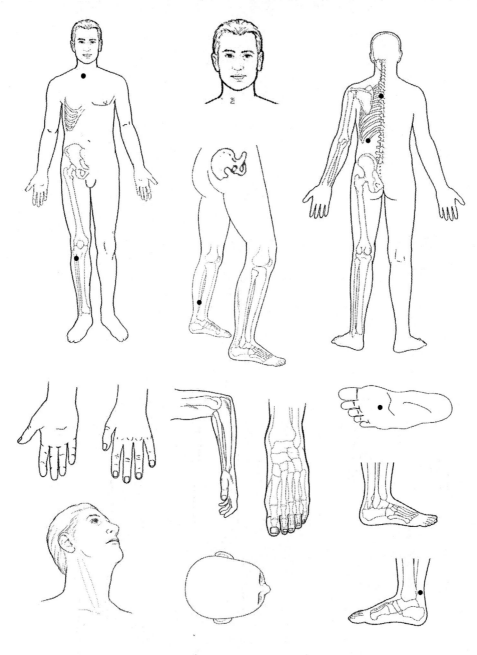

Hyperthyroidism

Daily Nutritional Crisis Program	Daily Nutritional Wellness Program
GlycoN*: 5 tsp & GlycoAO: 4 caps PhytoN: 1/2 tsp PreH: 3 tabs Cata: 4 tabs ImmS: 4 tabs MC: 3 caps	GlycoN*: ½ tsp & GlycoAO: 2 caps PhytoN: 1/4 tsp PreH: 3 tabs Cata: 4 tabs ImmS: 2 tabs MC: 2 caps

*For Adv.GlycoN see page 10. Product definitions are in Appendix A on page 381.

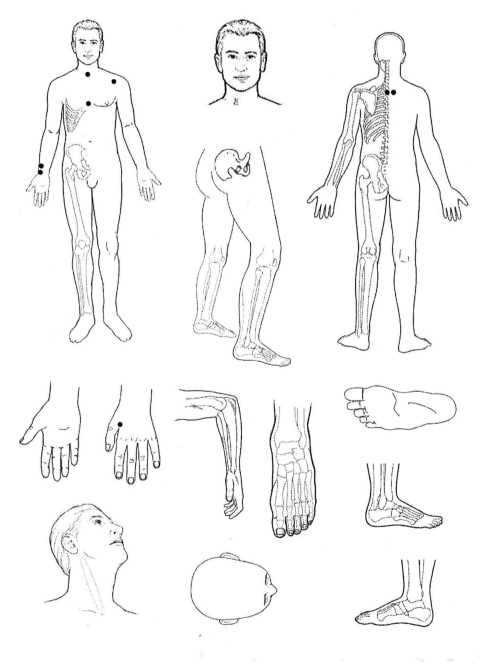

223

Hyperventilation

Daily Nutritional Crisis Program	Daily Nutritional Wellness Program
GlycoN*: 1 ½ tsp & GlycoAO: 3 caps PhytoN: 1/2 tsp PreH: 4 tabs GEssentials: 4 tabs MC: 4 caps SP: 4 caps	GlycoN*: ½ tsp & GlycoAO: 2 caps PhytoN: 1/4 tsp PreH: 3 tabs GEssentials: 4 tabs MC: 2 caps SP: 2 caps

*For Adv.GlycoN see page 10. Product definitions are in Appendix A on page 381.

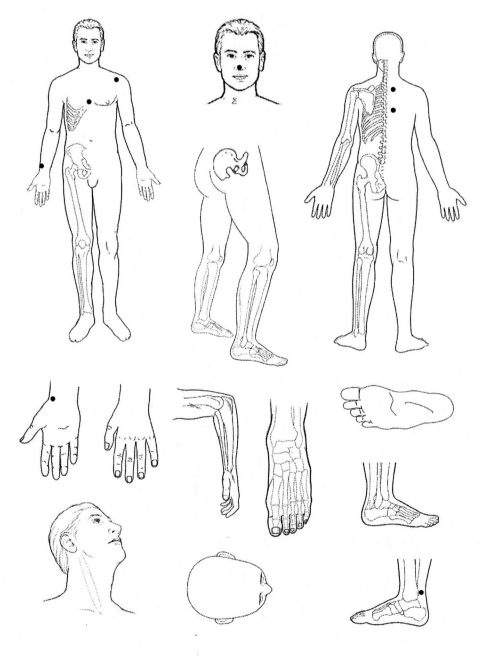

Hypoglycemia

Daily Nutritional Crisis Program	Daily Nutritional Wellness Program
GlycoN*: 2 ½ tsp & GlycoAO: 3 caps PhytoN: 1½ tsp PreH: 6 tabs GEssentials: 6 tabs	GlycoN*: ½ tsp & GlycoAO: 2 caps PhytoN: 3/4 tsp PreH: 3 tabs GEssentials: 4 tabs

*For Adv.GlycoN see page 10. Product definitions are in Appendix A on page 381.

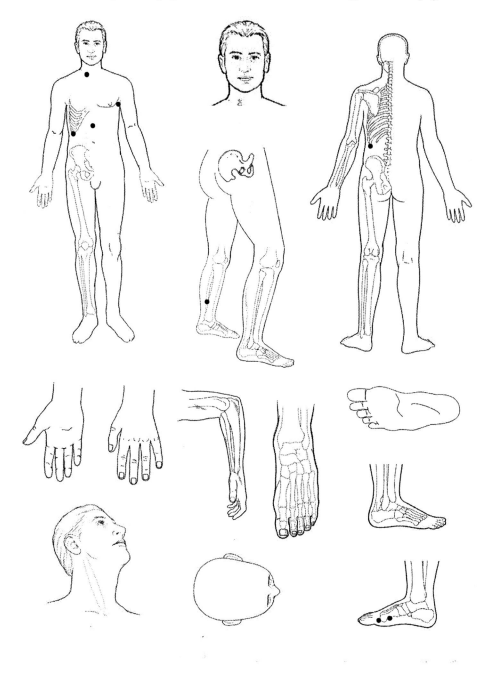

Hysterectomy

(order hormone panel with health care provider)

Daily Nutritional Crisis Program	Daily Nutritional Wellness Program
GlycoN*: 5 tsp & GlycoAO: 4 caps PhytoN: 1/2 tsp PreH: 6 tabs GEssentials: 4 tabs ImmS: 4 tabs MC: 4 caps	GlycoN*: ½ tsp & GlycoAO: 2 caps PhytoN: 1/4 tsp PreH: 3 tabs GEssentials: 4 tabs ImmS: 3 tabs MC: 3 caps

*For Adv.GlycoN see page 10. Product definitions are in Appendix A on page 381.

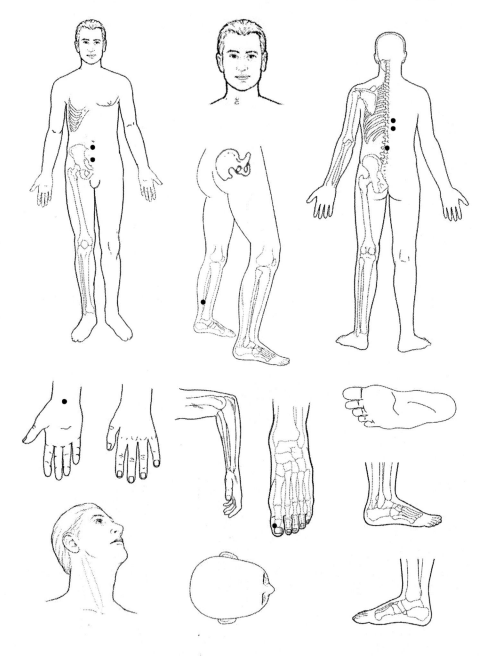

226

Ileitis

Daily Nutritional Crisis Program	Daily Nutritional Wellness Program
GlycoN*: 1 ½ tsp & GlycoAO: 3 caps PhytoN: 1/2 tsp PreH: 3 tabs GEssentials: 4 tabs Clean: 3 caps twice a day (2 weeks) MC: 4 caps & GstroP: 3 caps	GlycoN*: ½ tsp & GlycoAO: 2 caps PhytoN: 1/4 tsp PreH: 3 tabs GEssentials: 4 tabs Clean: 2 caps MC: 2 caps & GstroP: 1 cap

*For Adv.GlycoN see page 10. Product definitions are in Appendix A on page 381.

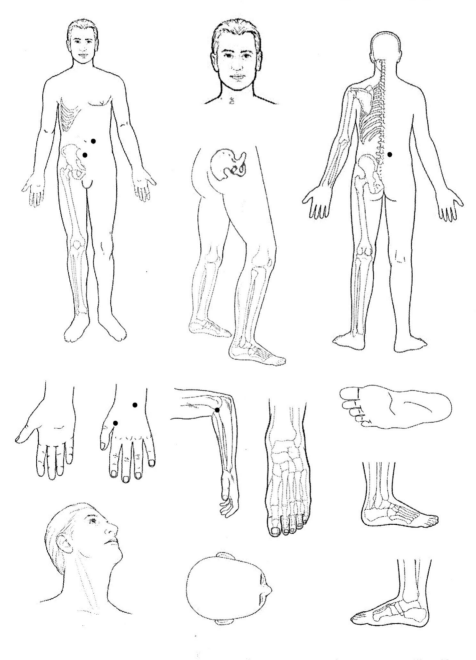

Immune Deficiency (Chronic)

Daily Nutritional Crisis Program	Daily Nutritional Wellness Program
GlycoN*: 8 tsp & GlycoAO: 5 caps PhytoN: 1 tsp PreH: 4 tabs Cata: 6 tabs ImmS: 6 tabs MC: 5 caps	GlycoN*: 2 ½ tsp & GlycoAO: 3 caps PhytoN: 1 tsp PreH: 3 tabs Cata: 6 tabs ImmS: 3 tabs MC: 3 caps

*For Adv.GlycoN see page 10. Product definitions are in Appendix A on page 381.

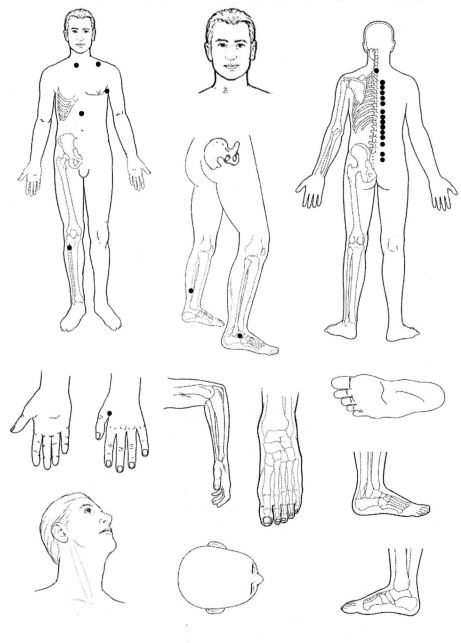

Immune System Support

Daily Nutritional Crisis Program	Daily Nutritional Wellness Program
GlycoN*: 6 tsp & GlycoAO: 5 caps PhytoN: 1 tsp PreH: 4 tabs Cata: 6 tabs ImmS: 5 tabs MC: 5 caps	GlycoN*: 2 ½ tsp & GlycoAO: 3 caps PhytoN: 1 tsp PreH: 3 tabs Cata: 6 tabs ImmS: 2 tabs MC: 3 caps

*For Adv.GlycoN see page 10. Product definitions are in Appendix A on page 381.

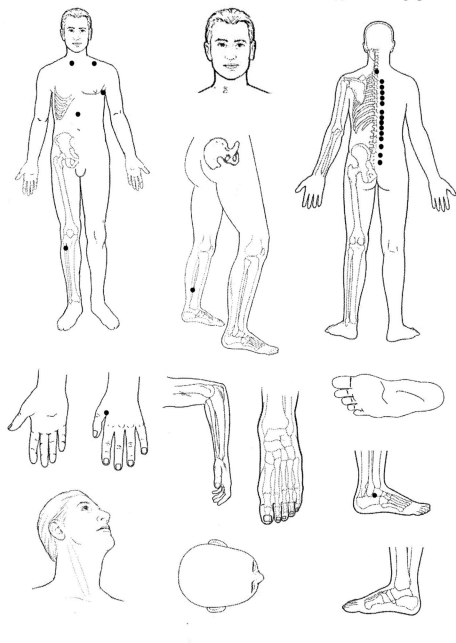

Impetigo

Daily Nutritional Crisis Program	Daily Nutritional Wellness Program
GlycoN*: 8 tsp & GlycoAO: 5 caps PhytoN: 1/2 tsp PreH: 3 tabs Cata: 4 tabs ImmS: 4 tabs MC: 4 caps	GlycoN*: ½ tsp & GlycoAO: 2 caps PhytoN: 1/4 tsp PreH: 3 tabs Cata: 4 tabs ImmS: 3 tabs MC: 3 caps

*For Adv.GlycoN see page 10. Product definitions are in Appendix A on page 381.

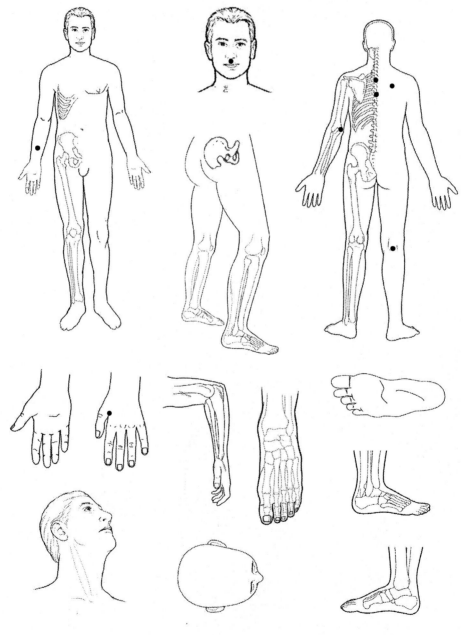

Impotence (Organic Erectile Dysfunction)

Daily Nutritional Crisis Program	Daily Nutritional Wellness Program
GlycoN*: 2 ½ tsp & GlycoAO: 3 caps PhytoN: 1 tsp PreH: 6 tabs Cata: 4 tabs ImmS: 4 tabs MC: 4 caps SP: 5 caps	GlycoN*: 1 ½ tsp & GlycoAO: 3 caps PhytoN: 1/2 tsp PreH: 4 tabs Cata: 4 tabs ImmS: 3 tabs MC: 3 caps SP: 3 caps

*For Adv.GlycoN see page 10. Product definitions are in Appendix A on page 381.

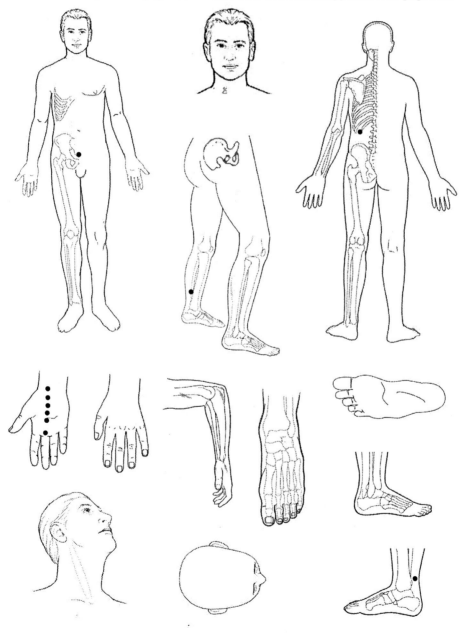

Incontinence Enuresis

Daily Nutritional Crisis Program	Daily Nutritional Wellness Program
GlycoN*: 2 ½ tsp & GlycoAO: 3 caps PhytoN: 1/2 tsp PreH: 4 tabs Cata: 4 tabs ImmS: 5 tabs MC: 5 caps	GlycoN*: ½ tsp & GlycoAO: 2 caps PhytoN: 1/4 tsp PreH: 3 tabs Cata: 4 tabs ImmS: 3 tabs MC: 3 caps

*For Adv.GlycoN see page 10. Product definitions are in Appendix A on page 381.

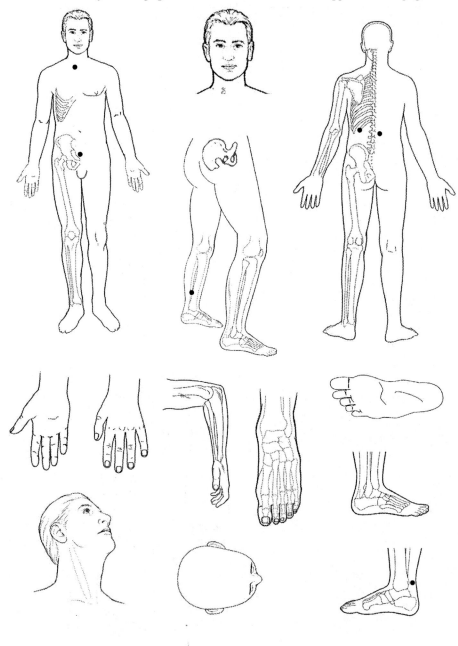

232

Infection (Systemic)

Daily Nutritional Crisis Program	Daily Nutritional Wellness Program
GlycoN*: 10 ¾ tsp & GlycoAO: 6 caps PhytoN: 1 tsp PreH: 6 tabs Cata: 6 tabs ImmS: 6 tabs MC: 6 caps SP: 4 caps	GlycoN*: 3 ½ tsp & GlycoAO: 3 caps PhytoN: 1/2 tsp PreH: 3 tabs Cata: 4 tabs ImmS: 3 tabs MC: 3 caps SP: 2 caps

*For Adv.GlycoN see page 10. Product definitions are in Appendix A on page 381.

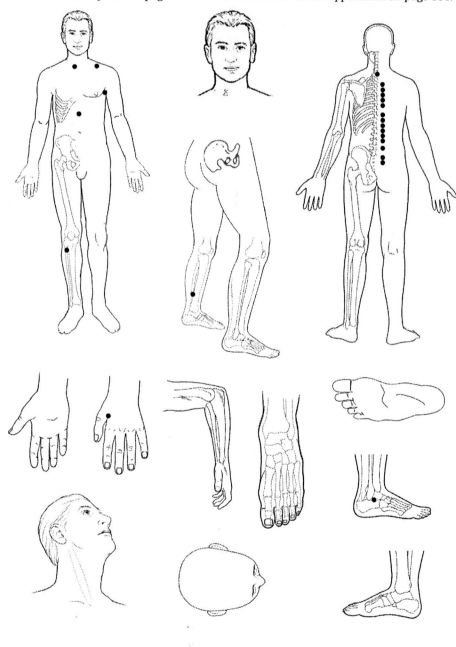

Infertility (Female)

Daily Nutritional Crisis Program	Daily Nutritional Wellness Program
GlycoN*: 2 ½ tsp & GlycoAO: 3 caps PhytoN: 1 tsp PreH: 6 tabs Cata: 4 tabs ImmS: 6 tabs MC: 5 caps SP: 5 caps	GlycoN*: 1 ½ tsp & GlycoAO: 3 caps PhytoN: 1/2 tsp PreH: 3 tabs Cata: 4 tabs ImmS: 4 tabs MC: 3 caps SP: 3 caps

*For Adv.GlycoN see page 10. Product definitions are in Appendix A on page 381.

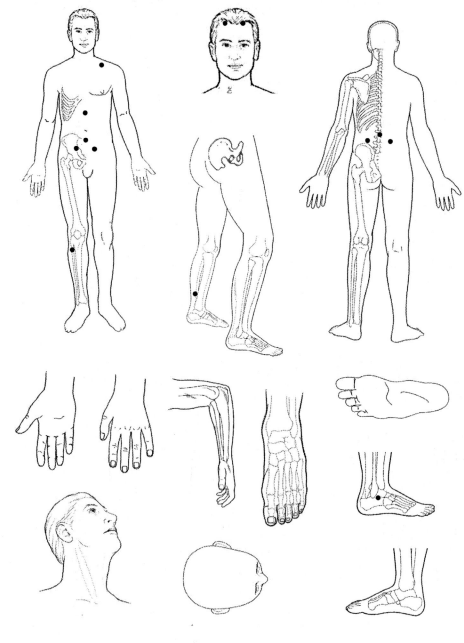

Infertility (Male)

Daily Nutritional Crisis Program	Daily Nutritional Wellness Program
GlycoN*: 2 ½ tsp & GlycoAO: 3 caps PhytoN: 1 tsp PreH: 6 tabs Cata: 4 tabs ImmS: 6 tabs MC: 5 caps SP: 5 caps	GlycoN*: 1 ½ tsp & GlycoAO: 3 caps PhytoN: 1/2 tsp PreH: 3 tabs Cata: 4 tabs ImmS: 4 tabs MC: 3 caps SP: 3 caps

*For Adv.GlycoN see page 10. Product definitions are in Appendix A on page 381.

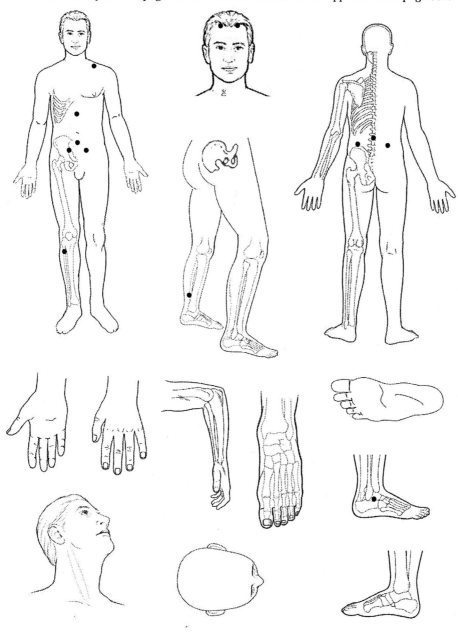

Inflammation (Systemic)

Daily Nutritional Crisis Program	Daily Nutritional Wellness Program
GlycoN*: 10 ¾ tsp & GlycoAO: 6 caps PhytoN: 1 tsp PreH: 6 tabs Cata: 6 tabs ImmS: 6 tabs MC: 6 caps SP: 4 caps	GlycoN*: 3 ½ tsp & GlycoAO: 3 caps PhytoN: 1/2 tsp PreH: 3 tabs Cata: 4 tabs ImmS: 4 tabs MC: 4 caps SP: 3 caps

*For Adv.GlycoN see page 10. Product definitions are in Appendix A on page 381.

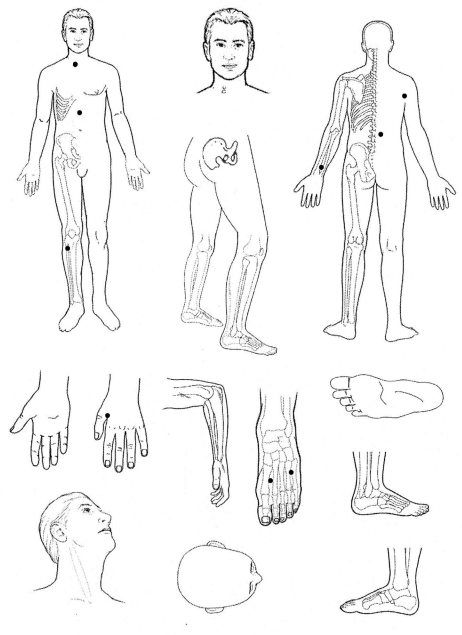

236

Influenza w/ Respiratory Manifestations

Daily Nutritional Crisis Program	Daily Nutritional Wellness Program
GlycoN*: 2 ½ tsp & GlycoAO: 3 caps PhytoN: 1 ¾ tsp PreH: 3 tabs GGEssentials : 6 tabs ImmS: 6 tabs MC: 6 caps	GlycoN*: ½ tsp & GlycoAO: 2 caps PhytoN: 1/4 tsp PreH: 3 tabs GGEssentials : 4 tabs ImmS: 3 tabs MC: 3 caps

*For Adv.GlycoN see page 10. Product definitions are in Appendix A on page 381.

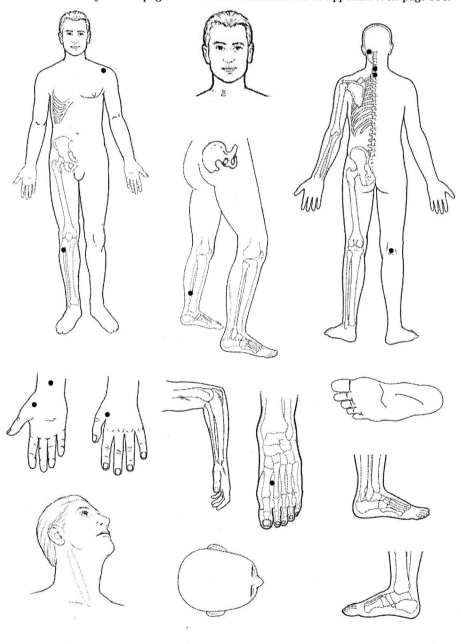

Insect Bite (venomous)
(apply SkZone to area)

Daily Nutritional Crisis Program	Daily Nutritional Wellness Program
GlycoN*: 10 ¾ tsp & GlycoAO: 6 caps	GlycoN*: 3 ½ tsp & GlycoAO: 2 caps
PhytoN: 1 tsp	PhytoN: 1/4 tsp
PreH: 6 tabs	PreH: 3 tabs
GEssentials : 4 tabs	GEssentials : 4 tabs
ImmS: 4 caps	ImmS: 3 caps
MC: 4 caps	MC: 3 caps
SP: 4 caps	SP: 3 caps

*For Adv.GlycoN see page 10. Product definitions are in Appendix A on page 381.

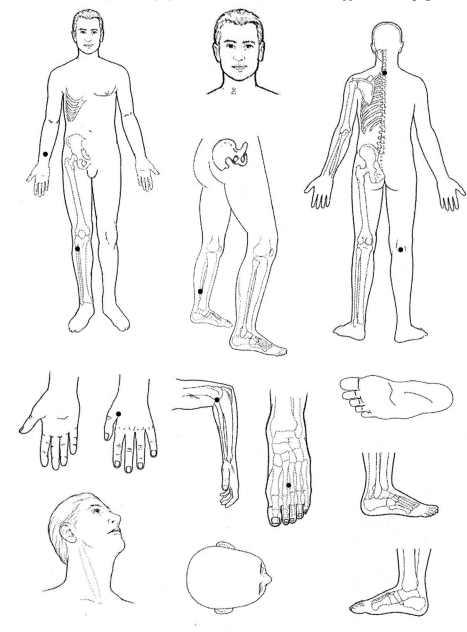

Insomnia

Daily Nutritional Crisis Program	Daily Nutritional Wellness Program
GlycoN*: 1 ½ tsp & GlycoAO: 3 caps PhytoN: 1/4 tsp PreH: 4 tabs GEssentials : 4 tabs MC: 4 caps	GlycoN*: ½ tsp & GlycoAO: 2 caps PhytoN: 1/4 tsp PreH: 3 tabs GEssentials : 4 tabs MC: 2 caps

*For Adv.GlycoN see page 10. Product definitions are in Appendix A on page 381.

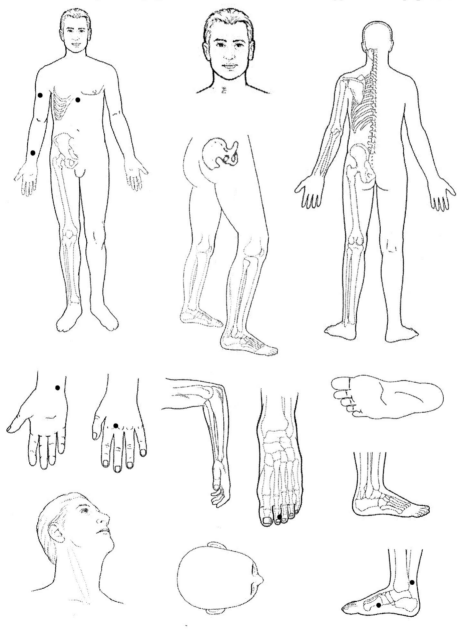

Intestinal Malabsorption

Daily Nutritional Crisis Program	Daily Nutritional Wellness Program
GlycoN*: 5 ¼ tsp & GlycoAO: 4 caps	GlycoN*: 1 ½ tsp & GlycoAO: 3 caps
PhytoN: 1 ¾ tsp	PhytoN: 3/4 tsp
PreH: 4 tabs	PreH: 3 tabs
Cata:4 tabs	Cata:4 tabs
ImmS: 4 tabs	ImmS: 2 tabs
MC: 4 caps & GstroP: 3 caps	MC: 2 caps & GstroP: 1 cap

*For Adv.GlycoN see page 10. Product definitions are in Appendix A on page 381.

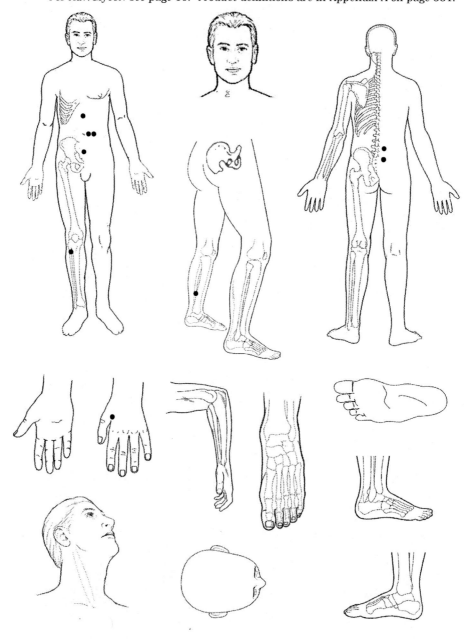

Irritable Bowel Syndrome (IBS)

Daily Nutritional Crisis Program	Daily Nutritional Wellness Program
GlycoN*: 5 ¼ tsp & GlycoAO: 4 caps	GlycoN*: 1 ½ tsp & GlycoAO: 3 caps
PhytoN: 1 ¾ tsp	PhytoN: 3/4 tsp
PreH: 4 tabs	PreH: 3 tabs
Cata:4 tabs	Cata:4 tabs
ImmS: 4 tabs	ImmS: 2 tabs
MC: 4 caps & GstroP: 3 caps	MC: 2 caps & GstroP: 1 cap

*For Adv.GlycoN see page 10. Product definitions are in Appendix A on page 381.

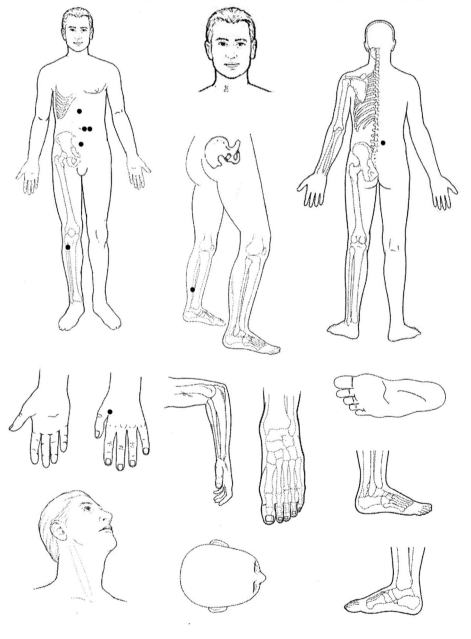

Ischemic Bowel Disease

Daily Nutritional Crisis Program	Daily Nutritional Wellness Program
GlycoN*: 5 ¼ tsp & GlycoAO: 4 caps PhytoN: 1 ¾ tsp PreH: 4 tabs Cata:4 tabs ImmS: 4 tabs MC: 4 caps & GstroP: 3 caps	GlycoN*: 1 ½ tsp & GlycoAO: 3 caps PhytoN: 3/4 tsp PreH: 3 tabs Cata:4 tabs ImmS: 2 tabs MC: 2 caps & GstroP: 1 cap

*For Adv.GlycoN see page 10. Product definitions are in Appendix A on page 381.

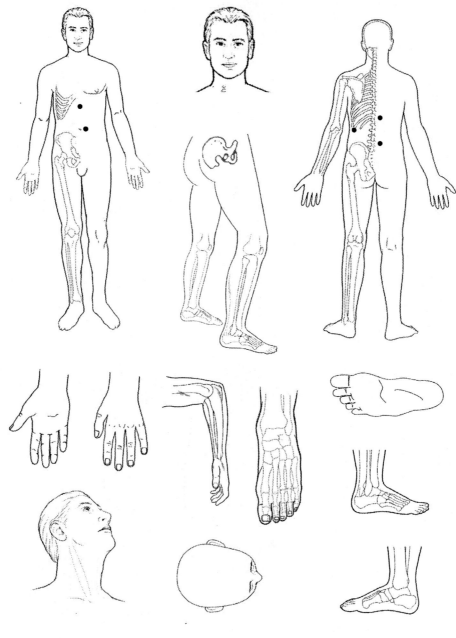

Itching (Pruritis)
(apply SkZone to areas)

Daily Nutritional Crisis Program	Daily Nutritional Wellness Program
GlycoN*: 1 ½ tsp & GlycoAO: 3 caps	GlycoN*: 1 ½ tsp & GlycoAO: 3 caps
PhytoN: 1/2 tsp	PhytoN: 1/2 tsp
PreH: 6 tabs	PreH: 3 tabs
GEssentials : 4 tabs	GEssentials : 4 tabs
ImmS: 4 tabs	ImmS: 3 tabs
MC: 4 caps	MC: 3 caps
SP: 3 caps	SP: 2 caps

*For Adv.GlycoN see page 10. Product definitions are in Appendix A on page 381.

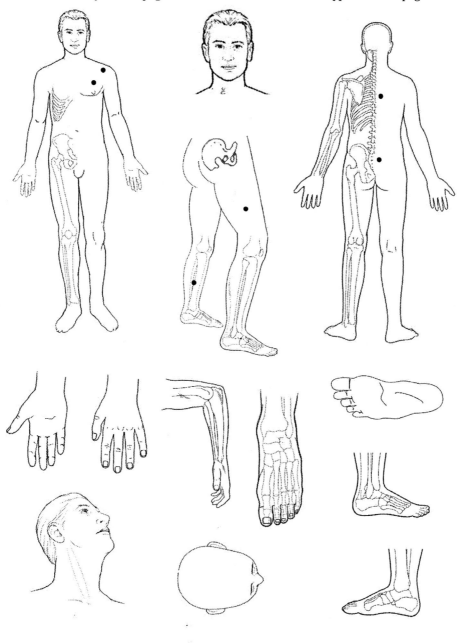

Jaundice

Daily Nutritional Crisis Program	Daily Nutritional Wellness Program
GlycoN*: 5 ¼ tsp & GlycoAO: 4 caps PhytoN: 1 tsp PreH: 6 tabs Cata: 4 tabs ImmS: 5 tabs MC: 5 caps Clean: 3 caps twice a day (2 weeks)	GlycoN*: 1 ½ tsp & GlycoAO: 3 caps PhytoN: 1/2 tsp PreH: 3 tabs Cata: 4 tabs ImmS: 4 tabs MC: 4 caps Clean: 2 caps

*For Adv.GlycoN see page 10. Product definitions are in Appendix A on page 381.

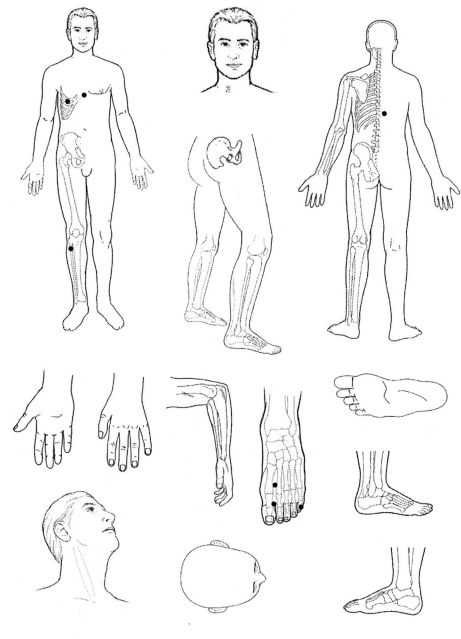

Jock Itch

Daily Nutritional Crisis Program	Daily Nutritional Wellness Program
GlycoN*: 1 ½ tsp & GlycoAO: 3 caps	GlycoN*: 1 ½ tsp & GlycoAO: 3 caps
PhytoN: 1/2 tsp	PhytoN: 1/2 tsp
PreH: 6 tabs	PreH: 3 tabs
GEssentials : 4 tabs	GEssentials : 4 tabs
ImmS: 4 tabs	ImmS: 3 tabs
MC: 4 caps	MC: 3 caps
SP: 3 caps	SP: 2 caps

*For Adv.GlycoN see page 10.   Product definitions are in Appendix A on page 381.

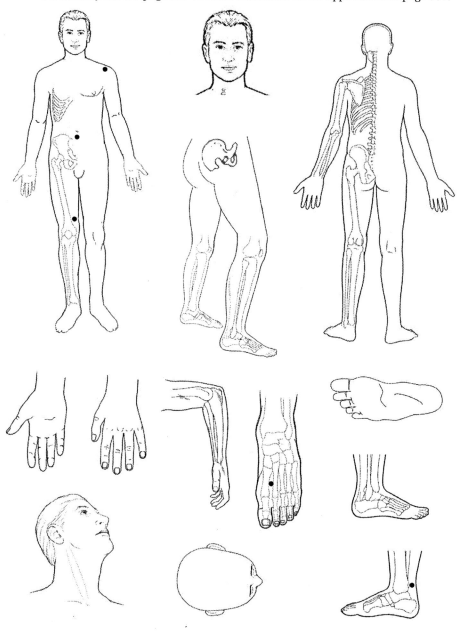

Joint Pain (Multiple Sites)

Daily Nutritional Crisis Program	Daily Nutritional Wellness Program
GlycoN*: 5¼ tsp & GlycoAO: 4 caps PhytoN: 1/2 tsp PreH: 6 tabs Cata: 4 tabs MC: 5 caps ImmS: 4 tabs SP: 4 caps	GlycoN*: 2½ tsp & GlycoAO: 2 caps PhytoN: 1/2 tsp PreH: 3 tabs Cata: 4 tabs MC: 3 caps ImmS: 3 tabs SP: 2 caps

*For Adv.GlycoN see page 10. Product definitions are in Appendix A on page 381.

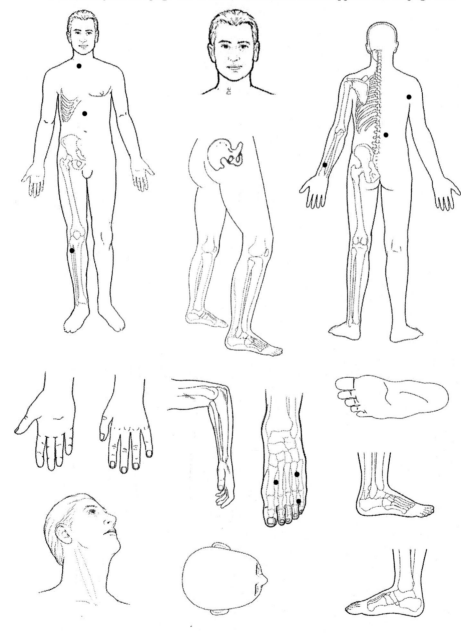

Juvenile Arthritis

Daily Nutritional Crisis Program	Daily Nutritional Wellness Program
GlycoN*: 5 ¼ tsp & GlycoAO: 4 caps PhytoN: 1 tsp PreH: 6 tabs Cata: 6 tabs Clean: 3 caps twice a day (2 weeks) MC: 4 caps	GlycoN*: 1 ½ tsp & GlycoAO: 3 caps PhytoN: 3/4 tsp PreH: 4 tabs Cata: 6 tabs Clean: 1 cap MC: 2 caps

*For Adv.GlycoN see page 10. Product definitions are in Appendix A on page 381.

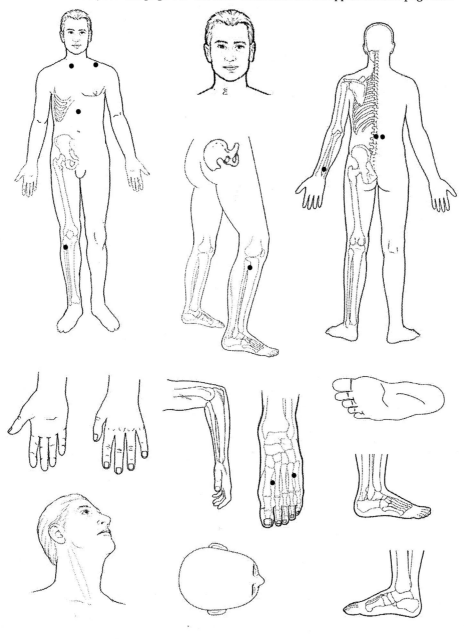

Kidney Detoxification

Daily Nutritional Crisis Program	Daily Nutritional Wellness Program
GlycoN*: 10 ¾ tsp & GlycoAO: 6 caps	GlycoN*: 3 ½ tsp & GlycoAO: 3 caps
PhytoN: 1 tsp	PhytoN: 1/2 tsp
PreH: 6 tabs	PreH: 3 tabs
Cata: 6 tabs	Cata: 4 tabs
ImmS: 6 tabs	ImmS: 3 tabs
MC: 6 caps	MC: 3 caps
SP: 4 caps	SP: 2 caps

*For Adv.GlycoN see page 10. Product definitions are in Appendix A on page 381.

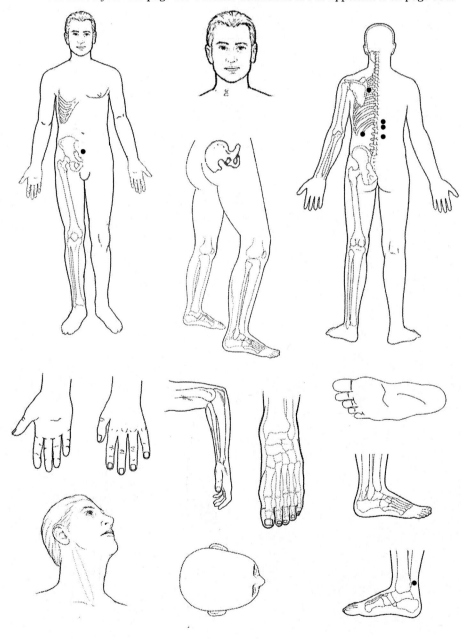

248

Kidney Infection

Daily Nutritional Crisis Program	Daily Nutritional Wellness Program
GlycoN*: 10 ¾ tsp & GlycoAO: 6 caps PhytoN: 1 tsp PreH: 6 tabs Cata: 6 tabs ImmS: 6 tabs MC: 6 caps SP: 4 caps	GlycoN*: 3 ½ tsp & GlycoAO: 3 caps PhytoN: 1/2 tsp PreH: 3 tabs Cata: 4 tabs ImmS: 3 tabs MC: 3 caps SP: 2 caps

*For Adv.GlycoN see page 10. Product definitions are in Appendix A on page 381.

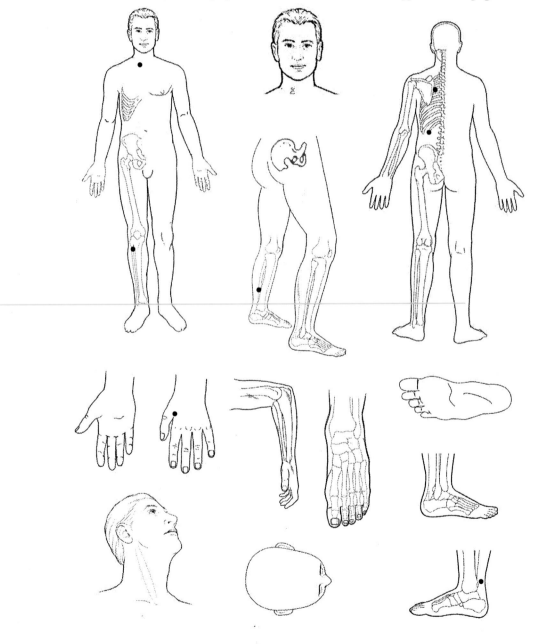

Labyrinthitis

Daily Nutritional Crisis Program	Daily Nutritional Wellness Program
GlycoN*: 2 ½ tsp & GlycoAO: 3 caps PhytoN: 3/4 tsp PreH: 3 tabs Cata:4 tabs ImmS: 5 tabs MC: 5 caps	GlycoN*: ½ tsp & GlycoAO: 2 caps PhytoN: 1/4 tsp PreH: 3 tabs Cata:4 tabs ImmS: 3 tabs MC: 3 caps

*For Adv.GlycoN see page 10. Product definitions are in Appendix A on page 381.

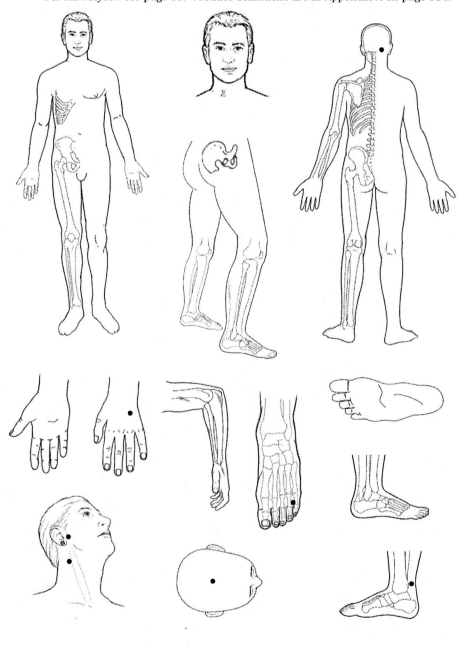

Laryngitis

Daily Nutritional Crisis Program	Daily Nutritional Wellness Program
GlycoN*: 2 tsp & GlycoAO: 3 caps PhytoN: 3/4 tsp PreH: 3 tabs GEssentials: 4 tabs ImmS: 5 tabs MC: 6 caps	GlycoN*: ½ tsp & GlycoAO: 2 caps PhytoN: 1/2 tsp PreH: 3 tabs GEssentials: 4 tabs ImmS: 3 tabs MC: 3 caps

*For Adv.GlycoN see page 10. Product definitions are in Appendix A on page 381.

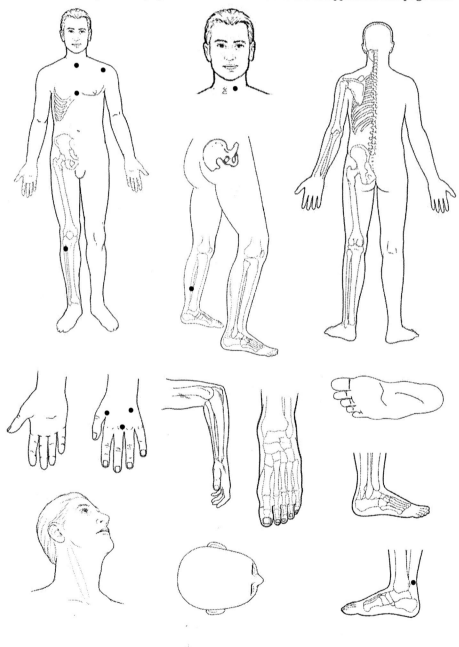

251

Leg Ulcers
apply soft laser to affected area

Daily Nutritional Crisis Program	Daily Nutritional Wellness Program
GlycoN*: 5 ¼ tsp & GlycoAO: 4 caps PhytoN: 1 tsp PreH: 4 tabs Cata: 6 tabs MC: 8 caps SkZone: apply to area	GlycoN*: 1 ½ tsp & GlycoAO: 3 caps PhytoN: 1 tsp PreH: 3 tabs Cata: 4 tabs MC: 4 caps SkZone: apply to area

*For Adv.GlycoN see page 10. Product definitions are in Appendix A on page 381.

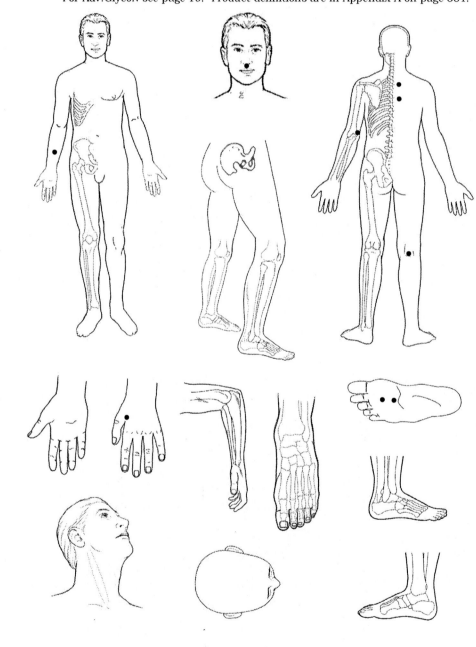

Leukemia

Daily Nutritional Crisis Program	Daily Nutritional Wellness Program
GlycoN*: 2 ½ tsp & GlycoAO: 3 caps PhytoN: 1 tsp PreH: 3 tabs GEssentials: 4 tabs MC: 3 caps	GlycoN*: 1 ½ tsp & GlycoAO: 3 caps PhytoN: 1 tsp PreH: 3 tabs GEssentials: 4 tabs MC: 2 caps

*For Adv.GlycoN see page 10. Product definitions are in Appendix A on page 381.

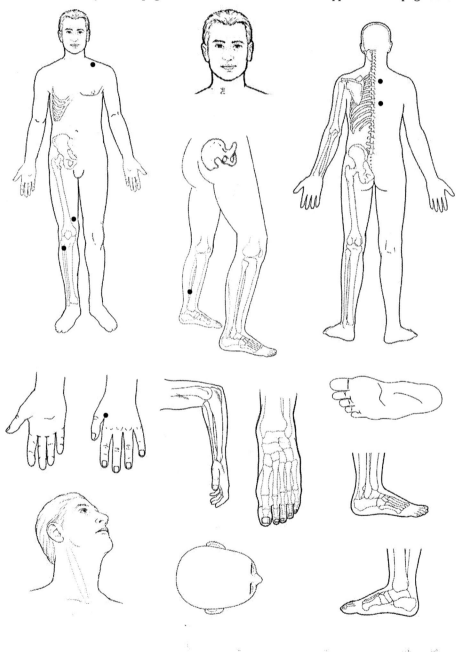

Liver Disease (Chronic)

Daily Nutritional Crisis Program	Daily Nutritional Wellness Program
GlycoN*: 1 ½ tsp & GlycoAO: 3 caps G	GlycoN*: ½ tsp & GlycoAO: 2 caps
PhytoN: 1/2 tsp	PhytoN: 1/4 tsp
PreH: 6 tabs	PreH: 3 tabs
Cata: 4 tabs	Cata: 4 tabs
Clean: 3 caps twice a day (2 weeks)	Clean: 1 cap
GstroZ: 2 caps before meals	GstroZ: 1 cap before meals

*For Adv.GlycoN see page 10. Product definitions are in Appendix A on page 381.

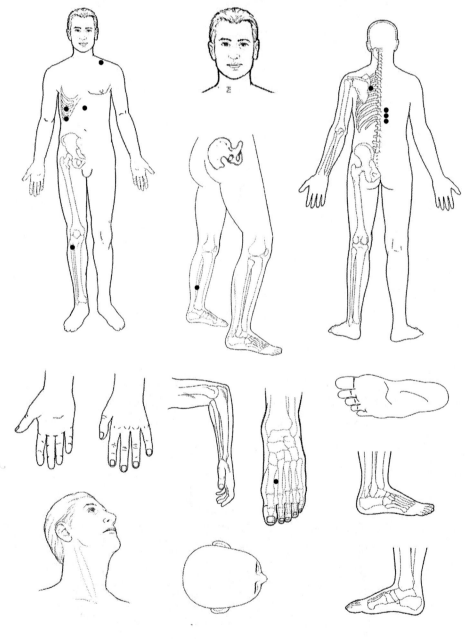

Lou Gehrig's Disease (ALS)

Daily Nutritional Crisis Program	Daily Nutritional Wellness Program
GlycoN*: 10 ¾ tsp & GlycoAO: 6 caps PhytoN: 3 tsp PreH: 6 tabs Cata: 6 tabs MC: 4 caps ImmS: 4 tabs	GlycoN*: 5 ¼ tsp & GlycoAO: 4 caps PhytoN: 1 tsp PreH: 4 tabs Cata: 6 tabs MC: 3 caps ImmS: 3 tabs

*For Adv.GlycoN see page 10. Product definitions are in Appendix A on page 381.

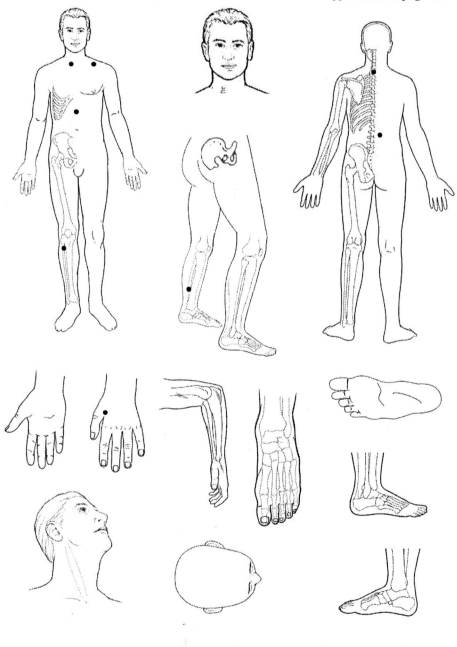

Low Blood Sugar

Daily Nutritional Crisis Program	Daily Nutritional Wellness Program
GlycoN*: 2 ½ tsp & GlycoAO: 3 caps G PhytoN: 1½ tsp PreH: 6 tabs GEssentials: 6 tabs	GlycoN*: ½ tsp & GlycoAO: 2 caps PhytoN: 3/4 tsp PreH: 3 tabs GEssentials: 4 tabs

*For Adv.GlycoN see page 10. Product definitions are in Appendix A on page 381.

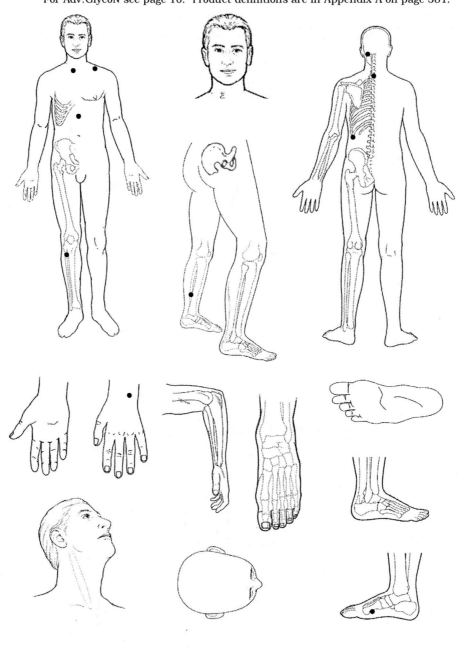

Lumbar Discitis

Daily Nutritional Crisis Program	Daily Nutritional Wellness Program
GlycoN*: 2 ½ tsp & GlycoAO: 3 caps	GlycoN*: 1 ½ tsp & GlycoAO: 3 caps
PhytoN: 3/4 tsp	PhytoN: 1/2 tsp
PreH: 3 tabs	PreH: 3 tabs
Cata:6 tabs	Cata:4 tabs
SP: 6 caps	SP: 4 caps
MC: 4 caps	MC: 2 caps

*For Adv.GlycoN see page 10. Product definitions are in Appendix A on page 381.

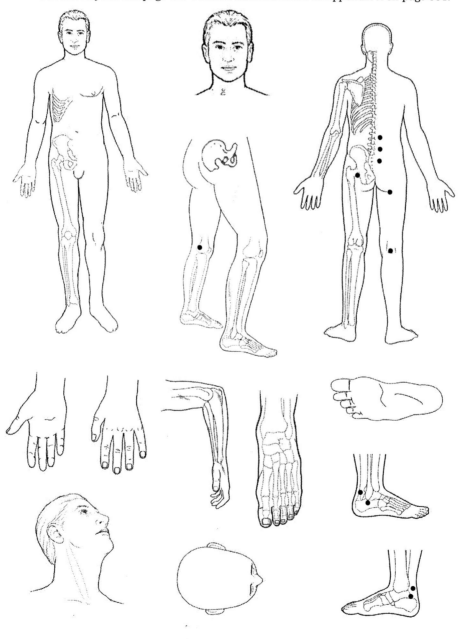

Lupus Erythematosis (SLE)

Daily Nutritional Crisis Program	Daily Nutritional Wellness Program
GlycoN*: 6 tsp & GlycoAO: 5 caps	GlycoN*: 2 ½ tsp & GlycoAO: 3 caps
PhytoN: 1 tsp	PhytoN: 1 tsp
PreH: 4 tabs	PreH: 3 tabs
Cata: 6 tabs	Cata: 6 tabs
ImmS: 5 tabs	ImmS: 2 tabs
MC: 5 caps	MC: 3 caps
SP: 4 caps	SP: 2 caps

*For Adv.GlycoN see page 10. Product definitions are in Appendix A on page 381.

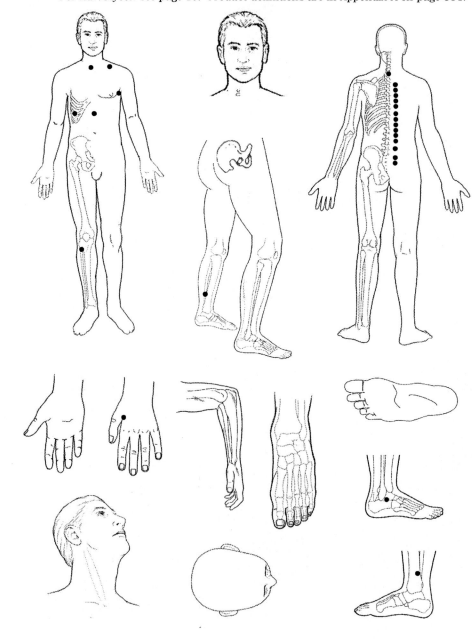

Lyme Disease

Daily Nutritional Crisis Program	Daily Nutritional Wellness Program
GlycoN*: 8 tsp & GlycoAO: 5 caps	GlycoN*: 2 tsp & GlycoAO: 2 caps
PhytoN: 2 tsp	PhytoN: 1/4 tsp
PreH: 6 tabs	PreH: 3 tabs
Cata: 6 tabs	Cata: 6 tabs
ImmS: 5 tabs	ImmS: 4 tabs
MC: 5 caps	MC: 4 caps
Clean: 3 caps twice a day (2 weeks)	Clean: 2 caps

*For Adv.GlycoN see page 10. Product definitions are in Appendix A on page 381.

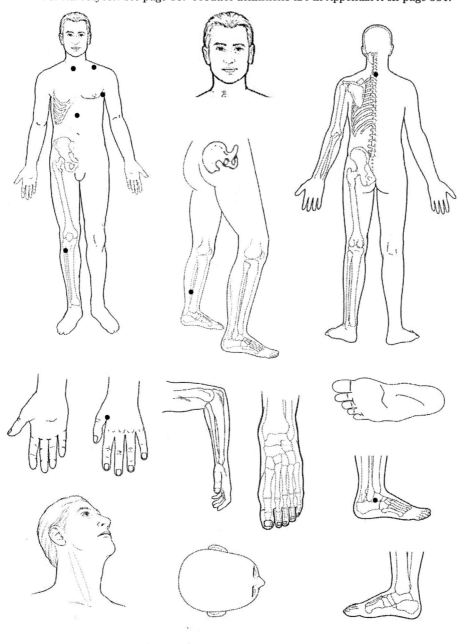

Lymph Nodes Swollen

Daily Nutritional Crisis Program	Daily Nutritional Wellness Program
GlycoN*: 10 ¾ tsp & GlycoAO: 6 caps PhytoN: 1 tsp PreH: 6 tabs Cata: 6 tabs ImmS: 6 tabs MC: 6 caps SP: 4 caps	GlycoN*: 3 ½ tsp & GlycoAO: 3 caps PhytoN: 1/2 tsp PreH: 3 tabs Cata: 4 tabs ImmS: 3 tabs MC: 3 caps SP: 2 caps

*For Adv.GlycoN see page 10. Product definitions are in Appendix A on page 381.

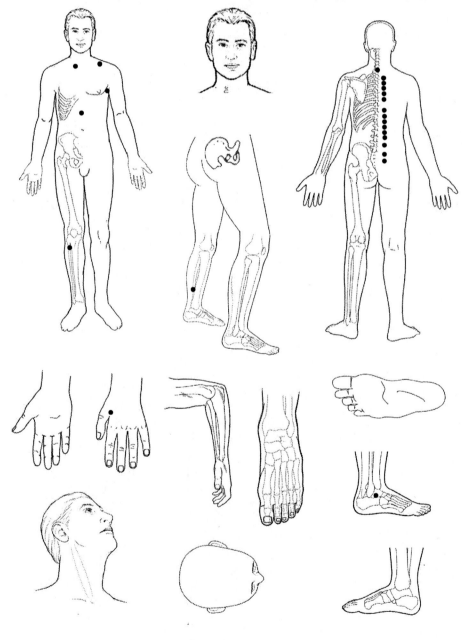

Lymphadenitis

Daily Nutritional Crisis Program	Daily Nutritional Wellness Program
GlycoN*: 10 ¾ tsp & GlycoAO: 6 caps PhytoN: 1 tsp PreH: 6 tabs Cata: 6 tabs ImmS: 6 tabs MC: 6 caps SP: 4 caps	GlycoN*: 3 ½ tsp & GlycoAO: 3 caps PhytoN: 1/2 tsp PreH: 3 tabs Cata: 4 tabs ImmS: 3 tabs MC: 3 caps SP: 2 caps

*For Adv.GlycoN see page 10. Product definitions are in Appendix A on page 381.

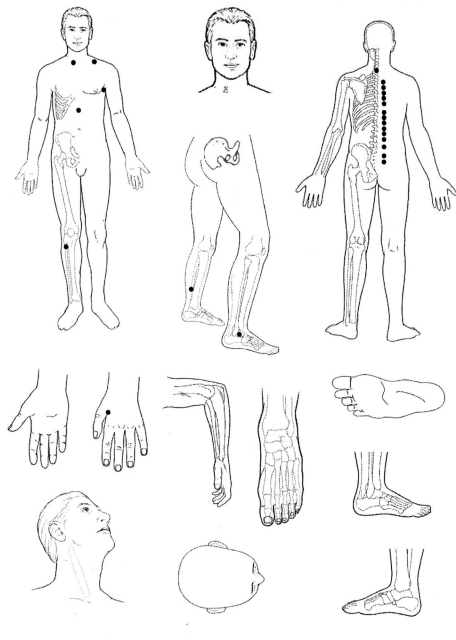

Lymphoma (Hodgkins)

Daily Nutritional Crisis Program	Daily Nutritional Wellness Program
GlycoN*: 10 ¾ tsp & GlycoAO: 6 caps	GlycoN*: 3 ½ tsp & GlycoAO: 3 caps
PhytoN: 1 tsp	PhytoN: 1/2 tsp
PreH: 6 tabs	PreH: 3 tabs
Cata: 6 tabs	Cata: 4 tabs
ImmS: 6 tabs	ImmS: 3 tabs
MC: 6 caps	MC: 3 caps
SP: 4 caps	SP: 2 caps

*For Adv.GlycoN see page 10. Product definitions are in Appendix A on page 381.

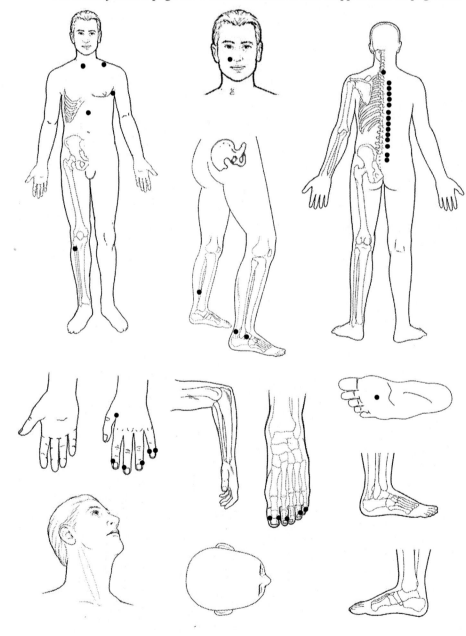

Macular Degeneration

Daily Nutritional Crisis Program	Daily Nutritional Wellness Program
GlycoN*: 2 tsp & GlycoAO: 3 caps	GlycoN*: ½ tsp & GlycoAO: 2 caps
PhytoN: 3/4 tsp	PhytoN: 1/4 tsp
PreH: 3 tabs	PreH: 3 tabs
GEssentials: 4 tabs	GEssentials: 4 tabs
MC: 4 caps	MC: 2 caps
SP: 4 caps	SP: 3 caps

*For Adv.GlycoN see page 10. Product definitions are in Appendix A on page 381.

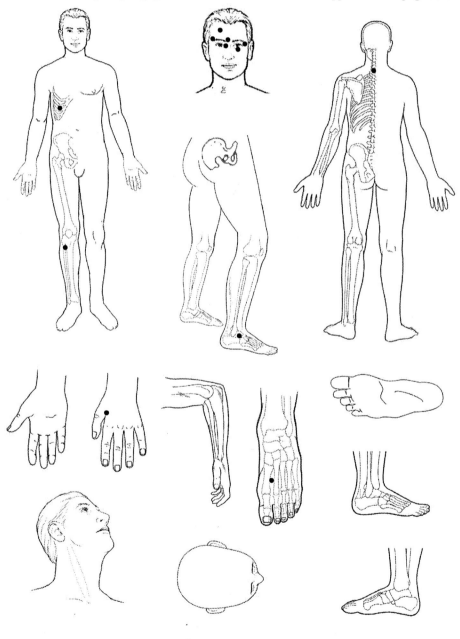

Malaria

Daily Nutritional Crisis Program	Daily Nutritional Wellness Program
GlycoN*: 8 tsp & GlycoAO: 5 caps	GlycoN*: 1 ½ tsp & GlycoAO: 3 caps
PhytoN: 2 tsp	PhytoN: 1/4 tsp
PreH: 6 tabs	PreH: 3 tabs
Cata: 6 tabs	Cata: 6 tabs
ImmS: 5 tabs	ImmS: 4 tabs
MC: 5 caps	MC: 4 caps
Clean: 3 caps twice a day (2 weeks)	Clean: 2 caps

*For Adv.GlycoN see page 10. Product definitions are in Appendix A on page 381.

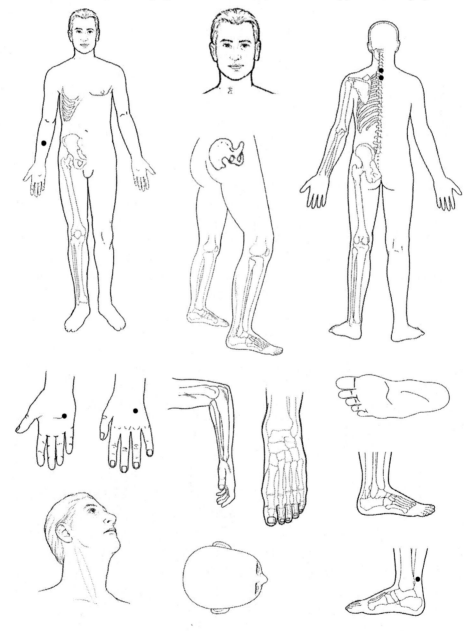

Malignant Melanoma

Daily Nutritional Crisis Program	Daily Nutritional Wellness Program
GlycoN*: 10 ¾ tsp & GlycoAO: 6 caps	GlycoN*: 2 ½ tsp & GlycoAO: 3 caps
PhytoN: 4 tsp	PhytoN: 2 tsp
PreH: 6 tabs	PreH: 4 tabs
Cata: 6 tabs	Cata: 6 tabs
ImmS: 6 tabs	ImmS: 3 tabs
MC: 6 caps	MC: 3 caps

*For Adv.GlycoN see page 10. Product definitions are in Appendix A on page 381.

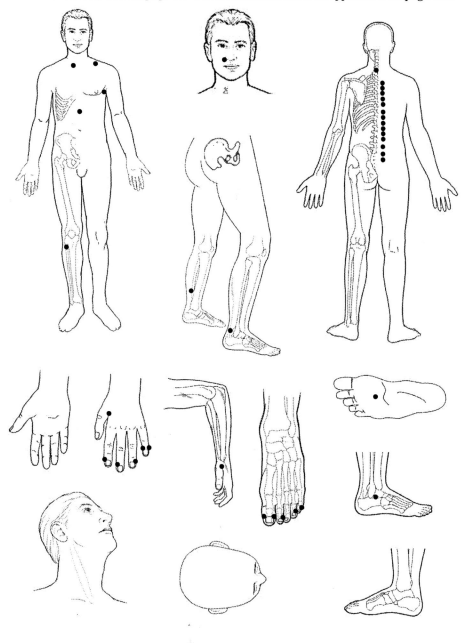

Mastitis

Daily Nutritional Crisis Program	Daily Nutritional Wellness Program
GlycoN*: 2 ½ tsp & GlycoAO: 3 caps PhytoN: 3/4 tsp PreH: 4 tabs GEssentials: 4 tabs ImmS: 5 tabs MC: 4 caps	GlycoN*: ½ tsp & GlycoAO: 2 caps PhytoN: 1/2 tsp PreH: 4 tabs GEssentials: 4 tabs ImmS: 3 tabs MC: 4 caps

*For Adv.GlycoN see page 10. Product definitions are in Appendix A on page 381.

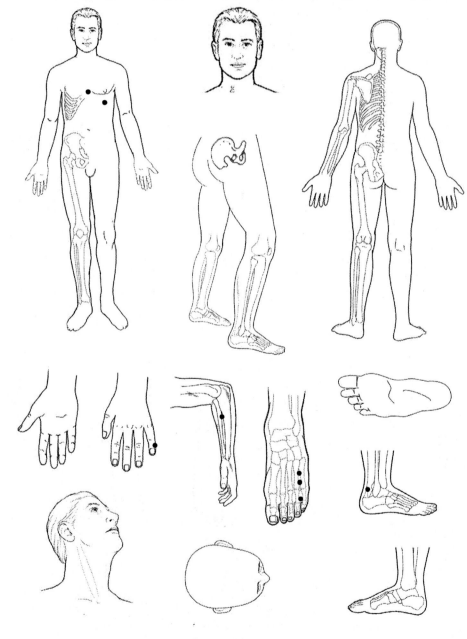

Measles

Daily Nutritional Crisis Program	Daily Nutritional Wellness Program
GlycoN*: 5 ¼ tsp & GlycoAO: 4 caps PhytoN: 1 tsp PreH: 4 tabs GEssentials: 4 tabs ImmS: 6 tabs MC: 4 tabs	GlycoN*: ½ tsp & GlycoAO: 2 caps PhytoN: 1/4 tsp PreH: 3 tabs GEssentials: 4 tabs ImmS: 3 tabs MC: 4 tabs

*For Adv.GlycoN see page 10. Product definitions are in Appendix A on page 381.

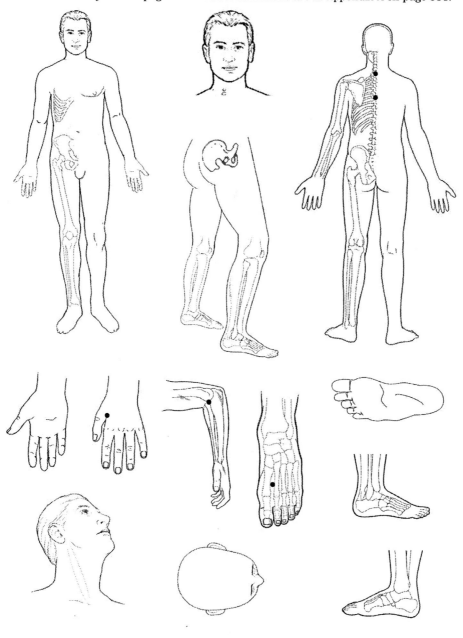

Meniere's Syndrome

Daily Nutritional Crisis Program	Daily Nutritional Wellness Program
GlycoN*: 2 ½ tsp & GlycoAO: 3 caps PhytoN: 3/4 tsp PreH: 3 tabs Cata:4 tabs ImmS: 5 tabs MC: 5 caps	GlycoN*: ½ tsp & GlycoAO: 2 caps PhytoN: 1/4 tsp PreH: 3 tabs Cata:4 tabs ImmS: 3 tabs MC: 3 caps

*For Adv.GlycoN see page 10. Product definitions are in Appendix A on page 381.

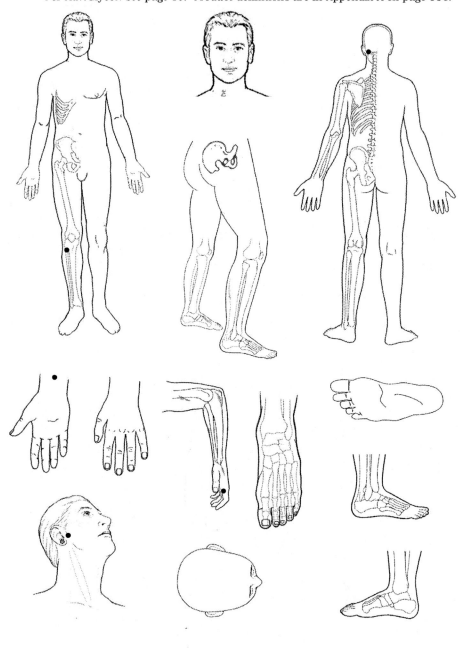

Meningitis

Daily Nutritional Crisis Program	Daily Nutritional Wellness Program
GlycoN*: 10 ¾ tsp & GlycoAO: 6 caps	GlycoN*: 3 ½ tsp & GlycoAO: 3 caps
PhytoN: 1 tsp	PhytoN: 1/2 tsp
PreH: 6 tabs	PreH: 3 tabs
Cata: 6 tabs	Cata: 4 tabs
ImmS: 6 tabs	ImmS: 3 tabs
MC: 6 caps	MC: 3 caps
SP: 4 caps	SP: 2 caps

*For Adv.GlycoN see page 10. Product definitions are in Appendix A on page 381.

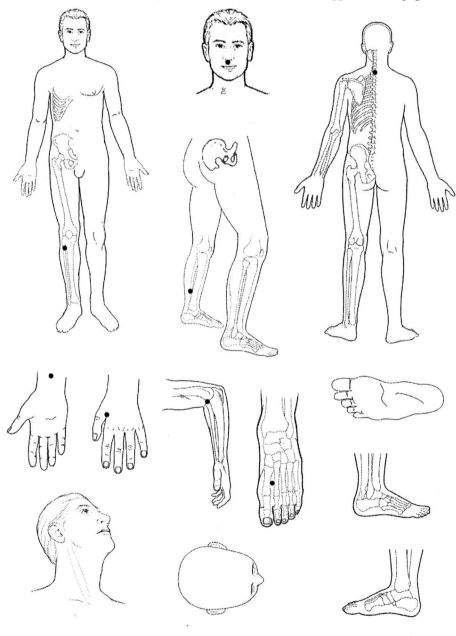

Menopausal Disorder

Daily Nutritional Crisis Program	Daily Nutritional Wellness Program
GlycoN*: 3 tsp & GlycoAO: 4 caps	GlycoN*: 1 ½ tsp & GlycoAO: 3 caps
PhytoN: 1 tsp	PhytoN: 1/2 tsp
PreH: 4 tabs	PreH: 3 tabs
GEssentials: 4 tabs	GEssentials: 4 tabs
ImmS: 6 tabs	ImmS: 3 tabs
MC: 4 caps	MC: 3 caps

*For Adv.GlycoN see page 10. Product definitions are in Appendix A on page 381.

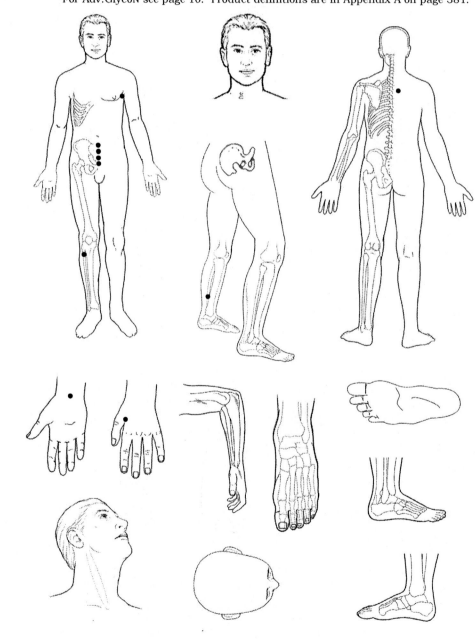

Menstrual Cramps (Dysmenorrhea)

Daily Nutritional Crisis Program	Daily Nutritional Wellness Program
GlycoN*: 3 tsp & GlycoAO: 4 caps	GlycoN*: 1 ½ tsp & GlycoAO: 3 caps
PhytoN: 1 tsp	PhytoN: 1/2 tsp
PreH: 4 tabs	PreH: 3 tabs
GEssentials: 4 tabs	GEssentials: 4 tabs
ImmS: 6 tabs	ImmS: 3 tabs
MC: 4 caps	MC: 3 caps

*For Adv.GlycoN see page 10. Product definitions are in Appendix A on page 381.

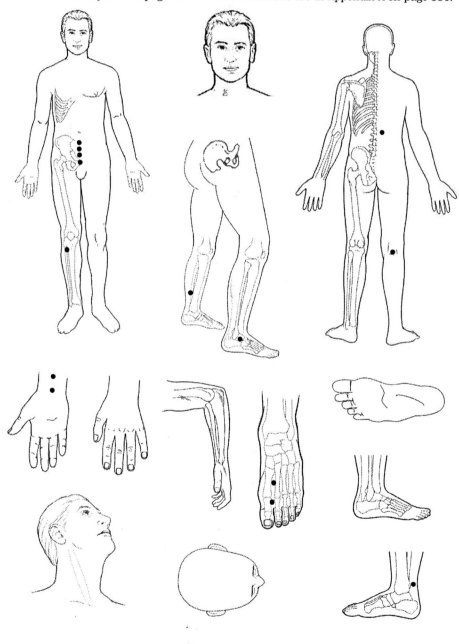

Mental Retardation

Daily Nutritional Crisis Program	Daily Nutritional Wellness Program
GlycoN*: 8 tsp & GlycoAO: 5 caps	GlycoN*: 1 ½ tsp & GlycoAO: 3 caps
PhytoN: 1 tsp	PhytoN: 1/4 tsp
PreH: 6 tabs	PreH: 4 tabs
Cata: 4 tabs	Cata: 4 tabs
SP: 4 caps	SP: 2 caps
ImmS: 4 tabs	ImmS: 2 tabs
MC: 4caps	MC: 2 caps

*For Adv.GlycoN see page 10. Product definitions are in Appendix A on page 381.

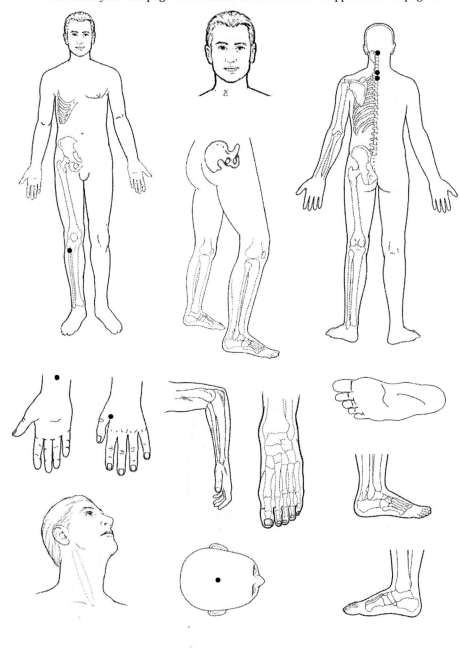

Mercury Detoxification

Daily Nutritional Crisis Program	Daily Nutritional Wellness Program
GlycoN*: 8 ¼ tsp & GlycoAO: 4 caps PhytoN: 1 tsp PreH: 3 tabs Cata: 6 tabs Clean: 3 caps twice a day (2 weeks) ImmS: 4 tabs	GlycoN*: 3 ½ tsp & GlycoAO: 3 caps PhytoN: 1/4 tsp PreH: 3 tabs Cata: 6 tabs Clean: 1 cap ImmS: 2 tabs

*For Adv.GlycoN see page 10. Product definitions are in Appendix A on page 381.

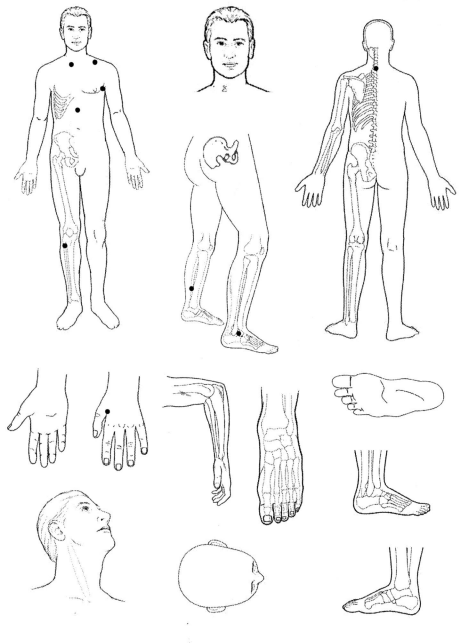

Metastatic Carcinoma

Daily Nutritional Crisis Program	Daily Nutritional Wellness Program
GlycoN*: 10 ¾ tsp & GlycoAO: 6 caps PhytoN: 4 tsp PreH: 6 tabs Cata: 6 tabs ImmS: 6 tabs MC: 6 caps	GlycoN*: 2 ½ tsp & GlycoAO: 3 caps PhytoN: 2 tsp PreH: 4 tabs Cata: 6 tabs ImmS: 3 tabs MC: 3 caps

*For Adv.GlycoN see page 10. Product definitions are in Appendix A on page 381.

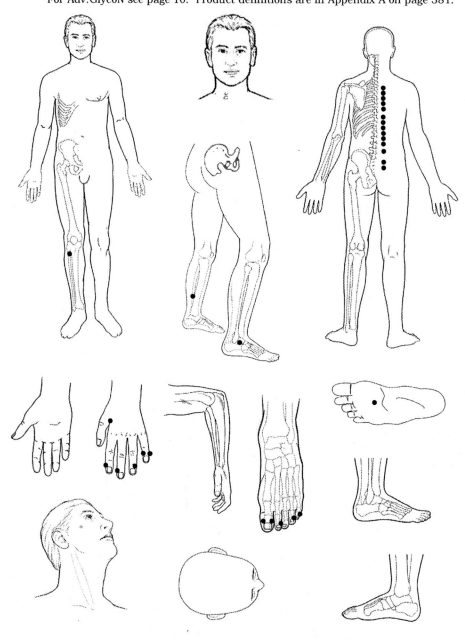

Migraine

Daily Nutritional Crisis Program	Daily Nutritional Wellness Program
GlycoN*: 8 tsp & GlycoAO: 5 caps PhytoN: 1/2 tsp PreH: 6 tabs GEssentials: 4 tabs SP: 4 caps ImmS: 4 tabs	GlycoN*: 1 tsp & GlycoAO: 2 caps PhytoN: 1/4 tsp PreH: 4 tabs GEssentials: 2 tabs SP: 2 caps ImmS: 2 tabs

*For Adv.GlycoN see page 10. Product definitions are in Appendix A on page 381.

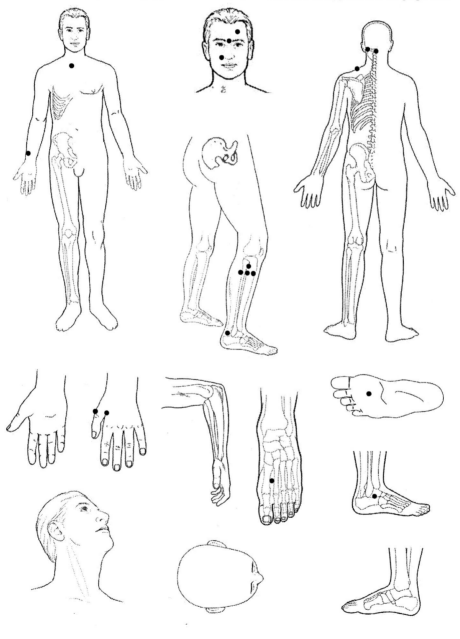

Mononucleosis

Daily Nutritional Crisis Program	Daily Nutritional Wellness Program
GlycoN*: 4 ½ tsp & GlycoAO: 3 caps PhytoN: 1 tsp PreH: 3 tabs GEssentials: 4 tabs MC: 3 caps	GlycoN*: 1 ½ tsp & GlycoAO: 3 caps PhytoN: 1 tsp PreH: 3 tabs GEssentials: 4 tabs MC: 2 caps

*For Adv.GlycoN see page 10. Product definitions are in Appendix A on page 381.

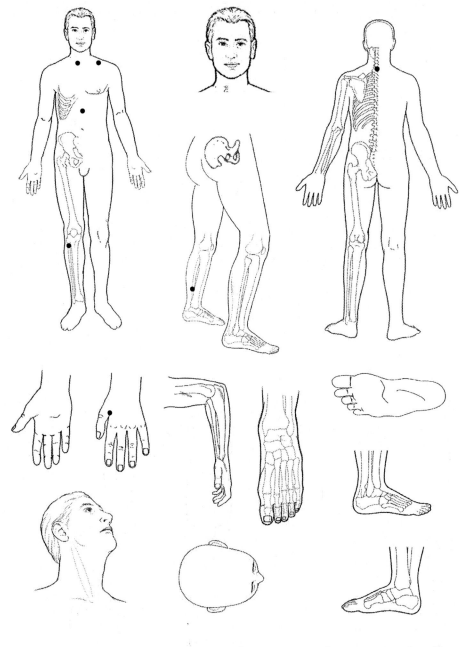

Mouth Sores
(apply soft laser to affect areas)

Daily Nutritional Crisis Program	Daily Nutritional Wellness Program
GlycoN*: 2 ½ tsp & GlycoAO: 3 caps PhytoN: 1/2 tsp PreH: 4 tabs GEssentials: 4 tabs ImmS: 5 tabs MC: 4 caps	GlycoN*: ½ tsp & GlycoAO: 2 caps PhytoN: 1/4 tsp PreH: 3 tabs GEssentials: 4 tabs ImmS: 3 tabs MC: 2 caps

*For Adv.GlycoN see page 10. Product definitions are in Appendix A on page 381.

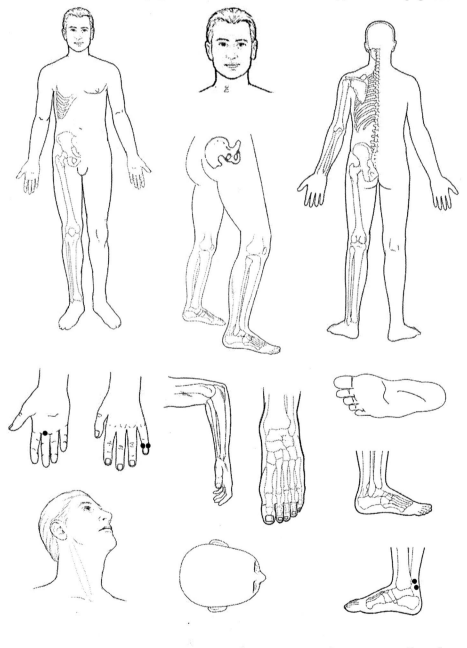

Multiple Myeloma

Daily Nutritional Crisis Program	Daily Nutritional Wellness Program
GlycoN*: 10 ¾ tsp & GlycoAO: 6 caps	GlycoN*: 2 ½ tsp & GlycoAO: 3 caps
PhytoN: 4 tsp	PhytoN: 2 tsp
PreH: 6 tabs	PreH: 4 tabs
Cata: 6 tabs	Cata: 6 tabs
ImmS: 6 tabs	ImmS: 3 tabs
MC: 6 caps	MC: 3 caps

*For Adv.GlycoN see page 10. Product definitions are in Appendix A on page 381.

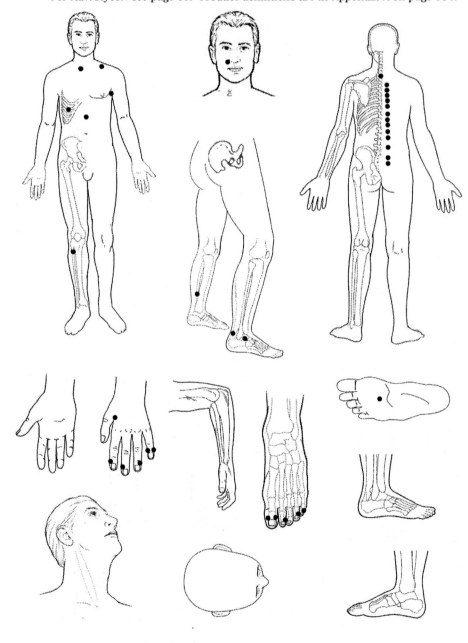

Multiple Sclerosis (MS)

Daily Nutritional Crisis Program	Daily Nutritional Wellness Program
GlycoN*: 10 ¾ tsp & GlycoAO: 6 caps	GlycoN*: 5 ¼ tsp & GlycoAO: 4 caps
PhytoN: 3 tsp	PhytoN: 1 tsp
PreH: 6 tabs	PreH: 4 tabs
Cata: 6 tabs	Cata: 6 tabs
MC: 4 caps	MC: 3 caps
ImmS: 4 tabs	ImmS: 3 tabs

*For Adv.GlycoN see page 10. Product definitions are in Appendix A on page 381.

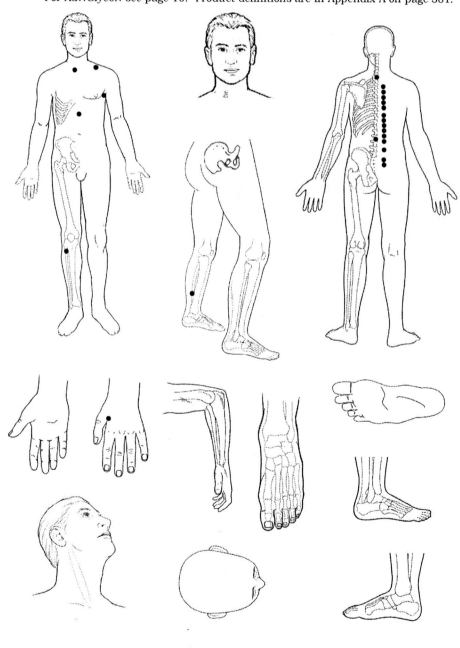

279

Mumps

Daily Nutritional Crisis Program	Daily Nutritional Wellness Program
GlycoN*: 4 ½ tsp & GlycoAO: 3 caps PhytoN: 1 tsp PreH: 3 tabs GEssentials: 4 tabs MC: 3 caps	GlycoN*: 1 ½ tsp & GlycoAO: 3 caps PhytoN: 1 tsp PreH: 3 tabs GEssentials: 4 tabs MC: 2 caps

*For Adv.GlycoN see page 10. Product definitions are in Appendix A on page 381.

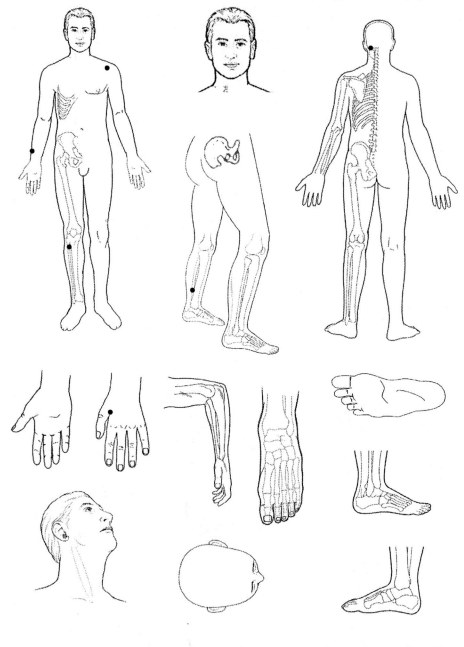

Myasthenia Gravis

Daily Nutritional Crisis Program	Daily Nutritional Wellness Program
GlycoN*: 8 tsp & GlycoAO: 5 caps	GlycoN*: 1 ½ tsp & GlycoAO: 3 caps
PhytoN: 1/4 tsp	PhytoN: 1/4 tsp
PreH: 4 tabs	PreH: 3 tabs
Cata: 4 tabs	Cata: 4 tabs
ImmS: 5 tabs	ImmS: 3 tabs
MC: 5 caps	MC: 3 caps
SP: 4 caps	SP: 2 caps

*For Adv.GlycoN see page 10. Product definitions are in Appendix A on page 381.

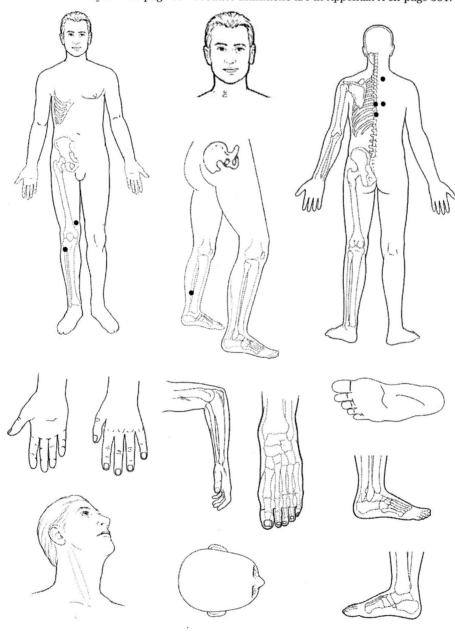

Myocardial Infarction (non-acute)

Daily Nutritional Crisis Program	Daily Nutritional Wellness Program
GlycoN*: 5 ¼ tsp & GlycoAO: 4 caps PhytoN: 1 tsp PreH: 4 tabs Cata: 6 tabs CB: 5 caps	GlycoN*: 1 ½ tsp & GlycoAO: 3 caps PhytoN: 3/4 tsp PreH: 3 tabs Cata: 6 tabs CB: 3 caps

*For Adv.GlycoN see page 10. Product definitions are in Appendix A on page 381.

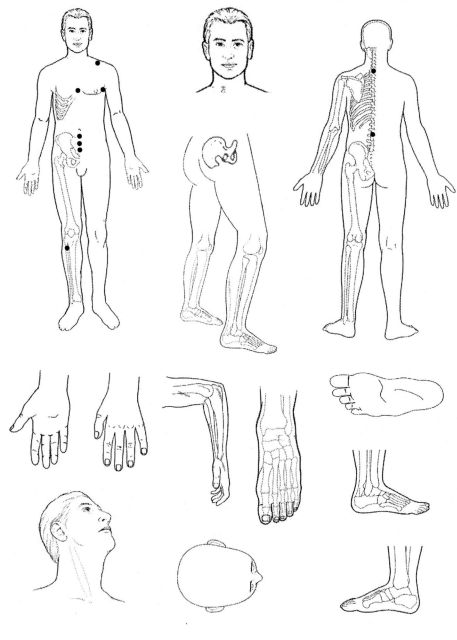

Myocarditis

Daily Nutritional Crisis Program	Daily Nutritional Wellness Program
GlycoN*: 5 ¼ tsp & GlycoAO: 4 caps PhytoN: 1 tsp PreH: 4 tabs Cata: 6 tabs CB: 5 caps	GlycoN*: 1 ½ tsp & GlycoAO: 3 caps PhytoN: 3/4 tsp PreH: 3 tabs Cata: 6 tabs CB: 3 caps

*For Adv.GlycoN see page 10. Product definitions are in Appendix A on page 381.

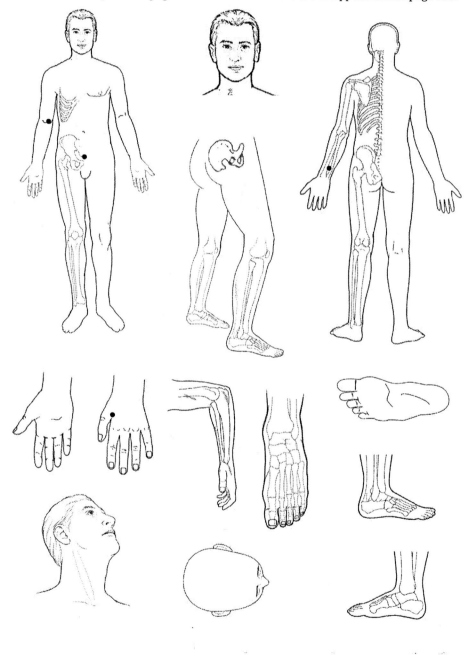

Myopathy

Daily Nutritional Crisis Program	Daily Nutritional Wellness Program
GlycoN*: 5 ¼ tsp & GlycoAO: 4 caps PhytoN: 1 tsp PreH: 4 tabs Cata: 6 tabs CB: 5 caps	GlycoN*: 1 ½ tsp & GlycoAO: 3 caps PhytoN: 3/4 tsp PreH: 3 tabs Cata: 6 tabs CB: 3 caps

*For Adv.GlycoN see page 10. Product definitions are in Appendix A on page 381.

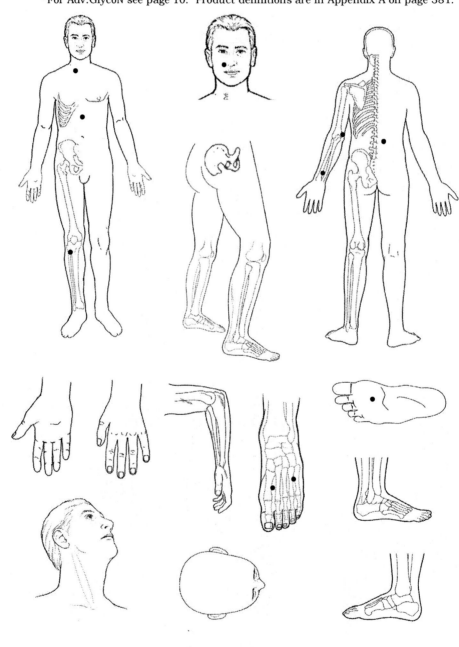

Narcolepsy

Daily Nutritional Crisis Program	Daily Nutritional Wellness Program
GlycoN*: 1 ½ tsp & GlycoAO: 3 caps PhytoN: 1/4 tsp PreH: 4 tabs GEssentials : 4 tabs MC: 4 caps	GlycoN*: ½ tsp & GlycoAO: 2 caps PhytoN: 1/4 tsp PreH: 3 tabs GEssentials : 4 tabs MC: 2 caps

*For Adv.GlycoN see page 10. Product definitions are in Appendix A on page 381.

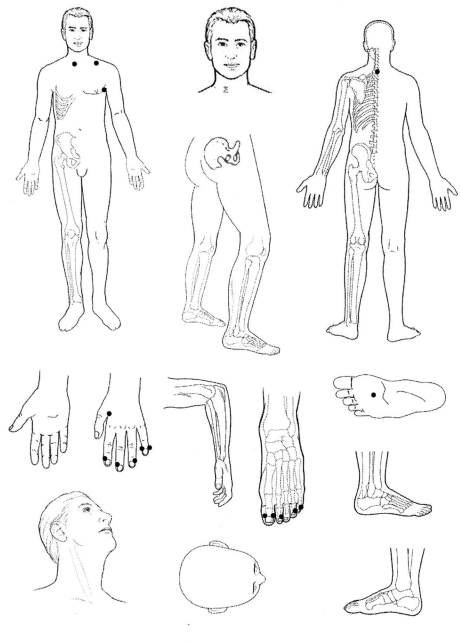

Nasal Polyp

Daily Nutritional Crisis Program	Daily Nutritional Wellness Program
GlycoN*: 2 ½ tsp & GlycoAO: 3 caps PhytoN: 1/2 tsp PreH: 3 tabs GEssentials: 4 tabs ImmS: 5 tabs MC: 3 caps	GlycoN*: ½ tsp & GlycoAO: 2 caps PhytoN: 1/4 tsp PreH: 3 tabs GEssentials: 4 tabs ImmS: 2 tabs MC: 2 caps

*For Adv.GlycoN see page 10. Product definitions are in Appendix A on page 381.

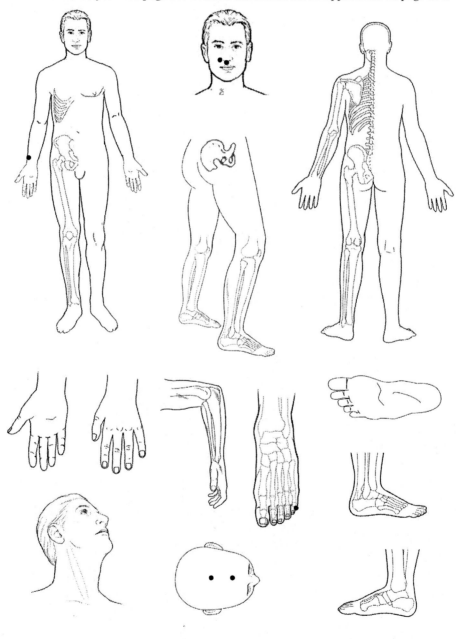

Nausea

Daily Nutritional Crisis Program	Daily Nutritional Wellness Program
GlycoN*: 2 ½ tsp & GlycoAO: 3 caps PhytoN: 1/2 tsp PreH: 3 tabs GEssentials: 4 tabs ImmS: 3 tabs MC: 3 caps	GlycoN*: ½ tsp & GlycoAO: 2 caps PhytoN: 1/2 tsp PreH: 3 tabs GEssentials: 4 tabs ImmS: 2 tabs MC: 3 caps

*For Adv.GlycoN see page 10. Product definitions are in Appendix A on page 381.

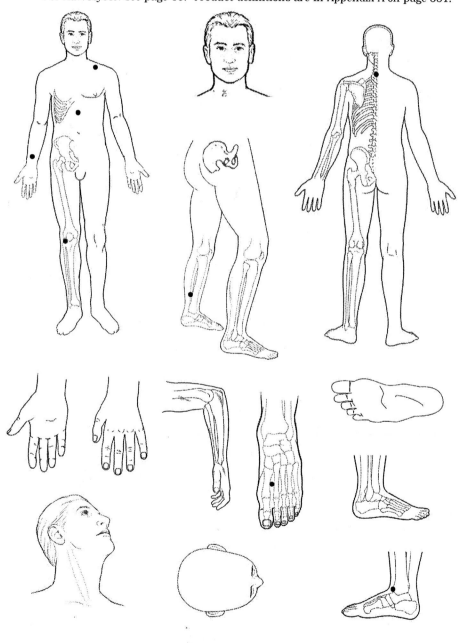

Nephritis

Daily Nutritional Crisis Program	Daily Nutritional Wellness Program
GlycoN*: 10 ¾ tsp & GlycoAO: 6 caps PhytoN: 1 tsp PreH: 6 tabs Cata: 6 tabs ImmS: 6 tabs MC: 6 caps SP: 4 caps	GlycoN*: 3 ½ tsp & GlycoAO: 3 caps PhytoN: 1/2 tsp PreH: 3 tabs Cata: 4 tabs ImmS: 3 tabs MC: 3 caps SP: 2 caps

*For Adv.GlycoN see page 10. Product definitions are in Appendix A on page 381.

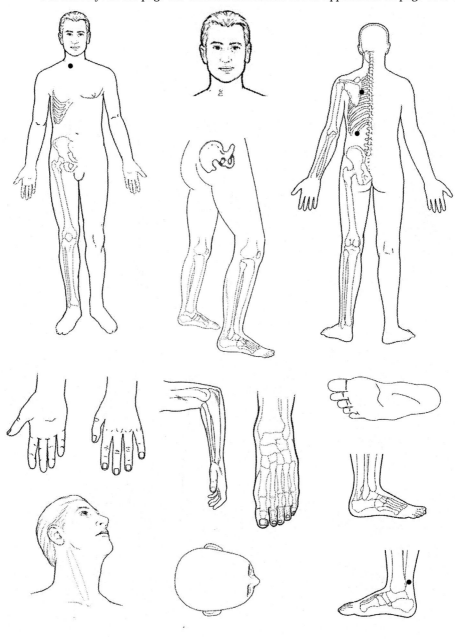

Neuralgia (Post-Herpetic)

Daily Nutritional Crisis Program	Daily Nutritional Wellness Program
GlycoN*: 8 tsp & GlycoAO: 5 caps PhytoN: 1/4 tsp PreH: 6 tabs Cata: 6 tabs ImmS: 5 tabs MC: 4 caps SP: 4 caps	Glyco: 1 tsp & GlycoAO: 3 caps PhytoN: 1/2 tsp PreH: 3 tabs Cata: 4 tabs ImmS: 3 tabs MC: 3 caps SP: 3 caps

*For Adv.GlycoN see page 10. Product definitions are in Appendix A on page 381.

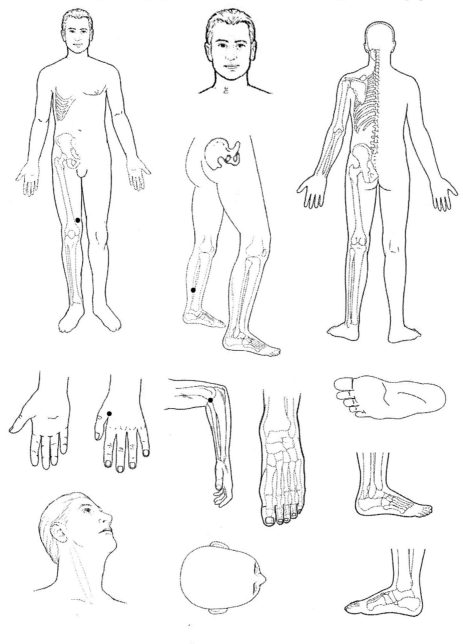

Neurogenic Bladder

Daily Nutritional Crisis Program	Daily Nutritional Wellness Program
GlycoN*: 2 ½ tsp & GlycoAO: 3 caps PhytoN: 1/2 tsp PreH: 3 tabs GEssentials: 4 tabs ImmS: 6 tabs MC: 4 caps	GlycoN*: ½ tsp & GlycoAO: 2 caps PhytoN: 1/4 tsp PreH: 3 tabs GEssentials: 4 tabs ImmS: 4 tabs MC: 2 caps

*For Adv.GlycoN see page 10. Product definitions are in Appendix A on page 381.

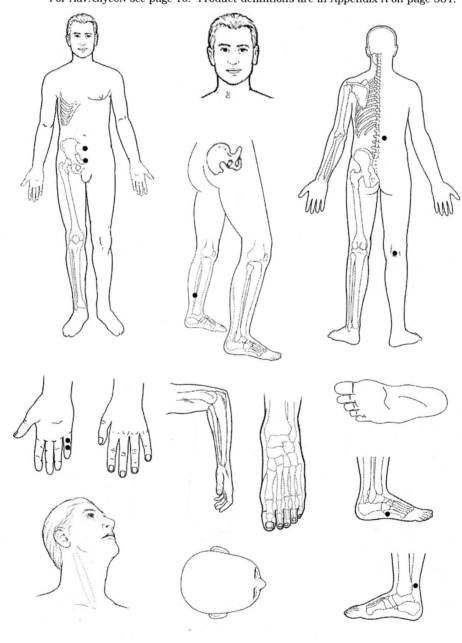

Neuromuscular Disorders

Daily Nutritional Crisis Program	Daily Nutritional Wellness Program
GlycoN*: 8 tsp & GlycoAO: 5 caps	GlycoN*: 1 ½ tsp & GlycoAO: 3 caps
PhytoN: 1/4 tsp	PhytoN: 1/4 tsp
PreH: 4 tabs	PreH: 3 tabs
Cata: 4 tabs	Cata: 4 tabs
ImmS: 5 tabs	ImmS: 3 tabs
MC: 5 caps	MC: 3 caps
SP: 4 caps	SP: 2 caps

*For Adv.GlycoN see page 10. Product definitions are in Appendix A on page 381.

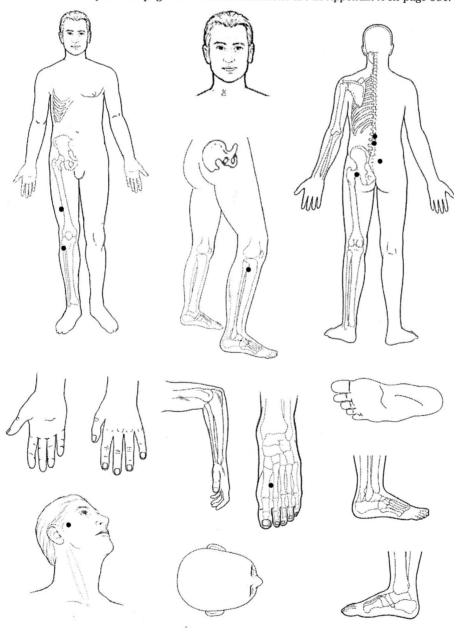

Night Sweats

Daily Nutritional Crisis Program	Daily Nutritional Wellness Program
GlycoN*: 5 tsp & GlycoAO: 4 caps	GlycoN*: 1 ½ tsp & GlycoAO: 3 caps
PhytoN: 1/2 tsp	PhytoN: 1/4 tsp
PreH: 6 tabs	PreH: 3 tabs
Cata: 4 tabs	Cata: 4 tabs
SP: 4 caps	SP: 4 caps
CB: 4 caps	CB: 3 caps

*For Adv.GlycoN see page 10. Product definitions are in Appendix A on page 381.

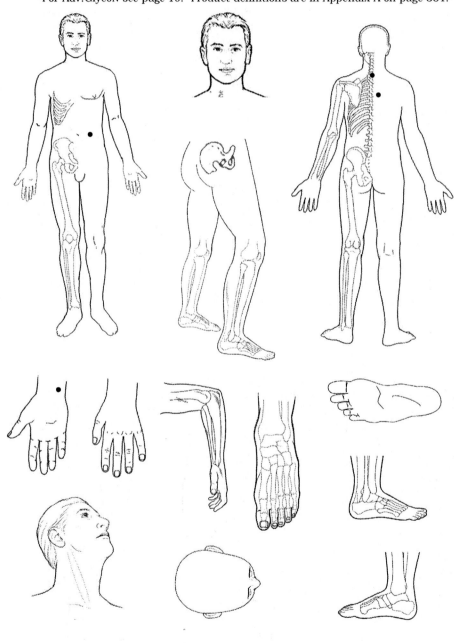

Obesity

Daily Nutritional Crisis Program	Daily Nutritional Wellness Program
GlycoN*:2 ½ tsp & GlycoAO: 3 caps PhytoN: 1/4 tsp PreH: 6 tabs GEssentials: 6 tabs ImmS: 4 tabs MC: 4 caps Clean: 3 caps twice a day (2 weeks)	GlycoN*:½ tsp & GlycoAO: 2 caps PhytoN: 1/4 tsp PreH: 4 tabs GEssentials: 4 tabs ImmS: 2 tabs MC: 2 caps Clean: 2 caps

*For Adv.GlycoN*see page 10. Product definitions are in Appendix A on page 381.

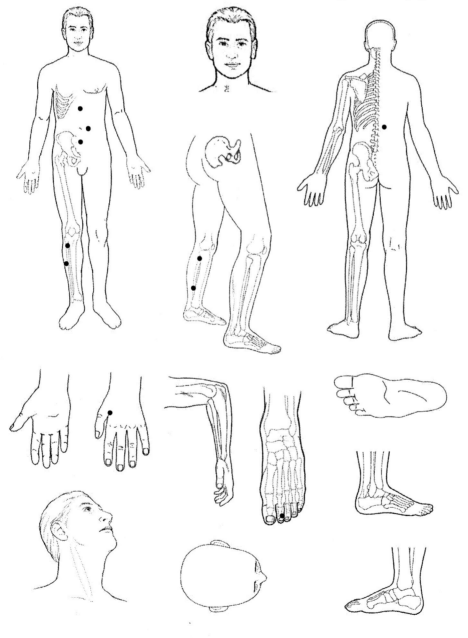

Optic Neuritis

Daily Nutritional Crisis Program	Daily Nutritional Wellness Program
GlycoN*:8 tsp & GlycoAO: 5 caps	GlycoN*:1 ½ tsp & GlycoAO: 3 caps
PhytoN: 1 tsp	PhytoN: 1/4 tsp
PreH: 4 tabs	PreH: 3 tabs
Cata: 6 tabs	Cata: 4 tabs
ImmS: 5 tabs	ImmS: 3 tabs
MC: 5 caps	MC: 3 caps

*For Adv.GlycoN*see page 10. Product definitions are in Appendix A on page 381.

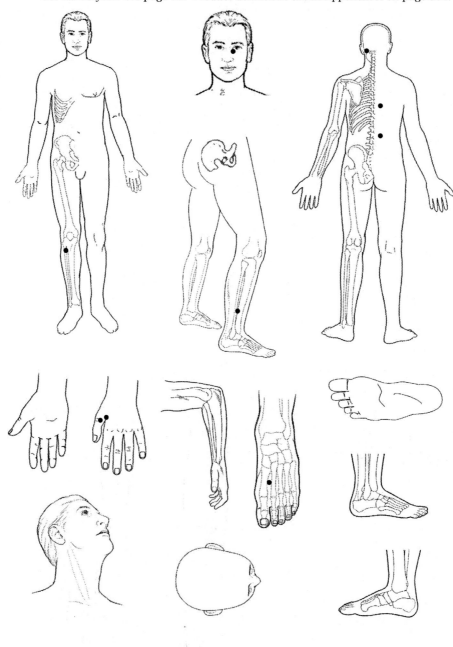

294

Osteoarthritis

Daily Nutritional Crisis Program	Daily Nutritional Wellness Program
GlycoN*:5 ¼ tsp & GlycoAO: 4 caps PhytoN: 1 tsp PreH: 6 tabs Cata: 6 tabs Clean: 3 caps twice a day (2 weeks) MC: 4 caps	GlycoN*:1 ½ tsp & GlycoAO: 3 caps PhytoN: 3/4 tsp PreH: 4 tabs Cata: 6 tabs Clean: 1 cap MC: 2 caps

*For Adv.GlycoN*see page 10. Product definitions are in Appendix A on page 381.

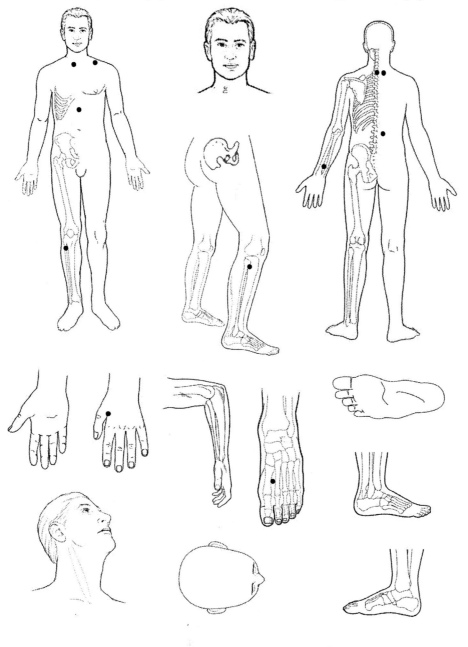

295

Osteomyelitis

Daily Nutritional Crisis Program	Daily Nutritional Wellness Program
GlycoN*:10 ¾ tsp & GlycoAO: 6 caps	GlycoN*:3 ½ tsp & GlycoAO: 3 caps
PhytoN: 1 tsp	PhytoN: 1/2 tsp
PreH: 6 tabs	PreH: 3 tabs
Cata: 6 tabs	Cata: 4 tabs
ImmS: 6 tabs	ImmS: 3 tabs
MC: 6 caps	MC: 3 caps
SP: 4 caps	SP: 2 caps

*For Adv.GlycoN*see page 10. Product definitions are in Appendix A on page 381.

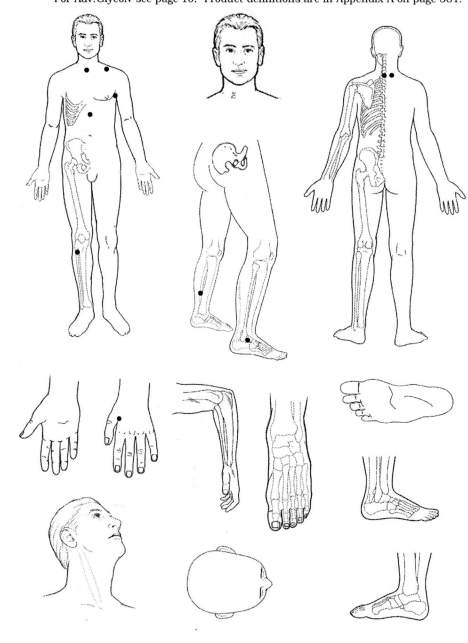

Osteoporosis

Daily Nutritional Crisis Program	Daily Nutritional Wellness Program
GlycoN*:2 ½ tsp & GlycoAO: 3 caps	GlycoN*:½ tsp & GlycoAO: 2 caps G
PhytoN: 1/4 tsp	PhytoN: 1/4 tsp
PreH: 6 tabs	PreH: 4 tabs
Cata: 4 tabs	Cata: 4 tabs
MC: 4 caps	MC: 3 caps
GstroZ: 2 caps before meals	GstroZ: 1 caps before meals

*For Adv.GlycoN*see page 10. Product definitions are in Appendix A on page 381.

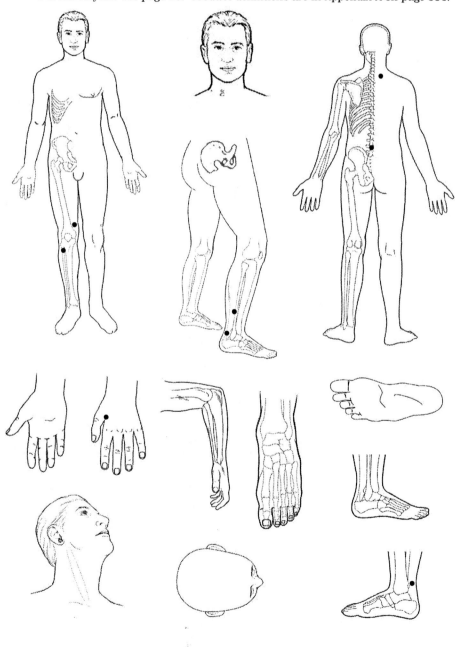

Otitis Media

Daily Nutritional Crisis Program	Daily Nutritional Wellness Program
GlycoN*:2 tsp & GlycoAO: 3 caps	GlycoN*:½ tsp & GlycoAO: 2 caps
PhytoN: 3/4 tsp	PhytoN: 1/4 tsp
PreH: 3 tabs	PreH: 3 tabs
GEssentials: 4 tabs	GEssentials: 4 tabs
ImmS: 6 tabs	ImmS: 3 tabs
MC: 5 caps	MC: 3 caps

*For Adv.GlycoN*see page 10. Product definitions are in Appendix A on page 381.

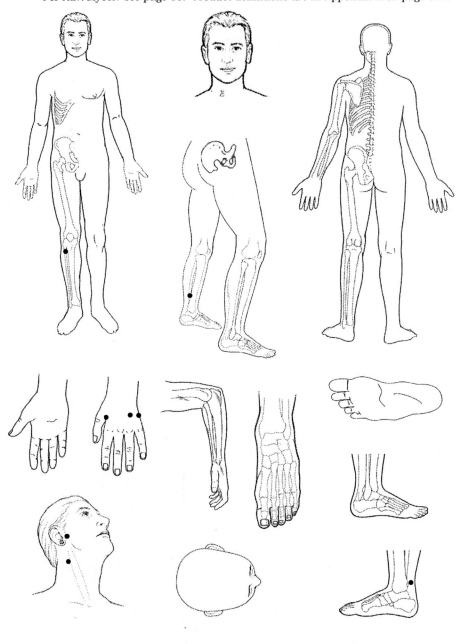

Ovaries (Infection)

Daily Nutritional Crisis Program	Daily Nutritional Wellness Program
GlycoN*:5 ¼ tsp & GlycoAO: 4 caps	GlycoN*:1 ½ tsp & GlycoAO: 3 caps
PhytoN: 1 tsp	PhytoN: 3/4 tsp
PreH: 4 tabs	PreH: 3 tabs
GEssentials: 4 tabs	GEssentials: 4 tabs
ImmS: 6 tabs	ImmS: 3 tabs
MC: 4 caps	MC: 3 caps

*For Adv.GlycoN*see page 10. Product definitions are in Appendix A on page 381.

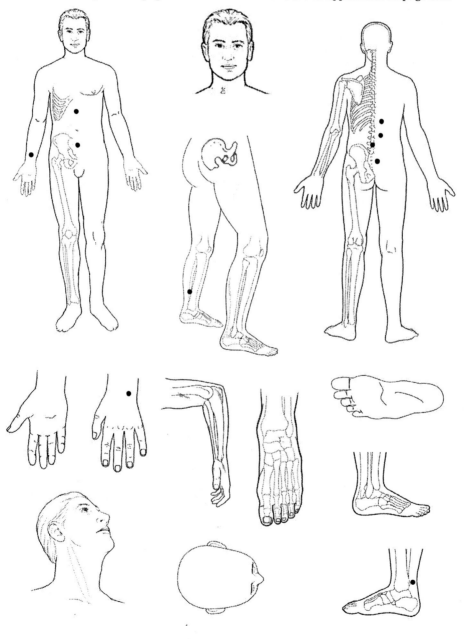

Pain (Generalized)

Daily Nutritional Crisis Program	Daily Nutritional Wellness Program
GlycoN*:5 ¼ tsp & GlycoAO: 4 caps	GlycoN*:1 ½ tsp & GlycoAO: 2 caps
PhytoN: 1/4 tsp	Phyto: 1/2 tsp
PreH: 6 tabs	PreH: 4 tabs
Cata: 4 tabs	Cata: 4 tabs
SP: 3 caps	SP: 2 caps
MC: 3 caps	MC: 2 caps

*For Adv.GlycoN*see page 10. Product definitions are in Appendix A on page 381.

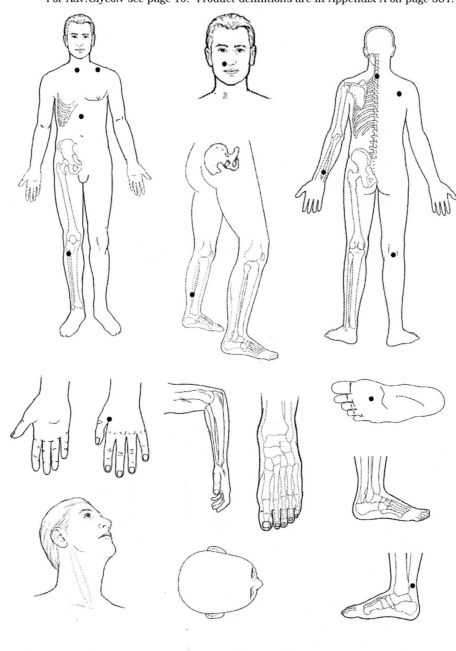

Pain (pleuritic)

Daily Nutritional Crisis Program	Daily Nutritional Wellness Program
GlycoN*:5 ¼ tsp & GlycoAO: 4 caps PhytoN: 1/4 tsp PreH: 6 tabs Cata: 4 tabs SP: 3 caps MC: 3 caps	GlycoN*:1½ tsp & GlycoAO: 2 caps Phyto: 1/2 tsp PreH: 4 tabs Cata: 4 tabs SP: 2 caps MC: 2 caps

*For Adv.GlycoN*see page 10. Product definitions are in Appendix A on page 381.

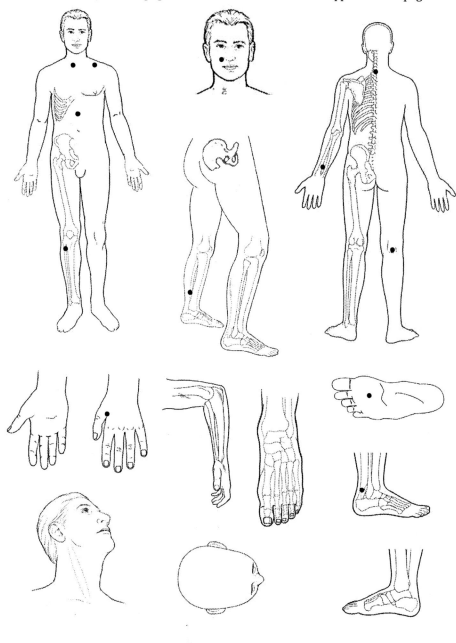

Palpitations

Daily Nutritional Crisis Program	Daily Nutritional Wellness Program
GlycoN*:5 ¼ tsp & GlycoAO: 4 caps PhytoN: 1 tsp PreH: 4 tabs Cata: 6 tabs CB: 5 caps	GlycoN*:1 ½ tsp & GlycoAO: 3 caps PhytoN: 3/4 tsp PreH: 3 tabs Cata: 6 tabs CB: 3 caps

*For Adv.GlycoN*see page 10. Product definitions are in Appendix A on page 381.

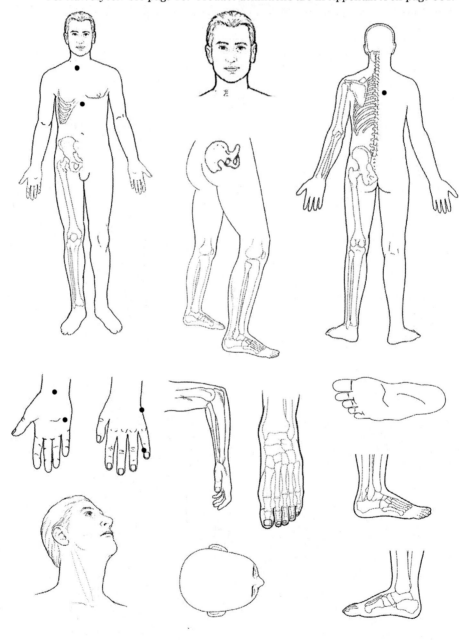

Pancreatitis (Chronic)

Daily Nutritional Crisis Program	Daily Nutritional Wellness Program
GlycoN*:5 ¼ tsp & GlycoAO: 4 caps PhytoN: 1/4 tsp PreH: 3 tabs Cata: 4 tabs ImmS: 4 tabs MC: 4 caps	GlycoN*:1 ½ tsp & GlycoAO: 3 caps PhytoN: 1/4 tsp PreH: 3 tabs Cata: 4 tabs ImmS: 2 tabs MC: 2 caps

*For Adv.GlycoN*see page 10. Product definitions are in Appendix A on page 381.

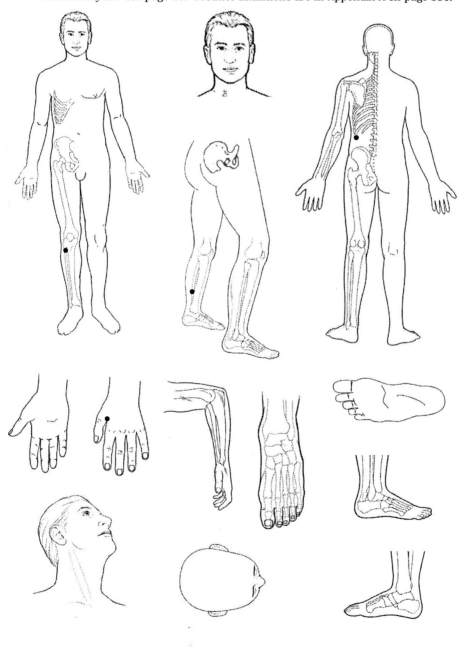

Panic Disorder

Daily Nutritional Crisis Program	Daily Nutritional Wellness Program
GlycoN*:2 ½ tsp & GlycoAO: 3 caps PhytoN: 1 tsp PreH: 6 tabs GEssentials: 4 tabs SP: 4 caps	GlycoN*:½ tsp & GlycoAO: 2 caps PhytoN: 1/4 tsp PreH: 3 tabs GEssentials: 4 tabs SP: 2 caps

*For Adv.GlycoN*see page 10. Product definitions are in Appendix A on page 381.

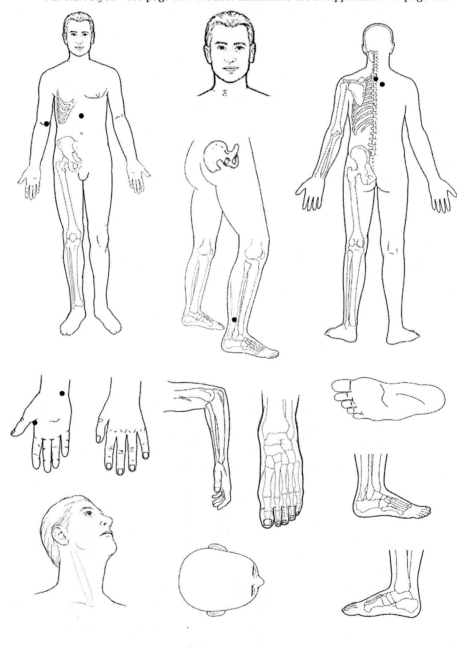

Paraplegia

(stimulate listed spinal points 2 vertebrae above and below injury)

Daily Nutritional Crisis Program	Daily Nutritional Wellness Program
GlycoN*:8 tsp & GlycoAO: 5 caps G PhytoN: 1 tsp PreH: 6 tabs Cata: 6 tabs ImmS: 4 tabs MC: 4 caps SP: 5 caps	GlycoN*:1 ½ tsp & GlycoAO: 3 caps PhytoN: 1/4 tsp PreH: 3 tabs Cata: 4 tabs ImmS: 2 tabs MC: 2 caps SP: 3 caps

*For Adv.GlycoN*see page 10. Product definitions are in Appendix A on page 381.

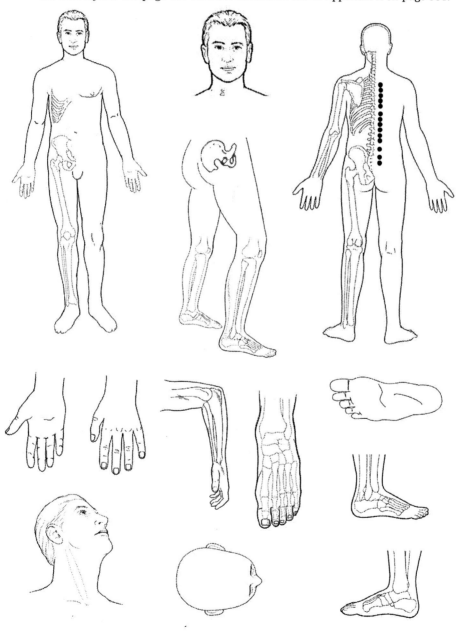

305

Parkinson's Disease

Daily Nutritional Crisis Program	Daily Nutritional Wellness Program
GlycoN*:3 ½ tsp & GlycoAO: 3 caps PhytoN: 1/2 tsp PreH: 6 tabs Cata: 4 tabs SP: 5 caps ImmS: 5 tabs MC: 5 caps	GlycoN*:2 ½ tsp & GlycoAO: 3 caps PhytoN: 1/4 tsp PreH: 3 tabs Cata: 4 tabs SP: 3 tabs ImmS: 3 tabs MC: 3 caps

*For Adv.GlycoN*see page 10. Product definitions are in Appendix A on page 381.

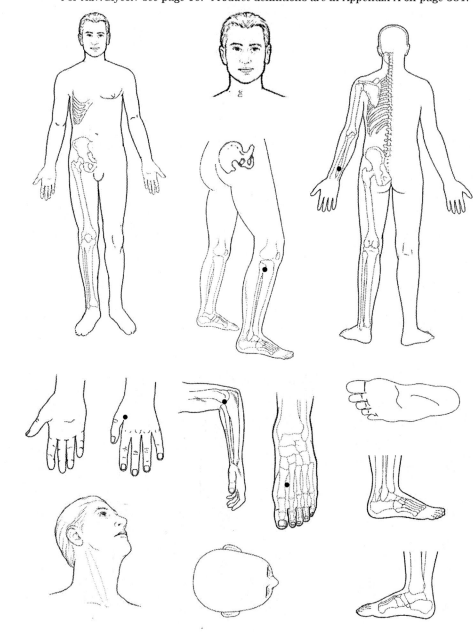

Pelvic Inflammatory Disease (PID)

Daily Nutritional Crisis Program	Daily Nutritional Wellness Program
GlycoN*:2 ½ tsp & GlycoAO: 3 caps PhytoN: 1/4 tsp PreH: 4 tabs Cata: 4 tabs ImmS: 4 tabs MC: 4 caps	GlycoN*:½ tsp & GlycoAO: 2 caps PhytoN: 1/4 tsp PreH: 3 tabs Cata: 4 tabs ImmS: 3 tabs MC: 3 caps

*For Adv.GlycoN*see page 10. Product definitions are in Appendix A on page 381.

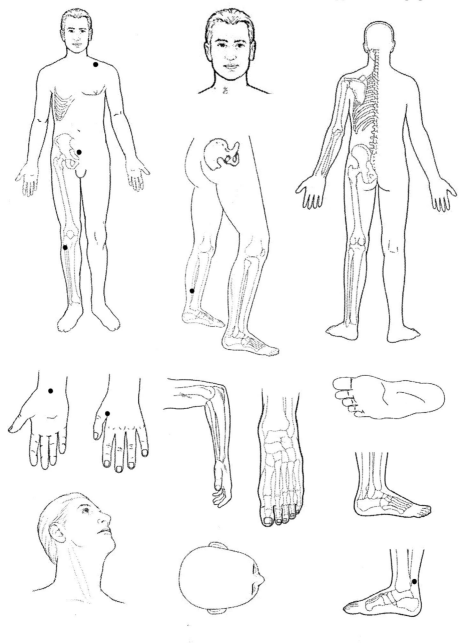

307

Peptic Ulcers

Daily Nutritional Crisis Program	Daily Nutritional Wellness Program
GlycoN*:1 ½ tsp & GlycoAO: 3 caps G	GlycoN*:½ tsp & GlycoAO: 2 caps
PhytoN: 1/2 tsp	PhytoN: 1/4 tsp
PreH: 3 tabs	PreH: 3 tabs
GEssentials: 4 tabs	GEssentials: 4 tabs
Clean: 3 caps twice a day (2 weeks)	Clean: 2 caps

*For Adv.GlycoN*see page 10.   Product definitions are in Appendix A on page 381.

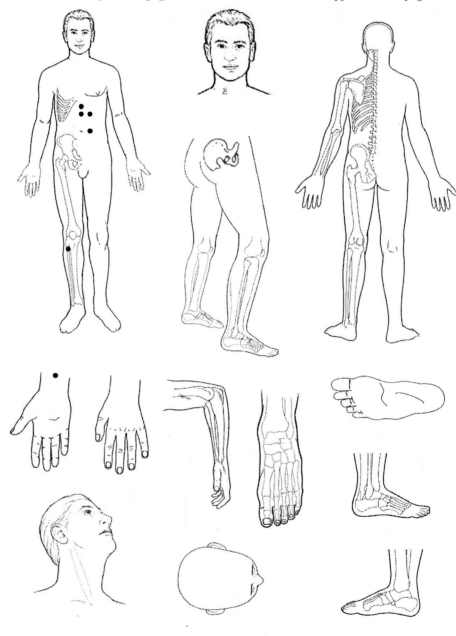

Peripheral Vascular Disease

Daily Nutritional Crisis Program	Daily Nutritional Wellness Program
GlycoN*:5 ¼ tsp & GlycoAO: 4 caps PhytoN: 1 ½ tsp PreH: 6 tabs Cata:6 tabs MC: 6 caps CB: 6 caps	GlycoN*:1 ½ tsp & GlycoAO: 3 caps PhytoN: 3/4 tsp PreH: 3 tabs Cata:4 tabs MC: 3 caps CB: 4 caps

*For Adv.GlycoN*see page 10. Product definitions are in Appendix A on page 381.

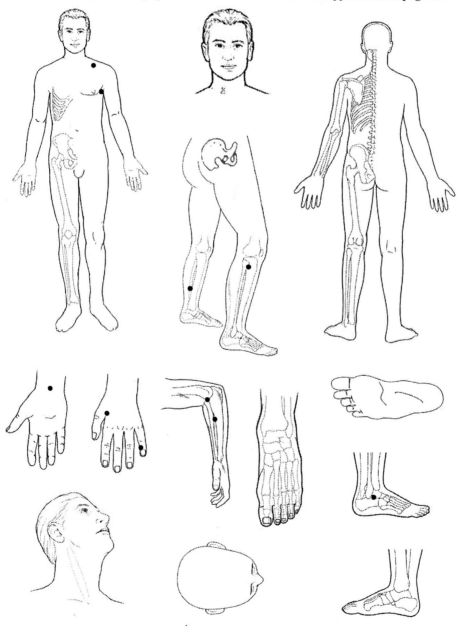

Pharyngitis (Sore Throat)

Daily Nutritional Crisis Program	Daily Nutritional Wellness Program
GlycoN*:2 tsp & GlycoAO: 3 caps	GlycoN*:½ tsp & GlycoAO: 2 caps
PhytoN: 3/4 tsp	PhytoN: 1/2 tsp
PreH: 3 tabs	PreH: 3 tabs
GEssentials: 4 tabs	GEssentials: 4 tabs
ImmS: 5 tabs	ImmS: 3 tabs
MC: 6 caps	MC: 3 caps

*For Adv.GlycoN*see page 10. Product definitions are in Appendix A on page 381.

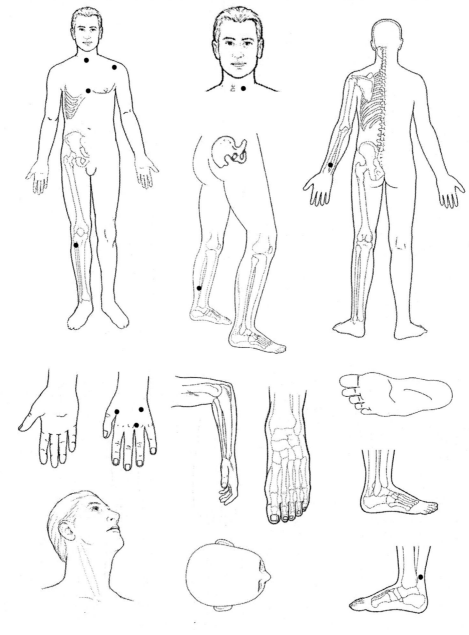

Pinkeye

Daily Nutritional Crisis Program	Daily Nutritional Wellness Program
GlycoN*:1 ½ tsp & GlycoAO: 3 caps PhytoN: 1/2 tsp PreH: 3 tabs GEssentials: 4 tabs ImmS: 6 tabs MC: 6 caps	GlycoN*:½ tsp & GlycoAO: 2 caps PhytoN: 1/4 tsp PreH: 3 tabs GEssentials: 4 tabs ImmS: 3 tabs MC: 3 caps

*For Adv.GlycoN*see page 10. Product definitions are in Appendix A on page 381.

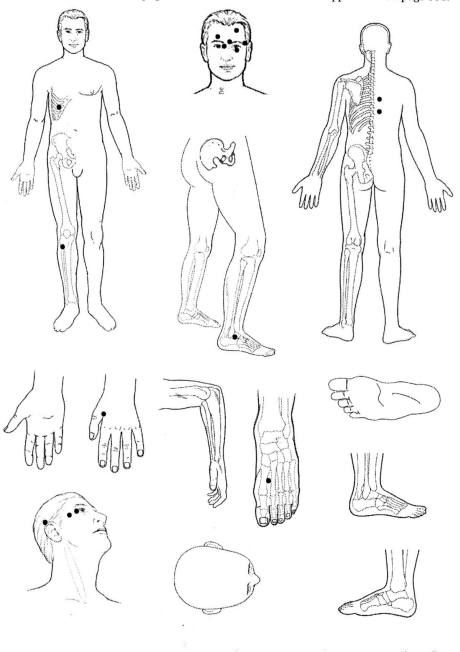

Pleurisy

Daily Nutritional Crisis Program	Daily Nutritional Wellness Program
GlycoN*:2 ½ tsp & GlycoAO: 3 caps	GlycoN*:1/2 tsp & GlycoAO: 2 caps
PhytoN: 1/4 tsp	Phyto: 1/2 tsp
PreH: 4 tabs	PreH: 3 tabs
GEssentials: 4 tabs	GEssentials: 4 tabs
ImmS: 4 tabs	ImmS: 3 tabs
MC: 4 caps	MC: 3 caps

*For Adv.GlycoN*see page 10. Product definitions are in Appendix A on page 381.

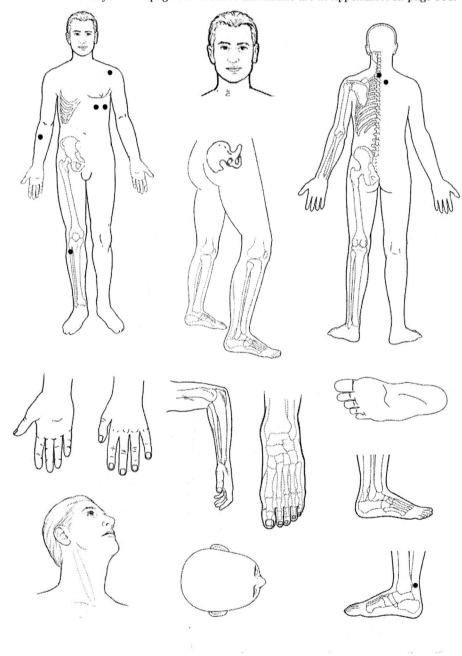

Pneumonia

Daily Nutritional Crisis Program	Daily Nutritional Wellness Program
GlycoN*:2 ½ tsp & GlycoAO: 3 caps PhytoN: 2 tsp PreH: 4 tabs Cata: 4 tabs ImmS: 6 tabs MC: 6 caps	GlycoN*:1 ½ tsp & GlycoAO: 3 caps PhytoN: 1 tsp PreH: 3 tabs Cata: 4 tabs ImmS: 4 tabs MC: 3 caps

*For Adv.GlycoN*see page 10. Product definitions are in Appendix A on page 381.

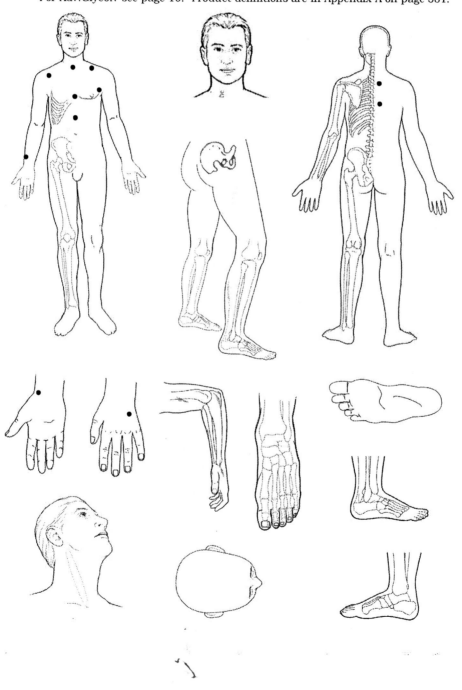

Polio

Daily Nutritional Crisis Program	Daily Nutritional Wellness Program
GlycoN*:8 tsp & GlycoAO: 5 caps PhytoN: 1 tsp PreH: 6 tabs Cata: 4 tabs SP: 4 caps ImmS: 4 tabs MC: 4 caps	GlycoN*:2 ½ tsp & GlycoAO: 3 caps PhytoN: 1 tsp PreH: 3 tabs Cata: 4 tabs SP: 3 caps ImmS: 3 tabs MC: 3 caps

*For Adv.GlycoN*see page 10. Product definitions are in Appendix A on page 381.

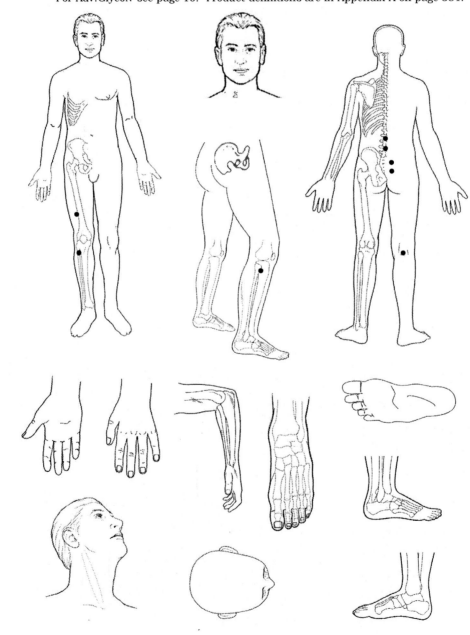

Polymyalgia Rheumatica

Daily Nutritional Crisis Program	Daily Nutritional Wellness Program
GlycoN*:10 ¾ tsp & GlycoAO: 6 caps PhytoN: 1 tsp PreH: 6 tabs Cata: 6 tabs SP: 4 caps ImmS: 5 tabs	GlycoN*:2 ½ tsp & GlycoAO: 3 caps PhytoN: 1 tsp PreH: 4 tabs Cata: 4 tabs SP: 3 caps ImmS: 3 tabs

*For Adv.GlycoN*see page 10. Product definitions are in Appendix A on page 381.

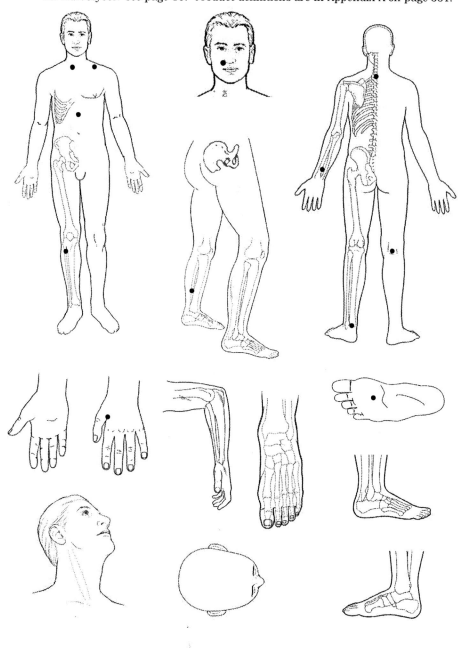

Premenstrual Syndrome (PMS)

Daily Nutritional Crisis Program	Daily Nutritional Wellness Program
GlycoN*:3 tsp & GlycoAO: 4 caps	GlycoN*:1 ½ tsp & GlycoAO: 3 caps
PhytoN: 1 tsp	PhytoN: 1/2 tsp
PreH: 4 tabs	PreH: 3 tabs
GEssentials: 4 tabs	GEssentials: 4 tabs
ImmS: 6 tabs	ImmS: 3 tabs
MC: 4 caps	MC: 3 caps

*For Adv.GlycoN*see page 10. Product definitions are in Appendix A on page 381.

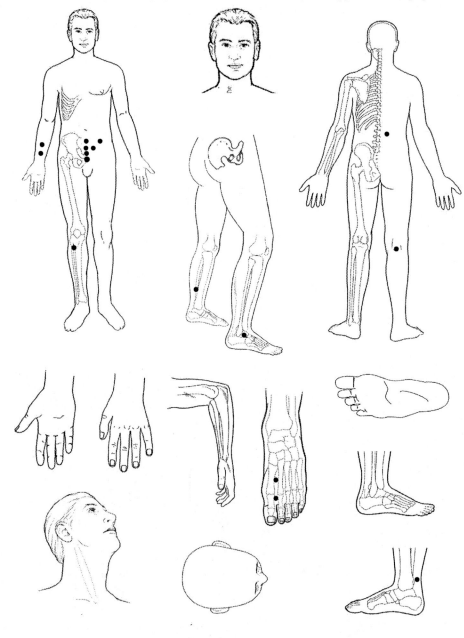

Prostatitis

Daily Nutritional Crisis Program	Daily Nutritional Wellness Program
GlycoN*:2 ½ tsp & GlycoAO: 3 caps	GlycoN*:½ tsp & GlycoAO: 2 caps
PhytoN: 1 tsp	PhytoN: 1/4 tsp
PreH: 4 tabs	PreH: 4 tabs
Cata: 4 tabs	Cata: 4 tabs
ImmS: 5 tabs	ImmS: 3 tabs
MC: 5 caps	MC: 3 caps
Clean: 3 caps twice a day (2 weeks)	Clean: 2 caps

*For Adv.GlycoN*see page 10. Product definitions are in Appendix A on page 381.

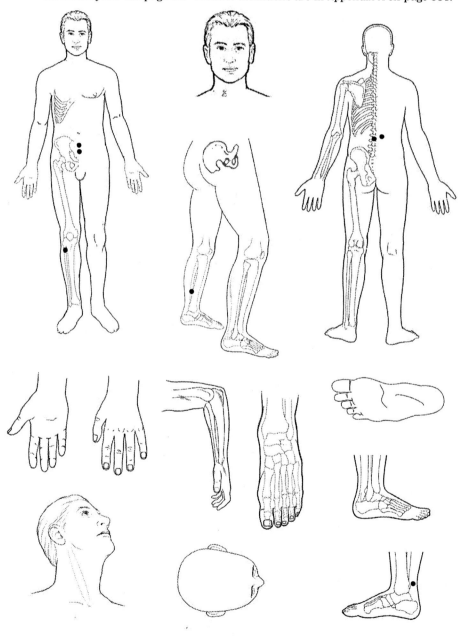

Pruritis

Daily Nutritional Crisis Program	Daily Nutritional Wellness Program
GlycoN*:1 ½ tsp & GlycoAO: 3 caps PhytoN: 1/2 tsp PreH: 6 tabs GEssentials : 4 tabs ImmS: 4 tabs MC: 4 caps SP: 3 caps	GlycoN*:1 ½ tsp & GlycoAO: 3 caps PhytoN: 1/2 tsp PreH: 3 tabs GEssentials : 4 tabs ImmS: 3 tabs MC: 3 caps SP: 2 caps

*For Adv.GlycoN*see page 10. Product definitions are in Appendix A on page 381.

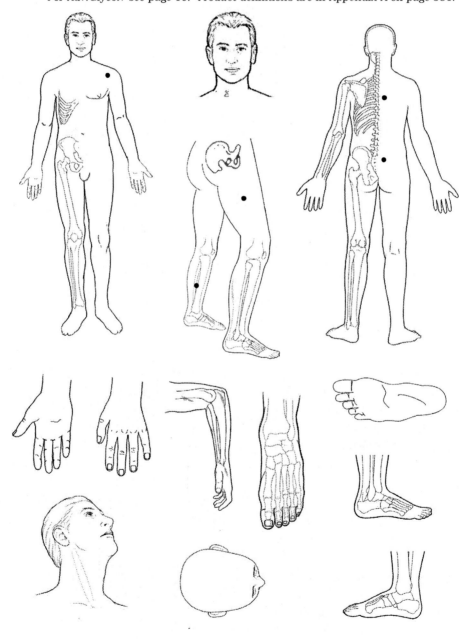

Psoriasis
(soft laser on affected areas)

Daily Nutritional Crisis Program	Daily Nutritional Wellness Program
GlycoN*:1 ½ tsp & GlycoAO: 3 caps PhytoN: 3/4 tsp PreH: 3 tabs GEssentials: 4 tabs Clean: 3 caps twice a day (2 weeks) GstroP: 4 caps	GlycoN*:½ tsp & GlycoAO: 2 caps PhytoN: 1/4 tsp PreH: 3 tabs GEssentials: 4 tabs Clean: 2 caps GstroP: 2 caps

*For Adv.GlycoN*see page 10. Product definitions are in Appendix A on page 381.

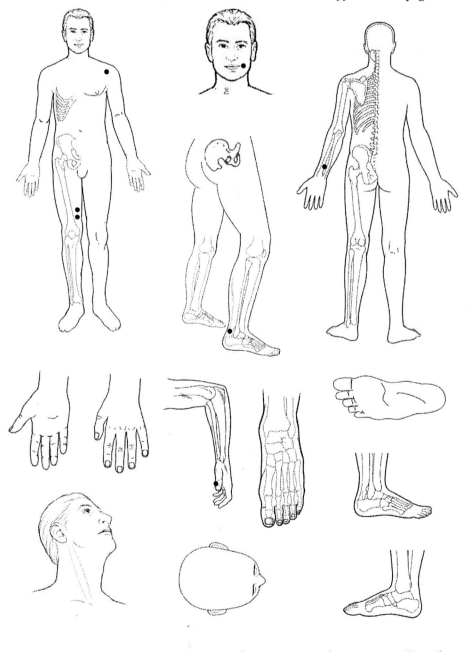

Psoriatic Arthritis

Daily Nutritional Crisis Program	Daily Nutritional Wellness Program
GlycoN*:5 ¼ tsp & GlycoAO: 4 caps PhytoN: 1 tsp PreH: 6 tabs Cata: 6 tabs Clean: 3 caps twice a day (2 weeks) MC: 4 caps	GlycoN*:1 ½ tsp & GlycoAO: 3 caps PhytoN: 3/4 tsp PreH: 4 tabs Cata: 6 tabs Clean: 1 cap MC: 2 caps

*For Adv.GlycoN*see page 10. Product definitions are in Appendix A on page 381.

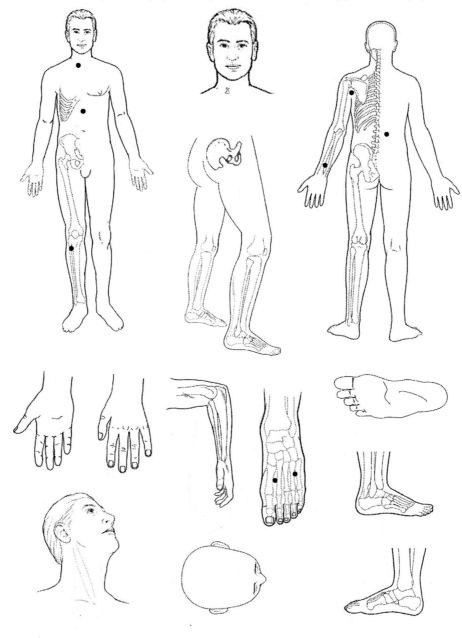

320

Pulmonary Fibrosis

Daily Nutritional Crisis Program	Daily Nutritional Wellness Program
GlycoN*:2 ½ tsp & GlycoAO: 3 caps PhytoN: 1½ tsp PreH: 4 tabs Cata: 4 tabs ImmS: 6 tabs MC: 6 caps	GlycoN*:1 ½ tsp & GlycoAO: 3 caps PhytoN: 3/4 tsp PreH: 3 tabs Cata: 4 tabs ImmS: 4 tabs MC: 3 caps

*For Adv.GlycoN*see page 10. Product definitions are in Appendix A on page 381.

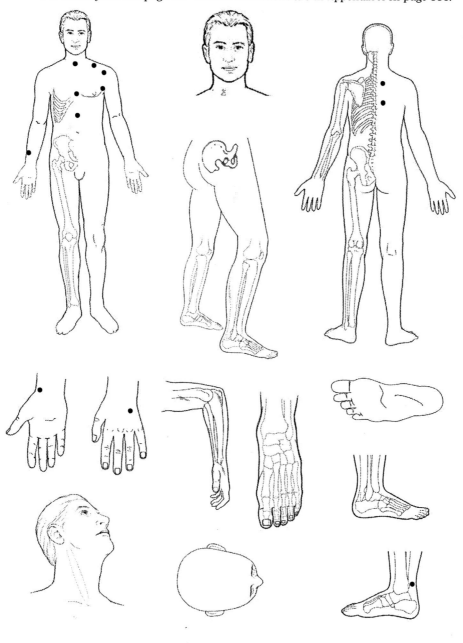

Pulmonary Hypertension

Daily Nutritional Crisis Program	Daily Nutritional Wellness Program
GlycoN*:5 ¼ tsp & GlycoAO: 4 caps PhytoN: 1 tsp PreH: 6 tabs Cata: 4 tabs CB: 4 caps	GlycoN*:1 ½ tsp & GlycoAO: 3 caps PhytoN: 3/4 tsp PreH: 3 tabs Cata: 4 tabs CB: 3 caps

*For Adv.GlycoN*see page 10. Product definitions are in Appendix A on page 381.

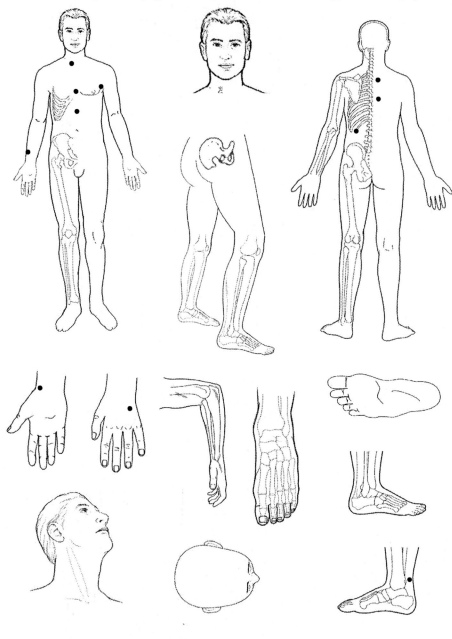

Pyelonephritis

Daily Nutritional Crisis Program	Daily Nutritional Wellness Program
GlycoN*:10 ¾ tsp & GlycoAO: 6 caps	GlycoN*:3 ½ tsp & GlycoAO: 3 caps
PhytoN: 1 tsp	PhytoN: 1/2 tsp
PreH: 6 tabs	PreH: 3 tabs
Cata: 6 tabs	Cata: 4 tabs
ImmS: 6 tabs	ImmS: 3 tabs
MC: 6 caps	MC: 3 caps
SP: 4 caps	SP: 2 caps

*For Adv.GlycoN*see page 10. Product definitions are in Appendix A on page 381.

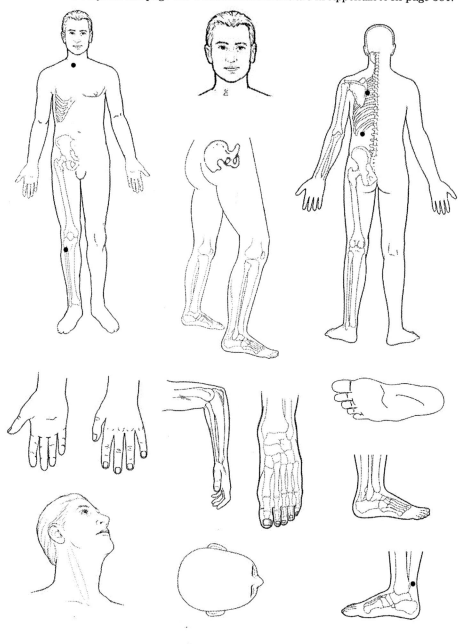

Rash

Daily Nutritional Crisis Program	Daily Nutritional Wellness Program
GlycoN*: 1 ½ tsp & GlycoAO: 3 caps PhytoN: 1/2 tsp PreH: 6 tabs GEssentials : 4 tabs ImmS: 4 tabs MC: 4 caps SP: 3 caps	GlycoN*: 1 ½ tsp & GlycoAO: 3 caps PhytoN: 1/2 tsp PreH: 3 tabs GEssentials : 4 tabs ImmS: 3 tabs MC: 3 caps SP: 2 caps

*For Adv.GlycoN see page 10. Product definitions are in Appendix A on page 381.

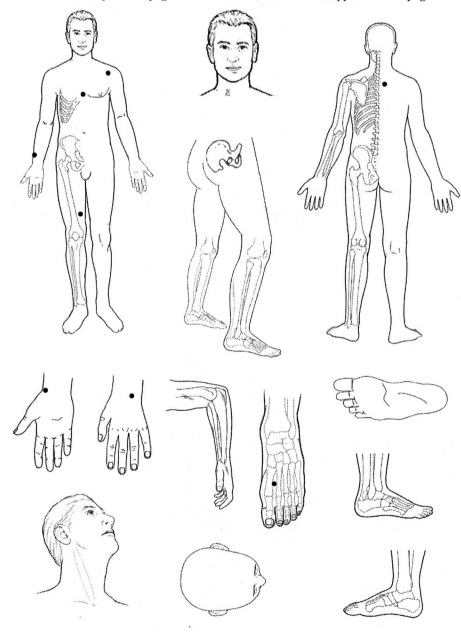

Raynaud's Syndrome

Daily Nutritional Crisis Program	Daily Nutritional Wellness Program
GlycoN*: 5 ¼ tsp & GlycoAO: 4 caps PhytoN: 1 ½ tsp PreH: 6 tabs Cata:6 tabs MC: 6 caps CB: 6 caps	GlycoN*: 1 ½ tsp & GlycoAO: 3 caps PhytoN: 3/4 tsp PreH: 3 tabs Cata:4 tabs MC: 3 caps CB: 4 caps

*For Adv.GlycoN see page 10. Product definitions are in Appendix A on page 381.

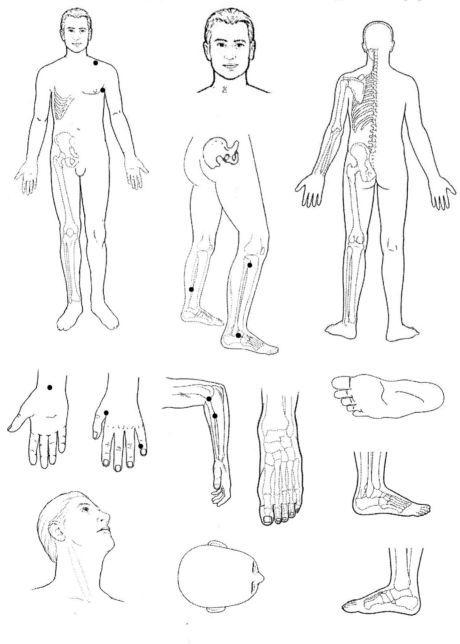

Reflex Sympathetic Dystrophy

Daily Nutritional Crisis Program	Daily Nutritional Wellness Program
GlycoN*: 5 ¼ tsp & GlycoAO: 4 caps PhytoN: 1 ½ tsp PreH: 6 tabs Cata:6 tabs MC: 6 caps CB: 6 caps	GlycoN*: 1 ½ tsp & GlycoAO: 3 caps PhytoN: 3/4 tsp PreH: 3 tabs Cata:4 tabs MC: 3 caps CB: 4 caps

*For Adv.GlycoN see page 10. Product definitions are in Appendix A on page 381.

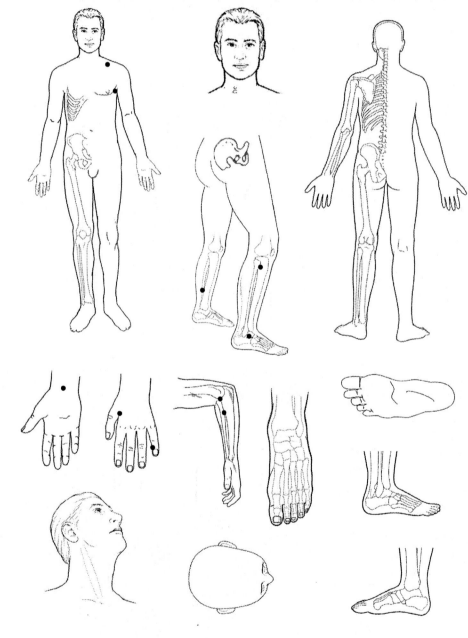

Renal Failure Chronic

Daily Nutritional Crisis Program	Daily Nutritional Wellness Program
GlycoN*: 10 ¾ tsp & GlycoAO: 6 caps	GlycoN*: 3 ½ tsp & GlycoAO: 3 caps
PhytoN: 1 tsp	PhytoN: 1/2 tsp
PreH: 6 tabs	PreH: 3 tabs
Cata: 6 tabs	Cata: 4 tabs
ImmS: 6 tabs	ImmS: 3 tabs
MC: 6 caps	MC: 3 caps
SP: 4 caps	SP: 2 caps

*For Adv.GlycoN see page 10. Product definitions are in Appendix A on page 381.

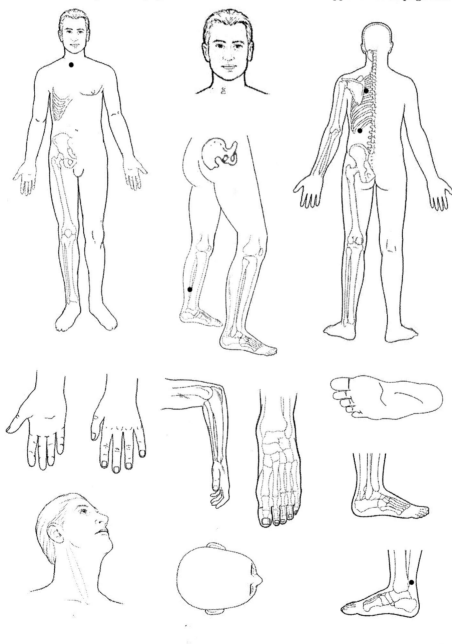

Restless Legs Syndrome

Daily Nutritional Crisis Program	Daily Nutritional Wellness Program
GlycoN*: 2 ½ tsp & GlycoAO: 3 caps PhytoN: 1/2 tsp PreH: 4 tabs Cata: 4 tabs SP: 4 caps MC: 4 caps	GlycoN*: ½ tsp & GlycoAO: 2 caps PhytoN: 1/4 tsp PreH: 3 tabs Cata: 4 tabs SP: 2 caps MC: 2 caps

*For Adv.GlycoN see page 10. Product definitions are in Appendix A on page 381.

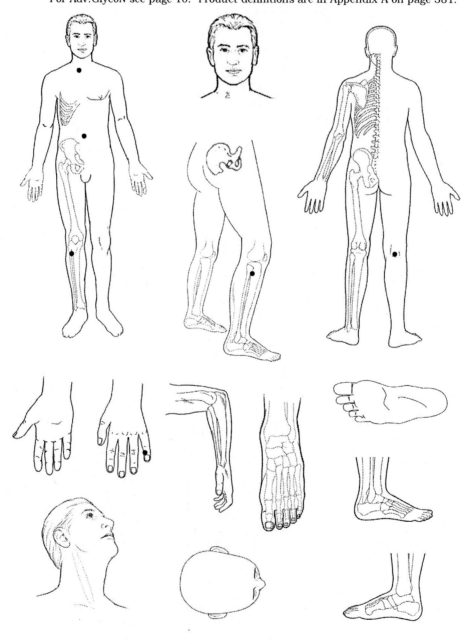

Retinitis

Daily Nutritional Crisis Program	Daily Nutritional Wellness Program
GlycoN*: 8 tsp & GlycoAO: 5 caps PhytoN: 1 tsp PreH: 4 tabs Cata: 6 tabs ImmS: 5 tabs MC: 5 caps	GlycoN*: 1 ½ tsp & GlycoAO: 3 caps PhytoN: 1/4 tsp PreH: 3 tabs Cata: 4 tabs ImmS: 3 tabs MC: 3 caps

*For Adv.GlycoN see page 10. Product definitions are in Appendix A on page 381.

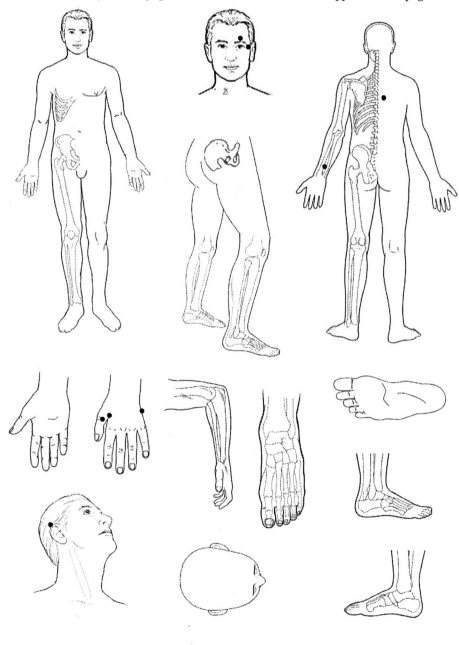

Rheumatoid Arthritis

Daily Nutritional Crisis Program	Daily Nutritional Wellness Program
GlycoN*: 5 ¼ tsp & GlycoAO: 4 caps PhytoN: 1 tsp PreH: 6 tabs Cata: 6 tabs Clean: 3 caps twice a day (2 weeks) MC: 4 caps	GlycoN*: 1 ½ tsp & GlycoAO: 3 caps PhytoN: 3/4 tsp PreH: 4 tabs Cata: 6 tabs Clean: 1 cap MC: 2 caps

*For Adv.GlycoN see page 10. Product definitions are in Appendix A on page 381.

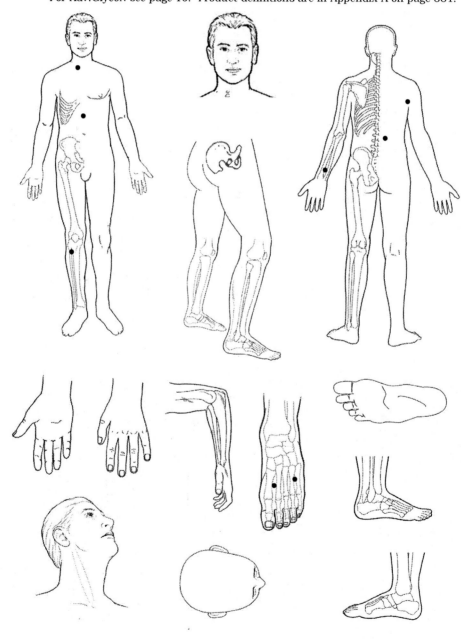

330

Rosacea
(apply soft laser to affect areas)

Daily Nutritional Crisis Program	Daily Nutritional Wellness Program
GlycoN*: 1 ½ tsp & GlycoAO: 3 caps	GlycoN*: 1 ½ tsp & GlycoAO: 3 caps
PhytoN: 1/2 tsp	PhytoN: 1/2 tsp
PreH: 6 tabs	PreH: 3 tabs
GEssentials : 4 tabs	GEssentials : 4 tabs
ImmS: 4 tabs	ImmS: 3 tabs
MC: 4 caps	MC: 3 caps
SP: 3 caps	SP: 2 caps

*For Adv.GlycoN see page 10. Product definitions are in Appendix A on page 381.

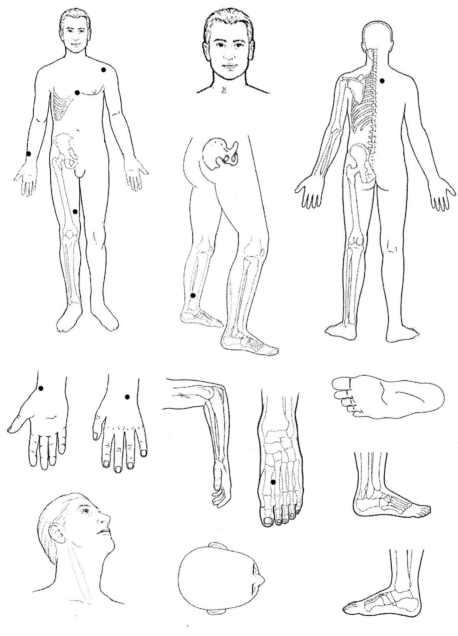

Sarcoidosis

Daily Nutritional Crisis Program	Daily Nutritional Wellness Program
GlycoN*: 2 ½ tsp & GlycoAO: 3 caps	GlycoN*: 1 ½ tsp & GlycoAO: 3 caps
PhytoN: 1½ tsp	PhytoN: 3/4 tsp
PreH: 4 tabs	PreH: 3 tabs
Cata: 4 tabs	Cata: 4 tabs
ImmS: 6 tabs	ImmS: 4 tabs
MC: 6 caps	MC: 3 caps

*For Adv.GlycoN see page 10. Product definitions are in Appendix A on page 381.

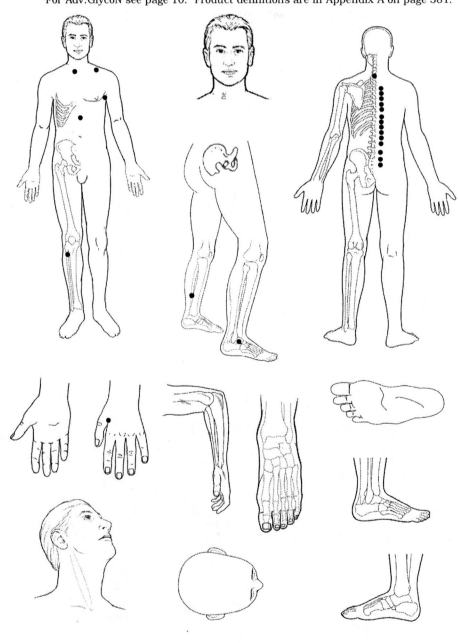

Seizure Disorder

Daily Nutritional Crisis Program	Daily Nutritional Wellness Program
GlycoN*: 8 tsp & GlycoAO: 5 caps PhytoN: 1/2 tsp PreH: 4 tabs Cata: 6 tabs SP: 4 caps MC: 4 caps	GlycoN*: 1 ½ tsp & GlycoAO: 3 caps PhytoN: 1/4 tsp PreH: 3 tabs Cata: 6 tabs SP: 2 caps MC: 3 caps

*For Adv.GlycoN see page 10. Product definitions are in Appendix A on page 381.

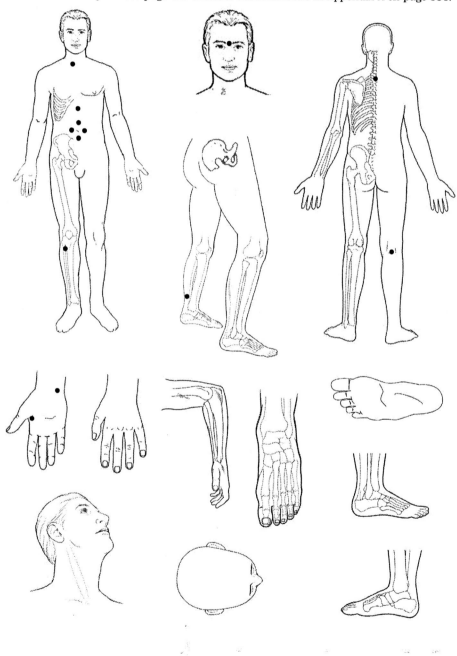

Sepsis

Daily Nutritional Crisis Program	Daily Nutritional Wellness Program
GlycoN*: 5 ¼ tsp & GlycoAO: 4 caps PhytoN: 1 tsp PreH: 6 tabs Cata: 4 tabs MC: 6 caps ImmS: 8 tabs	GlycoN*: 1 ½ tsp & GlycoAO: 2 caps PhytoN: 1/4 tsp PreH: 3 tabs Cata: 4 tabs MC: 3 caps ImmS: 4 tabs

*For Adv.GlycoN see page 10. Product definitions are in Appendix A on page 381.

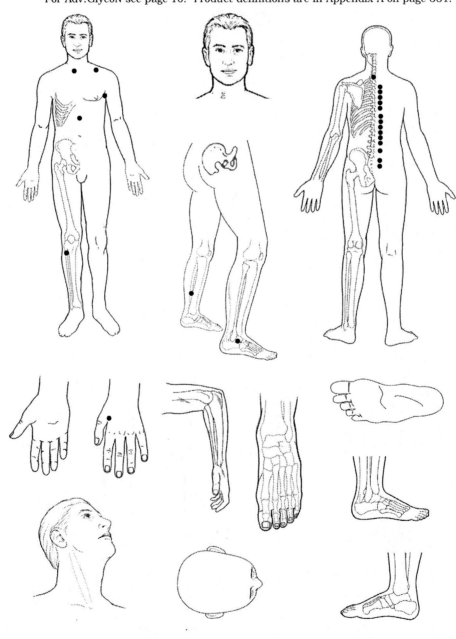

Shingles
(apply soft laser on affected areas)

Daily Nutritional Crisis Program	Daily Nutritional Wellness Program
GlycoN*: 1 ½ tsp & GlycoAO: 3 caps PhytoN: 1/2 tsp PreH: 6 tabs Cata: 4 tabs ImmS: 6 tabs MC: 5 caps SP: 4 caps	GlycoN*: ½ tsp & GlycoAO: 2 caps PhytoN: 1/4 tsp PreH: 3 tabs Cata: 4 tabs ImmS: 4 tabs MC: 4 caps SP: 2 caps

*For Adv.GlycoN see page 10. Product definitions are in Appendix A on page 381.

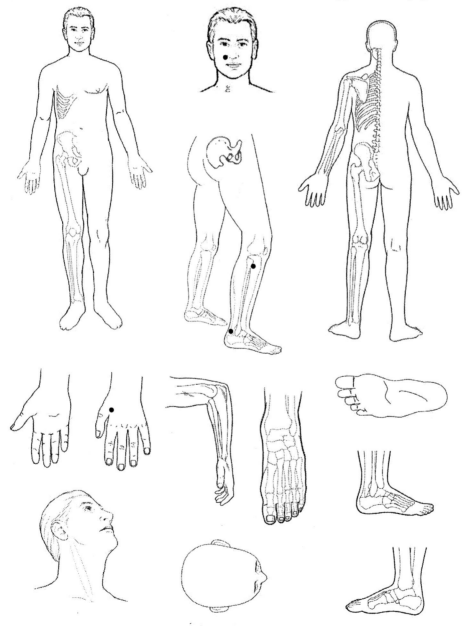

Shortness of Breath

Daily Nutritional Crisis Program	Daily Nutritional Wellness Program
GlycoN*: 5 ¼ tsp & GlycoAO: 4 caps	GlycoN*: ½ tsp & GlycoAO: 2 caps
PhytoN: 1/2 tsp	PhytoN: 1/4 tsp
PreH: 6 tabs	PreH: 3 tabs
GEssentials: 4 tabs	GEssentials: 4 tabs
ImmS: 5 tabs	ImmS: 3 tabs
MC: 4 caps	MC: 2 caps

*For Adv.GlycoN see page 10. Product definitions are in Appendix A on page 381.

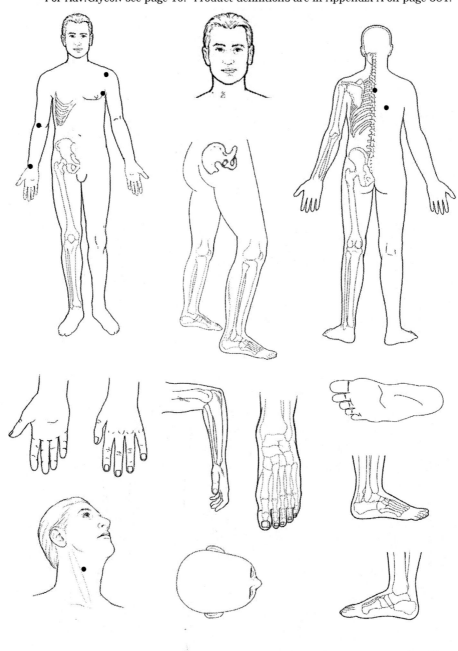

Sick Sinus Syndrome

Daily Nutritional Crisis Program	Daily Nutritional Wellness Program
GlycoN*: 2 ½ tsp & GlycoAO: 3 caps PhytoN: 1/4 tsp PreH: 3 tabs GEssentials: 4 tabs Clean: 3 caps twice a day (2 weeks) MC: 4 caps	GlycoN*: ½ tsp & GlycoAO: 2 caps PhytoN: 1/4 tsp PreH: 3 tabs GEssentials: 4 tabs Clean: 1 cap MC: 4 caps

*For Adv.GlycoN see page 10. Product definitions are in Appendix A on page 381.

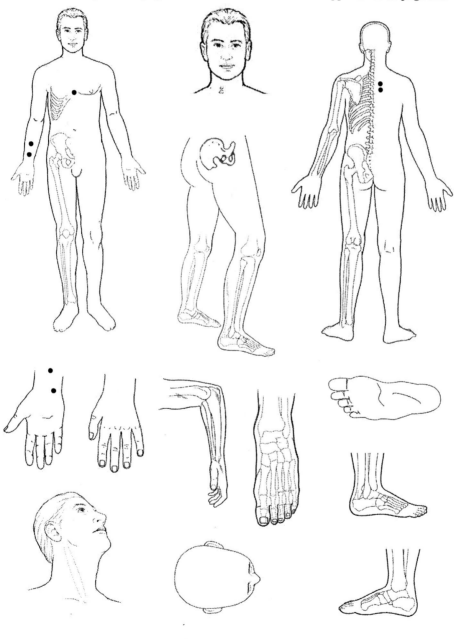

Sinusitis Chronic

Daily Nutritional Crisis Program	Daily Nutritional Wellness Program
GlycoN*: 2 ½ tsp & GlycoAO: 3 caps	GlycoN*: ½ tsp & GlycoAO: 2 caps
PhytoN: 1/4 tsp	PhytoN: 1/4 tsp
PreH: 3 tabs	PreH: 3 tabs
GEssentials: 4 tabs	GEssentials: 4 tabs
Clean: 3 caps twice a day (2 weeks)	Clean: 1 cap
MC: 4 caps	MC: 4 caps

*For Adv.GlycoN see page 10. Product definitions are in Appendix A on page 381.

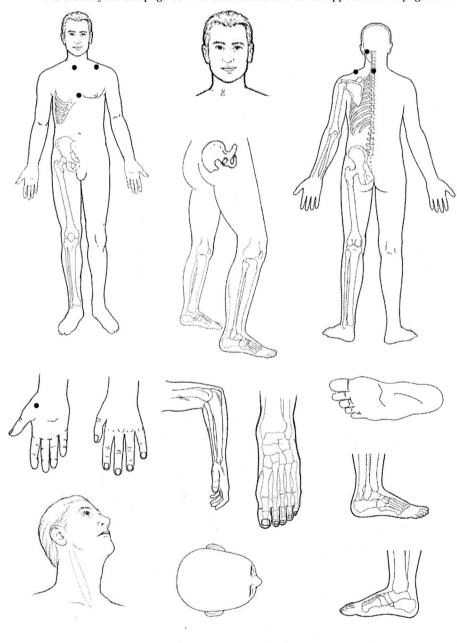

Sjogren's Syndrome

Daily Nutritional Crisis Program	Daily Nutritional Wellness Program
GlycoN*: 8 tsp & GlycoAO: 5 caps PhytoN: 1 tsp PreH: 6 tabs Cata: 6 tabs ImmS: 5 tabs MC: 4 caps	GlycoN*: 1 ½ tsp & GlycoAO: 3 caps PhytoN: 1/2 tsp PreH: 3 tabs Cata: 6 tabs ImmS: 3 tabs MC: 3 caps

*For Adv.GlycoN see page 10. Product definitions are in Appendix A on page 381.

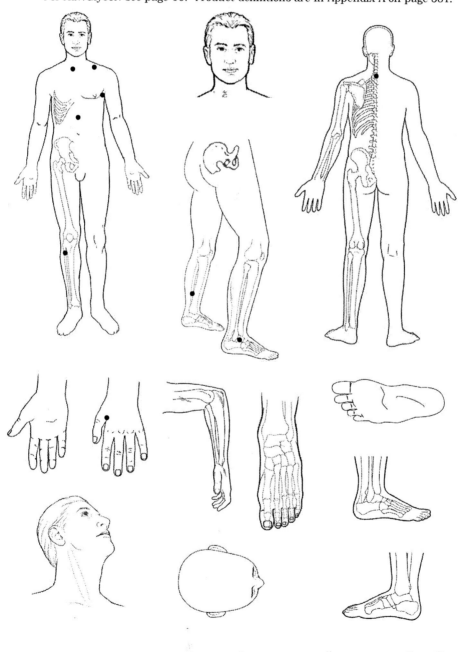

SLE (Systemic Lupus Erythematosis)

Daily Nutritional Crisis Program	Daily Nutritional Wellness Program
GlycoN*: 6 tsp & GlycoAO: 5 caps PhytoN: 1 tsp PreH: 4 tabs Cata: 6 tabs ImmS: 5 tabs MC: 5 caps SP: 4 caps	GlycoN*: 2 ½ tsp & GlycoAO: 3 caps PhytoN: 1 tsp PreH: 3 tabs Cata: 6 tabs ImmS: 2 tabs MC: 3 caps SP: 2 caps

*For Adv.GlycoN see page 10. Product definitions are in Appendix A on page 381.

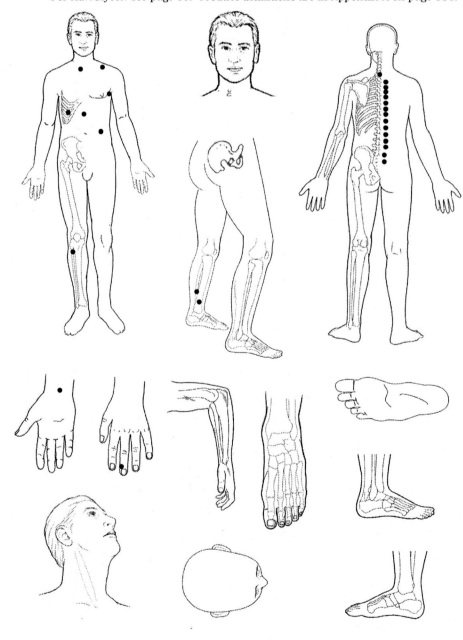

Sleep Apnea

Daily Nutritional Crisis Program	Daily Nutritional Wellness Program
GlycoN*: 2 ½ tsp & GlycoAO: 3 caps PhytoN: 1/2 tsp PreH: 4 tabs Cata: 4 tabs SP: 3 caps MC: 3 caps	GlycoN*: ½ tsp & GlycoAO: 2 caps PhytoN: 1/2 tsp PreH: 3 tabs Cata: 4 tabs SP: 3 caps MC: 3 caps

*For Adv.GlycoN see page 10. Product definitions are in Appendix A on page 381.

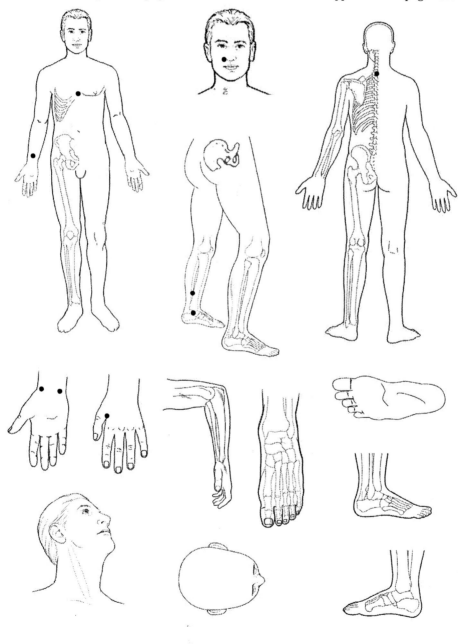

Smallpox

Daily Nutritional Crisis Program	Daily Nutritional Wellness Program
GlycoN*: 10 ¾ tsp & GlycoAO: 6 caps PhytoN: 1 tsp PreH: 6 tabs Cata: 6 tabs ImmS: 5 tabs MC: 4 caps	GlycoN*: 3 ½ tsp & GlycoAO: 3 caps PhytoN: 1/2 tsp PreH: 3 tabs Cata: 6 tabs ImmS: 3 tabs MC: 3 caps

*For Adv.GlycoN see page 10. Product definitions are in Appendix A on page 381.

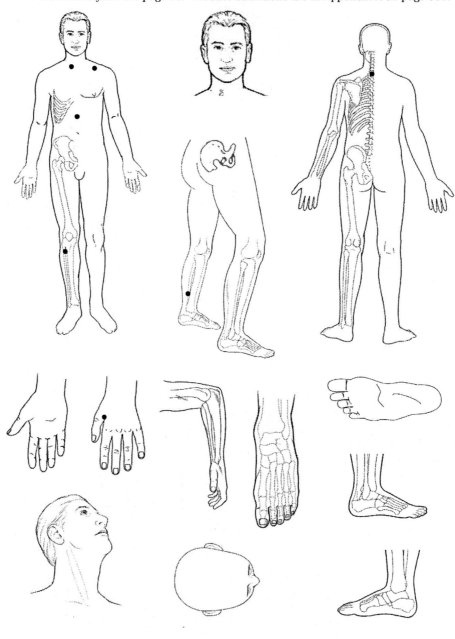

Sore Throat

Daily Nutritional Crisis Program	Daily Nutritional Wellness Program
GlycoN*: 2 tsp & GlycoAO: 3 caps	GlycoN*: ½ tsp & GlycoAO: 2 caps
PhytoN: 3/4 tsp	PhytoN: 1/2 tsp
PreH: 3 tabs	PreH: 3 tabs
GEssentials: 4 tabs	GEssentials: 4 tabs
ImmS: 5 tabs	ImmS: 3 tabs
MC: 6 caps	MC: 3 caps

*For Adv.GlycoN see page 10. Product definitions are in Appendix A on page 381.

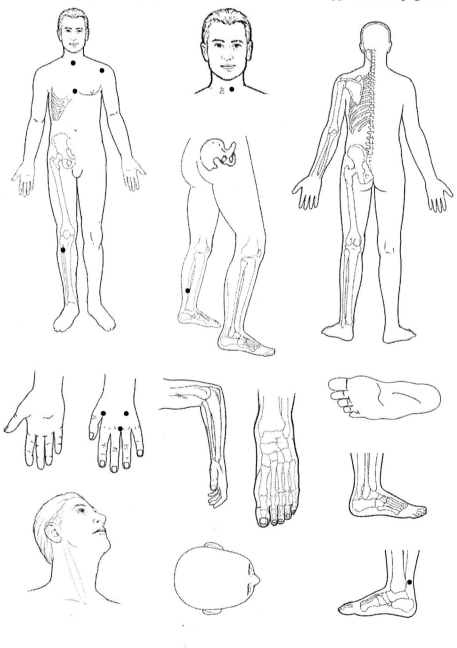

Spleen Infection

Daily Nutritional Crisis Program	Daily Nutritional Wellness Program
GlycoN*: 5 ¼ tsp & GlycoAO: 4 caps PhytoN: 1 tsp PreH: 6 tabs GEssentials: 4 tabs ImmS: 6 tabs MC: 5 caps	GlycoN*: ½ tsp & GlycoAO: 2 caps PhytoN: 1/2 tsp PreH: 3 tabs GEssentials: 4 tabs ImmS: 3 tabs MC: 4 caps

*For Adv.GlycoN see page 10. Product definitions are in Appendix A on page 381.

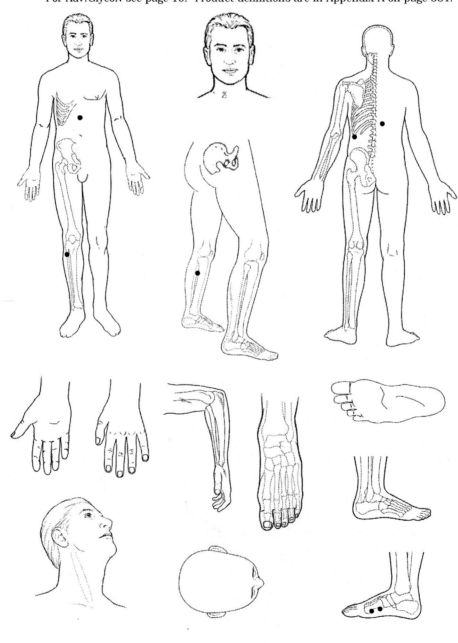

Splenomegaly

Daily Nutritional Crisis Program	Daily Nutritional Wellness Program
GlycoN*: 5 ¼ tsp & GlycoAO: 4 caps PhytoN: 1 tsp PreH: 6 tabs GEssentials: 4 tabs ImmS: 6 tabs MC: 5 caps	GlycoN*: ½ tsp & GlycoAO: 2 caps PhytoN: 1/2 tsp PreH: 3 tabs GEssentials: 4 tabs ImmS: 3 tabs MC: 4 caps

*For Adv.GlycoN see page 10. Product definitions are in Appendix A on page 381.

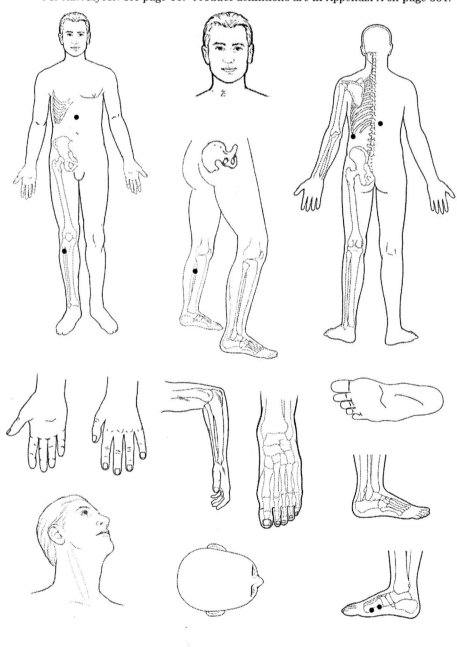

Staphylococcal Food Poisoning (Detoxification)

Daily Nutritional Crisis Program	Daily Nutritional Wellness Program
GlycoN*: 8 tsp & GlycoAO: 5 caps	GlycoN*: ½ tsp & GlycoAO: 2 caps
PhytoN: 1 tsp	PhytoN: 1/4 tsp
PreH: 4 tabs	PreH: 3 tabs
Cata: 4 tabs	Cata: 4 tabs
Clean: 3 caps twice a day (2 weeks)	Clean: 2 caps
ImmS: 6 tabs & GstroP: 4 caps	ImmS: 4 tabs & GstroP: 2 caps

*For Adv.GlycoN see page 10. Product definitions are in Appendix A on page 381.

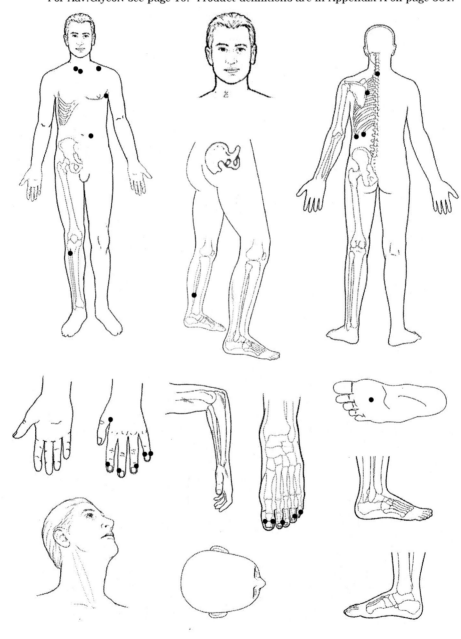

Stomach Problems

Daily Nutritional Crisis Program	Daily Nutritional Wellness Program
GlycoN*: 2 ½ tsp & GlycoAO: 3 caps PhytoN: 1/2 tsp PreH: 3 tabs GEssentials: 4 tabs ImmS: 3 tabs Clean: 3 caps twice a day (2 weeks) MC: 4 caps	GlycoN*: ½ tsp & GlycoAO: 2 caps PhytoN: 1/2 tsp PreH: 3 tabs GEssentials: 4 tabs ImmS: 2 tabs Clean: 2 caps MC: 3 caps

*For Adv.GlycoN see page 10. Product definitions are in Appendix A on page 381.

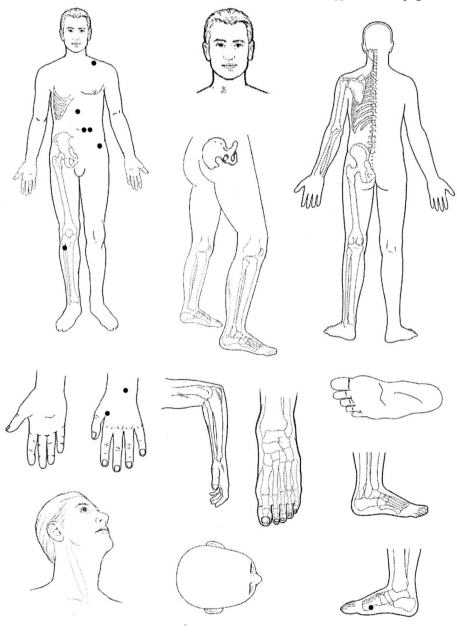

Stomatitis

Daily Nutritional Crisis Program	Daily Nutritional Wellness Program
GlycoN*: 2 ½ tsp & GlycoAO: 3 caps PhytoN: 1/2 tsp PreH: 4 tabs GEssentials: 4 tabs ImmS: 5 tabs MC: 4 caps	GlycoN*: ½ tsp & GlycoAO: 2 caps PhytoN: 1/4 tsp PreH: 3 tabs GEssentials: 4 tabs ImmS: 3 tabs MC: 2 caps

*For Adv.GlycoN see page 10. Product definitions are in Appendix A on page 381.

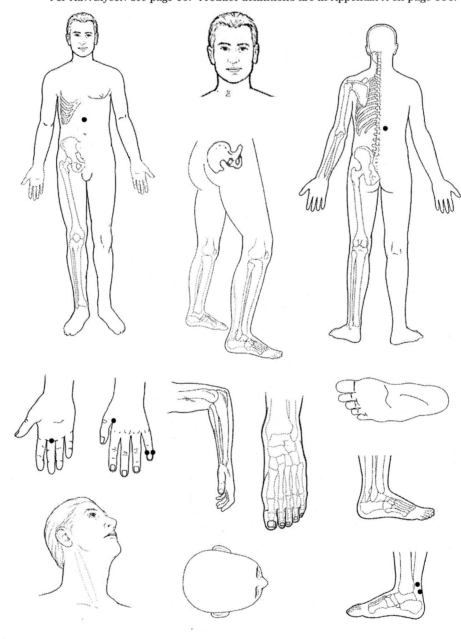

Strep Throat (Pharyngitis)

Daily Nutritional Crisis Program	Daily Nutritional Wellness Program
GlycoN*: 2 tsp & GlycoAO: 3 caps	GlycoN*: ½ tsp & GlycoAO: 2 caps
PhytoN: 3/4 tsp	PhytoN: 1/2 tsp
PreH: 3 tabs	PreH: 3 tabs
GEssentials: 4 tabs	GEssentials: 4 tabs
ImmS: 5 tabs	ImmS: 3 tabs
MC: 6 caps	MC: 3 caps

*For Adv.GlycoN see page 10. Product definitions are in Appendix A on page 381.

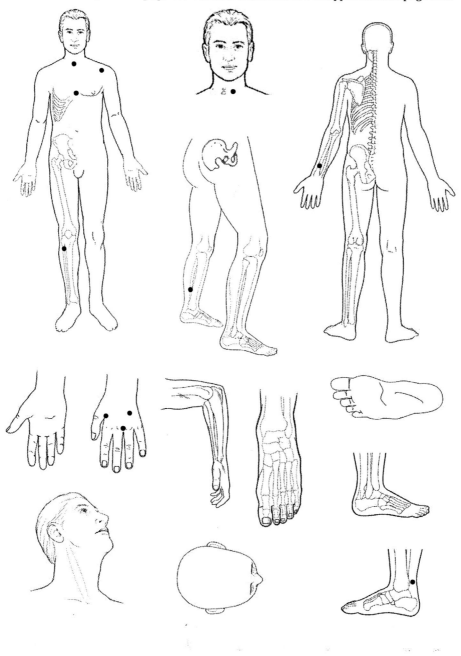

Stress (Physical or Emotional)

Daily Nutritional Crisis Program	Daily Nutritional Wellness Program
GlycoN*: 2 ½ tsp & GlycoAO: 3 caps PhytoN: 1 tsp PreH: 6 tabs GEssentials: 4 tabs SP: 4 caps	GlycoN*: ½ tsp & GlycoAO: 2 caps PhytoN: 1/4 tsp PreH: 3 tabs GEssentials: 4 tabs SP: 2 caps

*For Adv.GlycoN see page 10. Product definitions are in Appendix A on page 381.

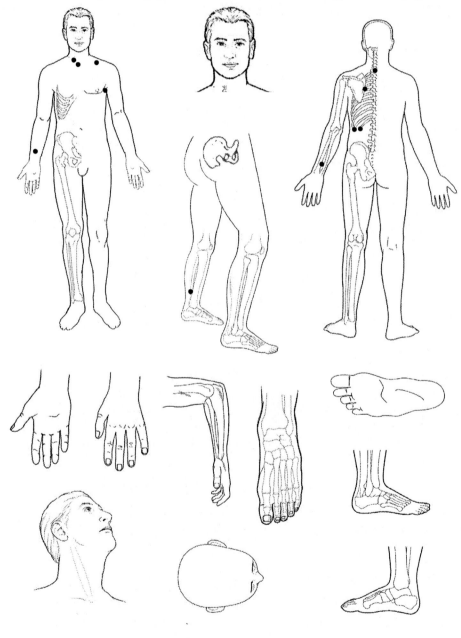

Sugar Craving

Daily Nutritional Crisis Program	Daily Nutritional Wellness Program
GlycoN*: 2 ½ tsp & GlycoAO: 3 caps PhytoN: 1½ tsp PreH: 6 tabs GEssentials: 6 tabs	GlycoN*: ½ tsp & GlycoAO: 2 caps PhytoN: 3/4 tsp PreH: 3 tabs GEssentials: 4 tabs

*For Adv.GlycoN see page 10. Product definitions are in Appendix A on page 381.

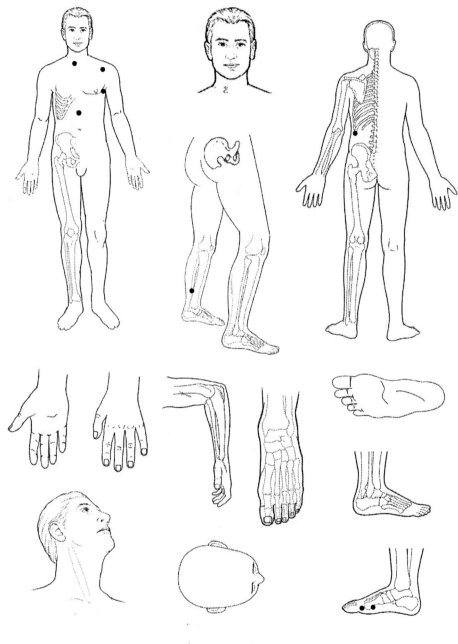

Surgery (During Recovery)

Daily Nutritional Crisis Program	Daily Nutritional Wellness Program
GlycoN*: 5 ¼ tsp & GlycoAO: 4 caps PhytoN: 1 tsp PreH: 6 tabs Cata: 6 tabs ImmS: 5 tabs MC: 5 caps SP: 4 caps	GlycoN*: 2 ¼ tsp & GlycoAO: 2 caps Phyto: 3/4 tsp PreH: 3 tabs Cata: 6 tabs ImmS: 3 tabs MC: 3 caps SP: 3 caps

*For Adv.GlycoN see page 10. Product definitions are in Appendix A on page 381.

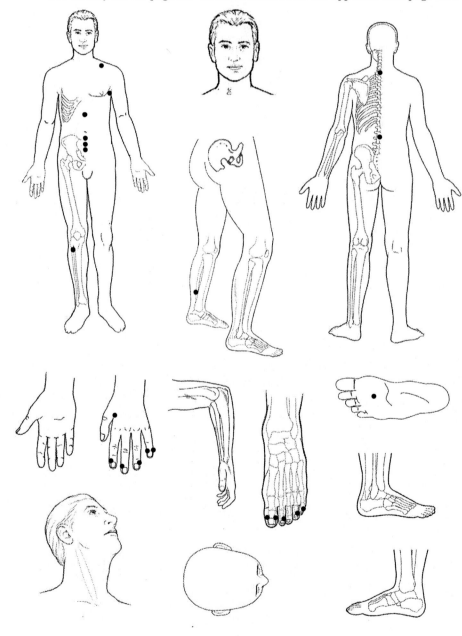

Systemic Lupus Erythematosis (SLE)

Daily Nutritional Crisis Program	Daily Nutritional Wellness Program
GlycoN*: 6 tsp & GlycoAO: 5 caps	GlycoN*: 2 ½ tsp & GlycoAO: 3 caps
PhytoN: 1 tsp	PhytoN: 1 tsp
PreH: 4 tabs	PreH: 3 tabs
Cata: 6 tabs	Cata: 6 tabs
ImmS: 5 tabs	ImmS: 2 tabs
MC: 5 caps	MC: 3 caps
SP: 4 caps	SP: 2 caps

*For Adv.GlycoN see page 10. Product definitions are in Appendix A on page 381.

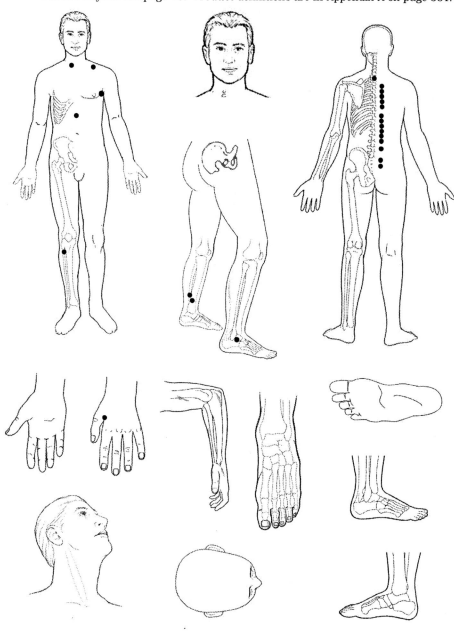

Temporal Arteritis

Daily Nutritional Crisis Program	Daily Nutritional Wellness Program
GlycoN*: 10 ¾ tsp & GlycoAO: 6 caps	GlycoN*: 1 ½ tsp & GlycoAO: 3 caps
PhytoN: 2 tsp	PhytoN: 3/4 tsp
PreH: 6 tabs	PreH: 3 tabs
Cata: 6 tabs	Cata: 6 tabs
MC: 5 caps	MC: 3 caps
ImmS: 4 tabs	ImmS: 3 tabs

*For Adv.GlycoN see page 10. Product definitions are in Appendix A on page 381.

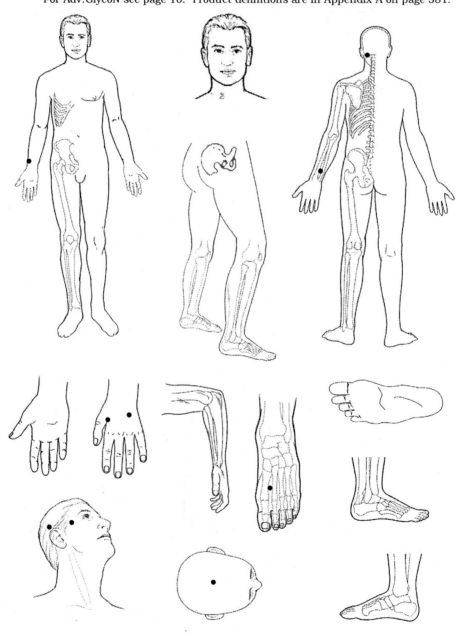

Tension Headache (Chronic)

Daily Nutritional Crisis Program	Daily Nutritional Wellness Program
GlycoN*: 1 ½ tsp & GlycoAO: 3 caps PhytoN: 1/2 tsp PreH: 6 tabs GEssentials: 4 tabs SP: 4 caps ImmS: 4 tabs	GlycoN*: ½ tsp & GlycoAO: 2 caps PhytoN: 1/2 tsp PreH: 3 tabs GEssentials: 4 tabs SP: 3 caps ImmS: 2 tabs

*For Adv.GlycoN see page 10. Product definitions are in Appendix A on page 381.

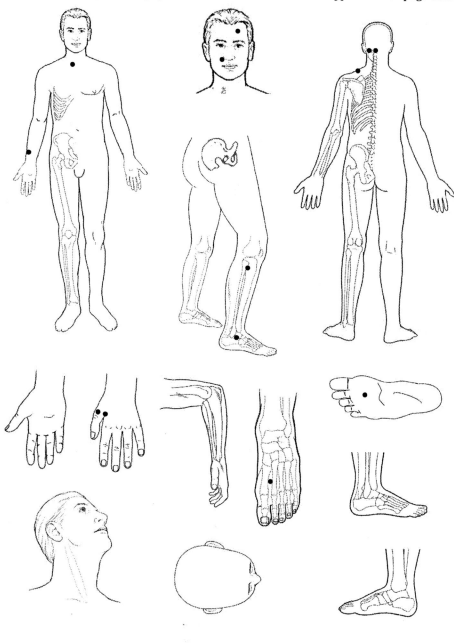

Thrombocytopenia

Daily Nutritional Crisis Program	Daily Nutritional Wellness Program
GlycoN*: 5 ¼ tsp & GlycoAO: 4 caps PhytoN: 3/4 tsp PreH: 4 tabs Cata: 4 tabs ImmS: 5 tabs MC: 4 caps	GlycoN*: ½ tsp & GlycoAO: 2 caps Phyto: 1/2 tsp PreH: 3 tabs Cata: 4 tabs ImmS: 3 tabs MC: 3 caps

*For Adv.GlycoN see page 10. Product definitions are in Appendix A on page 381.

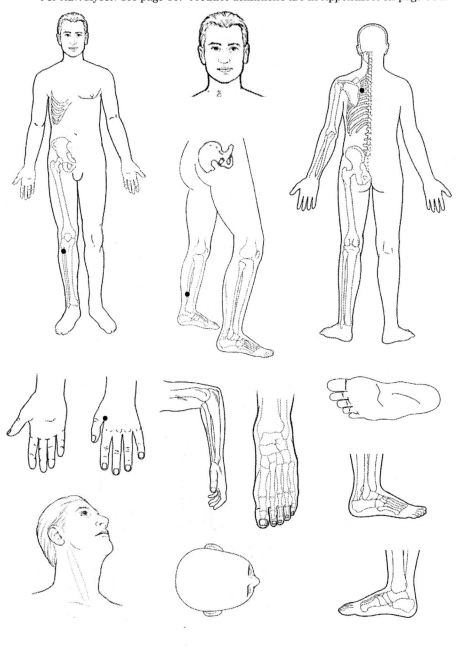

Thyroiditis (Acute)

Daily Nutritional Crisis Program	Daily Nutritional Wellness Program
GlycoN*: 5 tsp & GlycoAO: 4 caps PhytoN: 1/2 tsp PreH: 3 tabs Cata: 4 tabs ImmS: 4 tabs MC: 3 caps	GlycoN*: ½ tsp & GlycoAO: 2 caps PhytoN: 1/4 tsp PreH: 3 tabs Cata: 4 tabs ImmS: 2 tabs MC: 2 caps

*For Adv.GlycoN see page 10. Product definitions are in Appendix A on page 381.

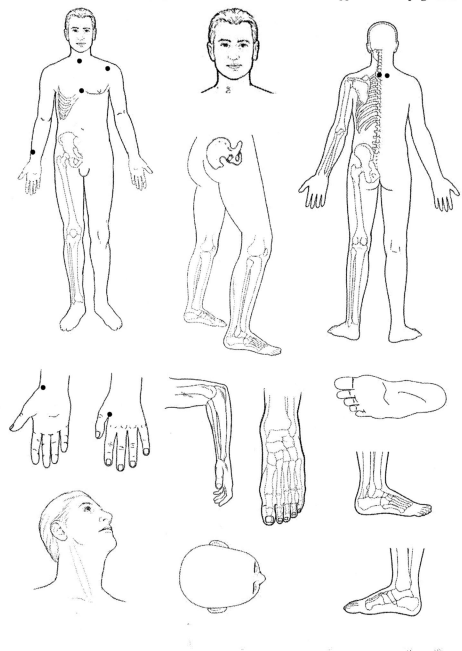

Tissue Trauma

Daily Nutritional Crisis Program	Daily Nutritional Wellness Program
GlycoN*: 10 ¾ tsp & GlycoAO: 6 caps PhytoN: 2 tsp PreH: 6 tabs Cata: 6 tabs ImmS: 5 tabs MC: 5 caps SP: 4 caps	GlycoN*: 1 ½ tsp & GlycoAO: 3 caps PhytoN: 3/4 tsp PreH: 3 tabs Cata: 6 tabs ImmS: 3 tabs MC: 3 caps SP: 3 caps

*For Adv.GlycoN see page 10. Product definitions are in Appendix A on page 381.

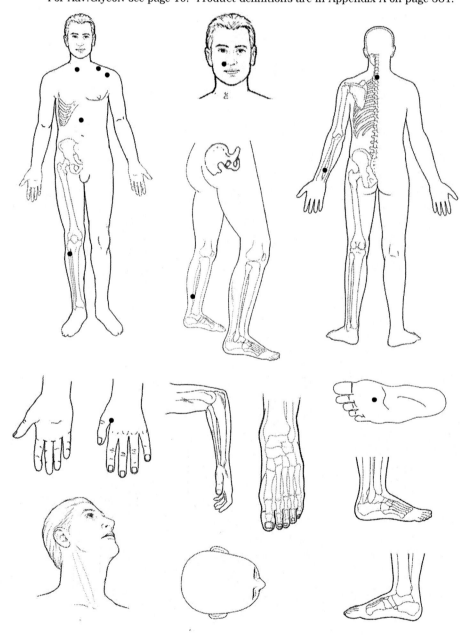

Tobacco Dependence

Daily Nutritional Crisis Program	Daily Nutritional Wellness Program
GlycoN*: 2½ tsp & GlycoAO: 3 caps PhytoN: 1/4 tsp PreH: 3 tabs Cata: 6 tabs ImmS: 5 tabs MC: 5 caps	GlycoN*: 1½ tsp & GlycoAO: 3 caps PhytoN: 1/4 tsp PreH: 3 tabs Cata: 6 tabs ImmS: 4 tabs MC: 4 caps

*For Adv.GlycoN see page 10. Product definitions are in Appendix A on page 381.

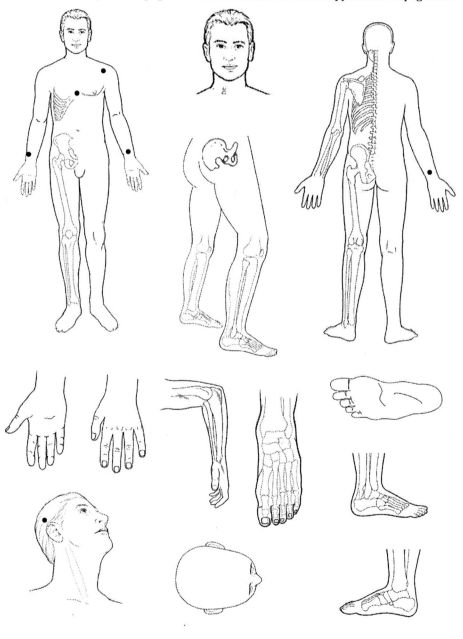

Tonsillitis

Daily Nutritional Crisis Program	Daily Nutritional Wellness Program
GlycoN*: 2 tsp & GlycoAO: 3 caps PhytoN: 3/4 tsp PreH: 3 tabs GEssentials: 4 tabs ImmS: 5 tabs MC: 6 caps	GlycoN*: ½ tsp & GlycoAO: 2 caps PhytoN: 1/2 tsp PreH: 3 tabs GEssentials: 4 tabs ImmS: 3 tabs MC: 3 caps

*For Adv.GlycoN see page 10. Product definitions are in Appendix A on page 381.

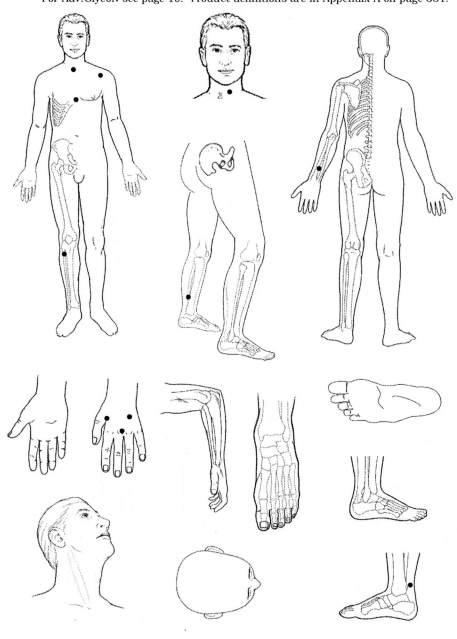

Tonsils (Swollen)

Daily Nutritional Crisis Program	Daily Nutritional Wellness Program
GlycoN*: 2 tsp & GlycoAO: 3 caps PhytoN: 3/4 tsp PreH: 3 tabs GEssentials: 4 tabs ImmS: 5 tabs MC: 6 caps	GlycoN*: ½ tsp & GlycoAO: 2 caps PhytoN: 1/2 tsp PreH: 3 tabs GEssentials: 4 tabs ImmS: 3 tabs MC: 3 caps

*For Adv.GlycoN see page 10. Product definitions are in Appendix A on page 381.

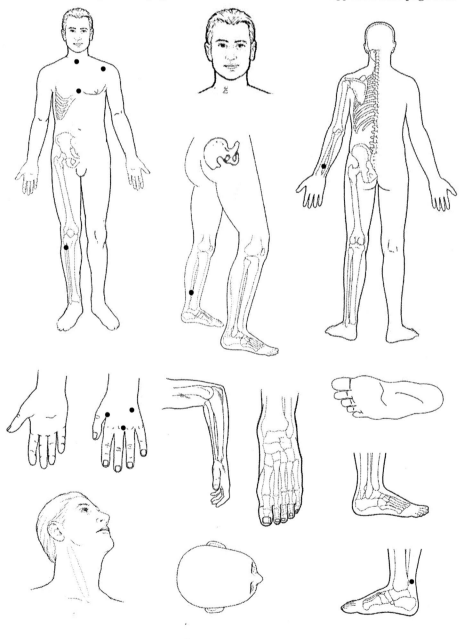

Ulcerative Colitis

Daily Nutritional Crisis Program	Daily Nutritional Wellness Program
GlycoN*: 5 ¼ tsp & GlycoAO: 4 caps	GlycoN*: 1 ½ tsp & GlycoAO: 3 caps
PhytoN: 1 ¾ tsp	PhytoN: 3/4 tsp
PreH: 4 tabs	PreH: 3 tabs
Cata:4 tabs	Cata:4 tabs
ImmS: 4 tabs	ImmS: 2 tabs
MC: 4 caps & GstroP: 3 caps	MC: 2 caps & GstroP: 1 cap

*For Adv.GlycoN see page 10. Product definitions are in Appendix A on page 381.

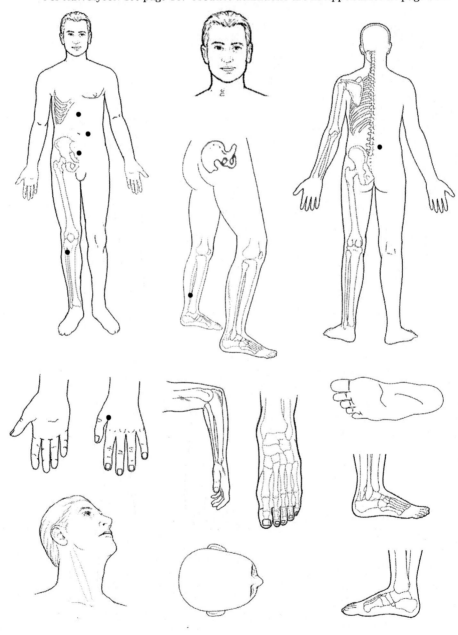

Ulcers- Diabetic
(apply soft laser over affected area)

Daily Nutritional Crisis Program	Daily Nutritional Wellness Program
GlycoN*: 5 ¼ tsp & GlycoAO: 4 caps PhytoN: 1 tsp PreH: 4 tabs Cata: 6 tabs MC: 8 caps SkZone: apply to area	GlycoN*: 1 ½ tsp & GlycoAO: 3 caps PhytoN: 1 tsp PreH: 3 tabs Cata: 4 tabs MC: 4 caps SkZone: apply to area

*For Adv.GlycoN see page 10. Product definitions are in Appendix A on page 381.

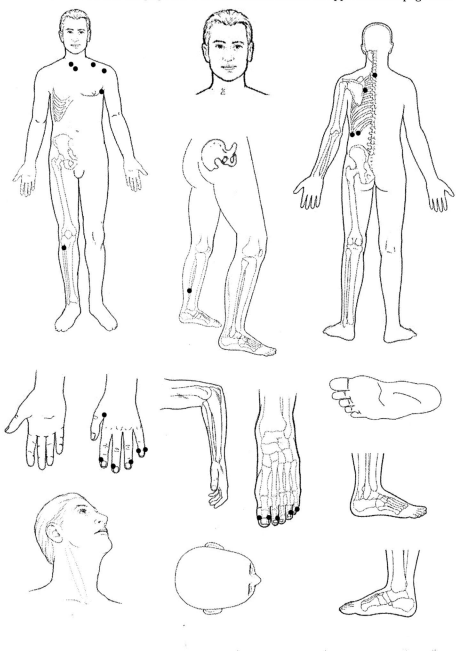

Urethritis

Daily Nutritional Crisis Program	Daily Nutritional Wellness Program
GlycoN*: 2 ½ tsp & GlycoAO: 3 caps PhytoN: 1/2 tsp PreH: 3 tabs GEssentials: 4 tabs ImmS: 6 tabs MC: 4 caps	GlycoN*: ½ tsp & GlycoAO: 2 caps PhytoN: 1/4 tsp PreH: 3 tabs GEssentials: 4 tabs ImmS: 4 tabs MC: 2 caps

*For Adv.GlycoN see page 10. Product definitions are in Appendix A on page 381.

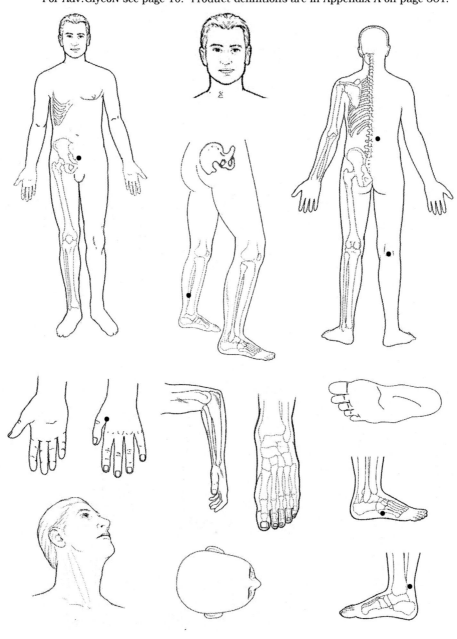

Urinary Tract Infection (UTI)

Daily Nutritional Crisis Program	Daily Nutritional Wellness Program
GlycoN*: 2 ½ tsp & GlycoAO: 3 caps	GlycoN*: ½ tsp & GlycoAO: 2 caps
PhytoN: 1/2 tsp	PhytoN: 1/4 tsp
PreH: 3 tabs	PreH: 3 tabs
GEssentials: 4 tabs	GEssentials: 4 tabs
ImmS: 6 tabs	ImmS: 4 tabs
MC: 4 caps	MC: 2 caps

*For Adv.GlycoN see page 10. Product definitions are in Appendix A on page 381.

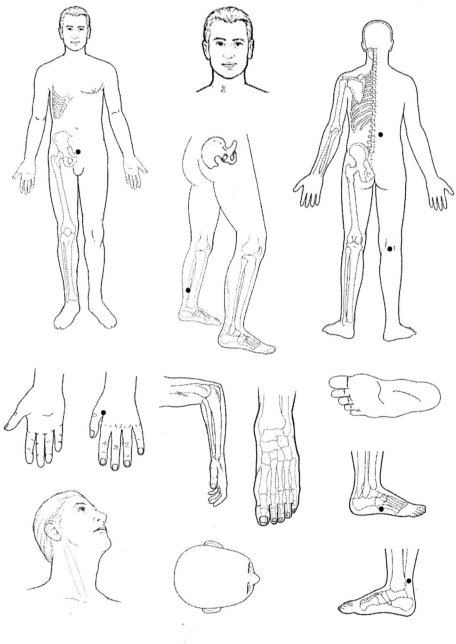

Uterine Fibroids

Daily Nutritional Crisis Program	Daily Nutritional Wellness Program
GlycoN*: 5 ¼ tsp & GlycoAO: 4 caps G	GlycoN*: 1 ½ tsp & GlycoAO: 3 caps
PhytoN: 1 tsp	PhytoN: 3/4 tsp
PreH: 4 tabs	PreH: 3 tabs
GEssentials: 4 tabs	GEssentials: 4 tabs
ImmS: 6 tabs	ImmS: 3 tabs
MC: 4 caps	MC: 3 caps

*For Adv.GlycoN see page 10. Product definitions are in Appendix A on page 381.

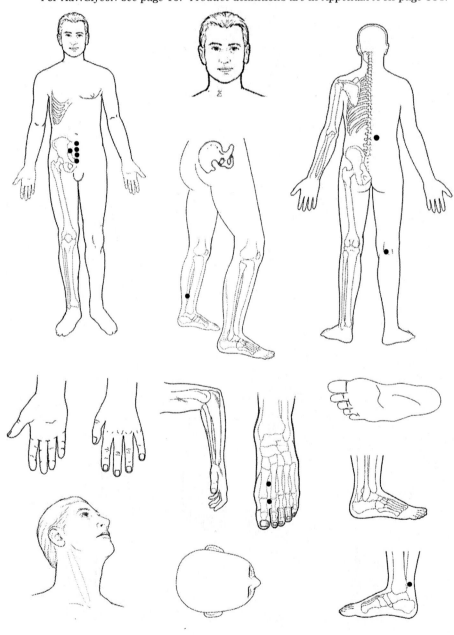

Vaginitis/Vulvitis (Candida)

Daily Nutritional Crisis Program	Daily Nutritional Wellness Program
GlycoN*: 5 ¼ tsp & GlycoAO: 4 caps PhytoN: 1 tsp PreH: 4 tabs Cata:4 tabs ImmS: 4 tabs GstroP: 3 caps	GlycoN*: 1 ½ tsp & GlycoAO: 3 caps PhytoN: 3/4 tsp PreH: 3 tabs Cata:4 tabs ImmS: 3 tabs GastroP: 1 cap

*For Adv.GlycoN see page 10. Product definitions are in Appendix A on page 381.

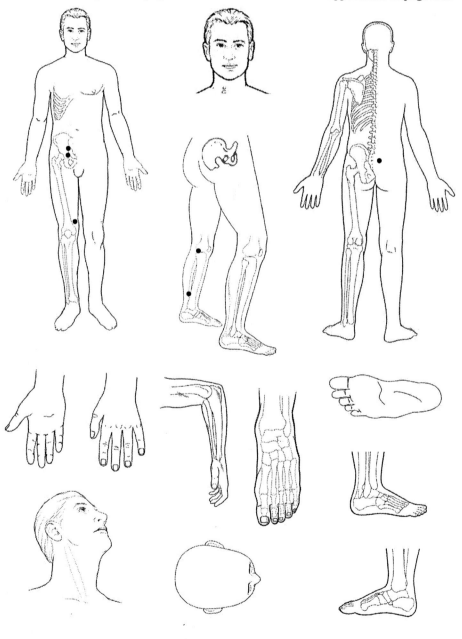

Varicella (Chickenpox)

Daily Nutritional Crisis Program	Daily Nutritional Wellness Program
GlycoN*: 5 ¼ tsp & GlycoAO: 4 caps PhytoN: 1 tsp PreH: 4 tabs GEssentials: 4 tabs ImmS: 6 tabs MC: 4 tabs	GlycoN*: ½ tsp & GlycoAO: 2 caps PhytoN: 1/4 tsp PreH: 3 tabs GEssentials: 4 tabs ImmS: 3 tabs MC: 4 tabs

*For Adv.GlycoN see page 10. Product definitions are in Appendix A on page 381.

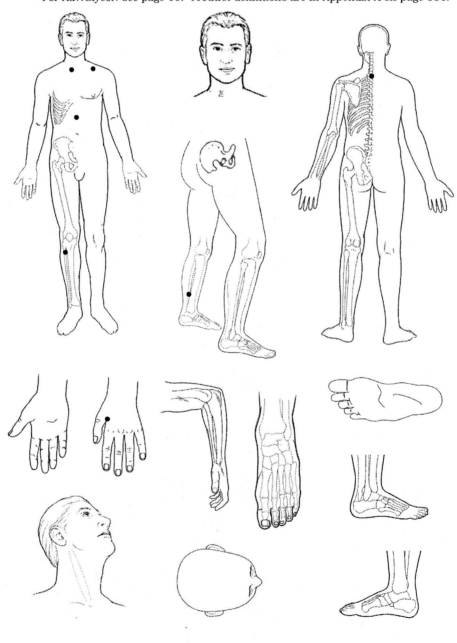

Vasculitis

Daily Nutritional Crisis Program	Daily Nutritional Wellness Program
GlycoN*: 10 ¾ tsp & GlycoAO: 6 caps Phyto: 2 tsp PreH: 6 tabs Cata: 6 tabs ImmS: 4 tabs MC: 4 caps CB: 4 caps	GlycoN*: 4 ½ tsp & GlycoAO: 2 caps PhytoN: 3/4 tsp PreH: 3 tabs Cata: 6 tabs ImmS: 3 tabs MC: 3 caps CB: 3 caps

*For Adv.GlycoN see page 10. Product definitions are in Appendix A on page 381.

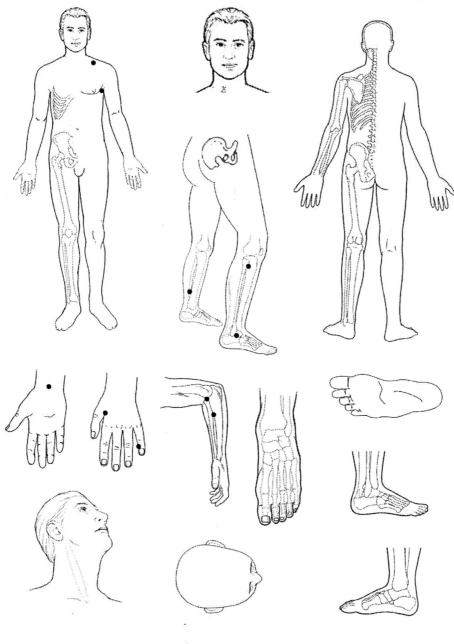

Venereal Disease

Daily Nutritional Crisis Program	Daily Nutritional Wellness Program
GlycoN*: 8 tsp & GlycoAO: 5 caps Phyto: 2 tsp PreH: 3 tabs GEssentials: 4 tabs ImmS: 5 tabs MC: 5 caps	GlycoN*: ½ tsp & GlycoAO: 2 caps PhytoN: 3/4 tsp PreH: 3 tabs GEssentials: 4 tabs ImmS: 3 tabs MC: 3 caps

*For Adv.GlycoN see page 10. Product definitions are in Appendix A on page 381.

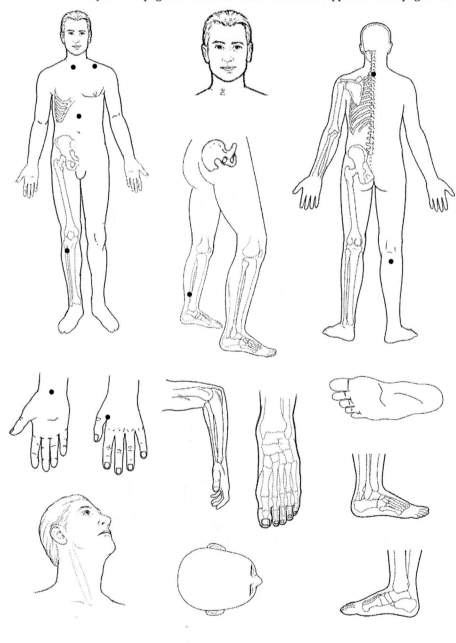

Vertigo (Dizziness)

Daily Nutritional Crisis Program	Daily Nutritional Wellness Program
GlycoN*: 2 ½ tsp & GlycoAO: 3 caps PhytoN: 3/4 tsp PreH: 3 tabs Cata: 4 tabs ImmS: 5 tabs MC: 5 caps	GlycoN*: ½ tsp & GlycoAO: 2 caps PhytoN: 1/4 tsp PreH: 3 tabs Cata: 4 tabs ImmS: 3 tabs MC: 3 caps

*For Adv.GlycoN see page 10. Product definitions are in Appendix A on page 381.

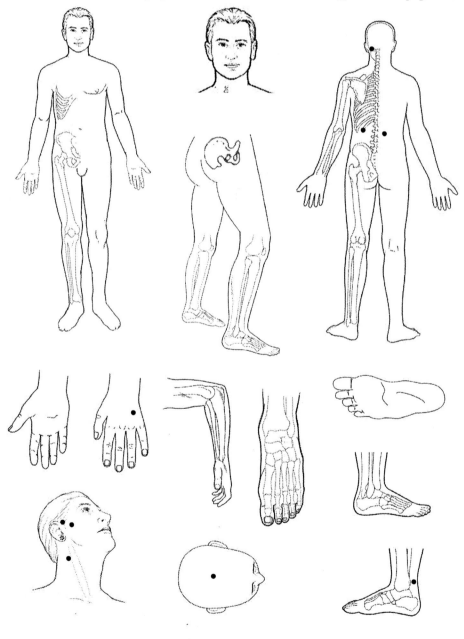

Viral Infection

Daily Nutritional Crisis Program	Daily Nutritional Wellness Program
GlycoN*: 5 ¼ tsp & GlycoAO: 4 caps Phyto: 2 tsp PreH: 4 tabs Cata: 4 tabs ImmS: 6 tabs MC: 5 caps	GlycoN*: ½ tsp & GlycoAO: 2 caps PhytoN: 1/4 tsp PreH: 3 tabs Cata: 4 tabs ImmS: 4 tabs MC: 4 caps

*For Adv.GlycoN see page 10. Product definitions are in Appendix A on page 381.

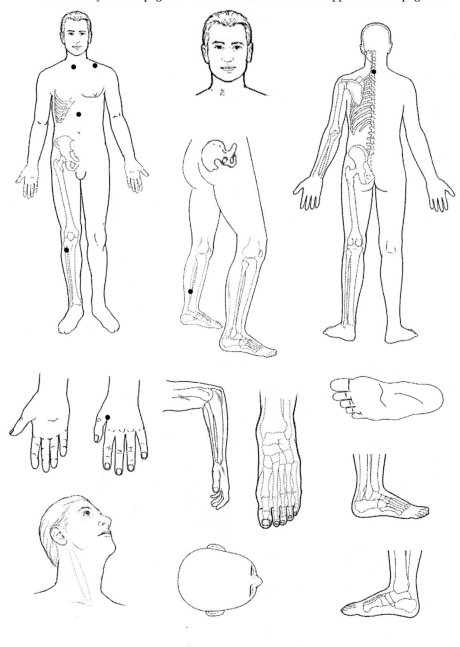

Warts

Daily Nutritional Crisis Program	Daily Nutritional Wellness Program
GlycoN*: 5 ¼ tsp & GlycoAO: 4 caps Phyto: 2 tsp PreH: 4 tabs Cata: 4 tabs ImmS: 6 tabs MC: 5 caps	GlycoN*: ½ tsp & GlycoAO: 2 caps PhytoN: 1/4 tsp PreH: 3 tabs Cata: 4 tabs ImmS: 4 tabs MC: 4 caps

*For Adv.GlycoN see page 10. Product definitions are in Appendix A on page 381.

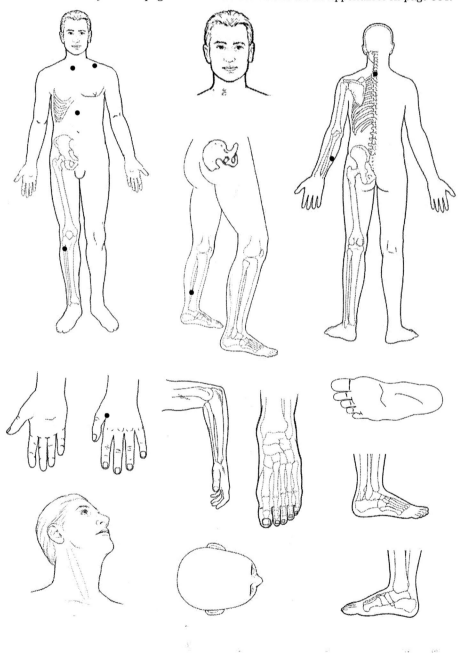

"No matter how many times you fail at something, you are never a failure until the day you quit trying."

~ Michael T. Vaisanen

Section II: Health Challenges Not Listed

God heals, and the doctor takes the fee.

- Benjamin Franklin

Health Challenges Not Listed
(see appendix A for product definitions)

GlycoN w/GlycoAO:
Maintenance*: 1/4 tsp & 1 capsule 2 times a day
Medical Challenge*: ½ tsp & 2 capsules 2 times a day
Severe Medical Challenge*: 3 ½ tsp & 3 capsules 2 times a day

PhytoN:
Maintenance*: 1 capsule 2 times a day
Medical Challenge*: 2 capsules 3x day
Severe Medical Challenge*: 2 to 4 capsules 2 times a day

Pre-H:
Maintenance*: 1 capsule 3 times a day.
Medical Challenge*: Serving Size: 2 capsules 3 times a day
Severe Medical Challenge*: 3 capsules 3 times a day

GEssentials:
Maintenance*: 2 capsules 2 times a day
Medical Challenge*: 2 capsules 3 times day
Severe Medical Challenge*: 2 capsules 3 times a day

Cata:
Maintenance*: 2 capsules 2 times a day
Medical Challenge*: 2 capsules 3 times day
Severe Medical Challenge*: 2 capsules 3 times a day

CB:
Maintenance*: 1 capsules 3 times a day
Medical Challenge*: 2 capsules 3 times day
Severe Medical Challenge*: 2 capsules 3 times a day

Clean:
Maintenance*: 2 capsules 2 times a day
Medical Challenge*: 2 capsules 3 times day
Severe Medical Challenge*: 2 capsules 3 times a day

GstroZ:
Maintenance*: 1 capsules 1 times a day
Medical Challenge*: 2 capsules 3 times day
Severe Medical Challenge*: 2 capsules 3 times a day

GstroP
Maintenance*: 1 capsule per day
Medical Challenge*: 2 capsules per day
Severe Medical Challenge*: 2 capsules 3 times a day

MC:
Maintenance*: 2 capsules a day
Medical Challenge*: 2 capsules 3 times day
Severe Medical Challenge*: 2 capsules 3 times a day

ImmS:
Maintenance*: 1 tablet 2 times a day
Medical Challenge*: 2 tablets 3 times day
Severe Medical Challenge*: 2 tablets 3 times a day

SP:
Maintenance*: 2 capsules following exercise
Medical Challenge*: 3 capsules following exercise

AdvGlycoN with GlycoAO:
Maintenance*: 1/4 tsp & 1 capsule 2 times a day
Medical Challenge*: ½ tsp & 2 capsules 2 times a day
Severe Medical Challenge*: 1 ½ tsp & 3 capsules 2 times a day

Key to Terms
*Maintenance: Prevention
*Medical Challenge: Current illness not an immediate threat to life
*Severe Medical Challenge: illness with possible compromise to life

See Appendix A for Product Definitions

Section III: Appendix

"Our own physical body possesses a wisdom
which we who inhabit the body lack.
We give it orders which make no sense.

- Henry Miller

380

Appendix A

Product Definitions

GlycoN:
Ambrotose™
Company: Mannatech, Inc.
www.mannatech.com
Phone: see directory

GlycoAO:
Ambrotose AO™
Company: Mannatech, Inc.
www.mannatech.com
Phone: see directory

PhytoN:
Phytaloe®
Company: Mannatech, Inc.
www.mannatech.com
Phone: see directory

PreH:
Plus™
Company: Mannatech, Inc.
www.mannatech.com
Phone: see directory

GEssentials
Glycentials™
Company: Mannatech, Inc.
www.mannatech.com
Phone: see directory

Cata:
Catalyst™
Company: Mannatech, Inc.
www.mannatech.com
Phone: see directory

ImmS:
ImmunoStart®
Company: Mannatech, Inc.
www.mannatech.com
Phone: see directory

SP:
Sport™
Company: Mannatech, Inc.
www.mannatech.com
Phone: see directory

Clean:
MannaCleanse™
Company: Mannatech, Inc.
www.mannatech.com
Phone: see directory

MC:
Manna-C™
Company: Mannatech, Inc.
www.mannatech.com
Phone: see directory

GstroP & GstroZ:
GI-Pro™ & GI-Zyme™
Company: Mannatech, Inc.
www.mannatech.com
Phone: see directory

CB:
CardioBalance™:
Company: Mannatech, Inc.
www.mannatech.com
Phone: see directory

SkZone:
Emprizone®
Company: Mannatech, Inc.
www.mannatech.com
Phone: see directory

AdvGlycoN:
Advanced Ambrotose®
Company: Mannatech, Inc.
www.mannatech.com
Phone: see directory

Appendix B

RESOURCES

VEGETARIANS

The material presented on this site comes from individuals with years of hard-won experience either practicing alternative diets or observing those who do. As you'll find, no two writers will necessarily agree on all topics. A unifying theme, however, is the intent to squarely acknowledge and discuss the sometimes serious problems that can occur on alternative diets but often go unreported, and to go beyond the simplistic dogmas readily available elsewhere--in fact almost everywhere--to "explain them away."

www.beyondveg.com

PRICE-POTTENGER NUTRITION FOUNDATION

A non-profit educational resource with a unique library of over 10,000 books and publications on health and nutrition.

www.price-pottenger.org

THE WESTON A. PRICE FOUNDATION

A nonprofit, tax-exempt charity founded in 1999 to disseminate the research of nutrition pioneer Dr. Weston Price, whose studies of isolated nonindustrialized peoples established the parameters of human health and determined the optimum characteristics of human diets.

www.westonaprice.org

HAY HOUSE RADIO

A free online radio link to popular authors and speakers on a variety of topics.

www.hayhouseradio.com

THE SPIRITUAL CINEMA CIRCLE

Brings you hours of inspiring entertainment each month at a remarkably low cost. You get new movies you won't see anywhere else. "Soul-nourishing entertainment".

www.cinemacircle.com

ORGANIC CONSUMERS ASSOCIATION

An online resource for listings of where to find organic retailers in your area. Also contains a multitude of information and the latest news regarding organic standards, genetically engineered foods, rBHT, Mad Cow Disease, irradiation and food safety.

www.organicconsumers.org

Coalition for Natural Health

Their mission is to protect every citizen's right to natural health freedom of choice. This includes the practitioner's right to practice and the consumer's right to access natural health options. CNH actively opposes legislation that would restrict or revoke a practitioner's right to provide consultation and make recommendations aimed at educating the consumer about natural health-related techniques and choices that promote a healthier lifestyle. CNH actively supports legislation that protects rights of natural healers and practitioners of holistic health modalities to practice. CNH also diligently attempts to educate consumers and legislators alike, regarding the role of natural health modalities in promoting wellness.

www.naturalhealth.org

Test Your Drinking Water
American Environmental Health Foundation
8345 Walnut Hill Ln
Dallas, TX 75231
Phone: 1-800-428-2343

www.ehcd.com

Spring Water (glass bottles) Mountain Valley
Mountain Valley Spring Co.
PO Box 1610
Hot Spr. National Park
AR 71902
Phone: 1-800-643-1501

www.mountainvalleyspring.com

Natural Lifestyle

A wonderful resource for a variety of organic foods, natural cookware, cleaning products, organic cotton clothing, teas and more. Order their catalogue by mail – it is easier to see all of their products than on their website.

16 Lookout Drive
Asheville, NC 28804-3330
Phone: 1-800-752-2775

www.natural-lifestyle.com

Eat Wild

A source to learn more about grass-fed beef and even find a local producer.

www.eatwild.com

Mac Nut Oil

A healthy, monounsaturated oil that is wonderful on salads, and because it can withstand high temperatures without developing dangerous trans fatty acids, it can even be used for cooking. It is a nutritious and delicious alternative to other oils.

PO Box 864066
Plano, TX 75086-4066
Phone: 1-866-462-2688

www.macnutoil.com

ORGANIC HERBS, SEASONINGS, FACIAL PRODUCTS

Mountain Rose Herbs

Online source for many herbs like Red Clover, Uva Ursi, Black Cohosh, Chaste Tree Berry; as well as herbal seasonings; face and body products; woman's products; bulk cosmetic ingredients like clay, beeswax or vegetable glycerin and even glass jars for storing your homemade beauty products.

85472 Dilley Lane
Eugene, OR 97405
Phone: 1-541-741-7341
Phone: 1-800-879-3337
Fax: 1-510-217-4012
e-mail: info@mountainroseherbs.com

www.mountainroseherbs.com

Organic Cotton and Female Products

Natracare

Organic 100% cotton feminine care products.

Phone: 1-303-617-3476
Fax: 1-303-617-3495

www.natracare.com

Organic Essentials

Source for organic cotton products including cotton balls, swabs and nursing pads.

822 Baldridge Street
O'Donnell, Texas 79351
Phone: 1-806-428-3486
Fax: 1-806-428-3475

www.organicessentials.com

Hormone Testing

Rhein Consulting Laboratories

This company endeavors to provide clinicians and their patients with a rational and cost-effective approach to assessing steroid hormone levels. As opposed to saliva testing, measuring hormones in urine is widely accepted in medical and academic scientific circles as well as by clinical laboratory professionals. Results are accurate, relevant and reproducible. The relatively minor inconvenience involved in collecting specimen is a small price to pay for the security of knowing that results obtained are meaningful.

Rhein Consulting Laboratories
4475 SW Scholls Ferry Road • Suite 101
Portland, OR 97225

www.rheinlabs.com

HEALING SUPPLIES

Taris Products
This company offers a full range of physician recommended products to support the healing process in an office, hospital or home setting. Included are soft lasers and teisheins for meridian point and scar tissue stimulation. Product line also includes Qi Gong machine, Guasha tools, Five-Element Music and Homeopathy.

www.tarisproducts.com

FULL SPECTRUM LIGHTS

Bio-Light Group
Apply the therapeutic benefits of sunlight indoors. These full spectrum lights simulate natural sunlight. Highly recommended for hospitalized patients or those bedridden or confined to indoor environment for an extended period of time.

Biologically beneficial lighting pioneers
Phone: 1-800-234-3724; 805-564-3467
Fax: 1-805-564-2147

www.biolightgroup.com

The Q-Link
Q-Link is the most advanced personal energy system available today. A quarter century of frontier research has given birth to the Q-Link, a sleek pendant that tunes your being for optimal living: More energy, less stress, greater focus, and enhanced well being. No matter what you do, the Q-Link simply helps you feel better and gives you a creative edge by helping harmonizing your mind and body.

Clarus Products International
80 East Sir Francis Drake Blvd, Suite 3G
Larkspur, CA 94939 1-800-246-2765

www.clarus.com

Natural Cosmetics and Skin Care

Dr. Hauschka
Highly recommended natural skin care and cosmetic company. Their products contain no chemical preservatives.

59C North Street
Hatfield, MA 01038
Phone: 1-800-247-9907
Fax: 1-413-247-5633

www.drhauschka.com

Beeswork
A great source of natural face, body and bath products, as well as lip balm and candles.

122 Hamilton Drive, Suite D
Novato, Ca 94949
Phone: 1-415-883-5660
Fax: 1-415-883-6038

www.beeswork.comSUPPLEMENTS

Carlson Laboratories
A Source of Vitamin E (ask for E-Gems Elite), Fish Oil and Cod Liver Oil.

Phone: 888-234-5656

www.carlsonlabs.com

Mannatech Corporation
Mannatech is a fast-growing company delivering wellness solutions to the marketplace through its proprietary and internationally patented new glyconutrient technology. Mannatech is a company of hope, offering the potential of optimal health and wellness, and providing an unparalleled opportunity to fulfill your purposes and dreams by helping others.

www.mannatech.com

Bach Flower Essences

These are gentle homeopathic remedies that work in conjunction with any other healing modality without interaction or side effects. Many health care practitioners including naturopaths, chiropractors, dentists, and other alternative healers use them. They work by energetically helping to improve our coping mechanisms to reduce stress, alleviate worry and anxiety, and feel an increased sense of well-being.

100 Research Drive
Wilmington, MA 01887
Phone:1-800-319-9191
      1-800-338-0843
      1-978-988-3833

www.nelsonbach.com

Organic Teas

St. Dalfour Organic Teas offer certified organic black and green teas in bags. In addition to Classic Breakfast and Earl Grey teas, they have a wide range of flavored teas. Flavors include: Golden Peach, Lemon tea, Strawberry, Black Cherry, Peppermint, Cinnamon Apple Green, Golden Mango Green, Ginger Honey Green, Strawberry Rose Green, Mandarin Orange Green, and Spring Mint Green. Believe it or not, these organic tea bags can also be found at grocery stores.

www.stdalfour.com

ON-LINE HEALTH EDUCATION

Glyconutrients

The most in depth, coherent and complete compilation of the science of glyconutrients, the essential sugars necessary for the maintenance of health.

www.glycoscience.com

Council for Responsible Nutrition

Founded in 1973, is a Washington-based trade association representing ingredient suppliers and manufacturers in the dietary supplement industry. CRN members adhere to a strong code of ethics, comply with dosage limits and manufacture dietary supplements to high quality standards under good manufacturing practices.

www.crnusa.org

Dairy – Not Milk
Information regarding _controversial_ issues surrounding milk and other dairy products.

www.notmilk.com

Institute for Health Freedom
An honest source for information about policies that affect your freedom to choose your health care treatments and providers and to maintain your health privacy including genetic privacy.

www.forhealthfreedom.org

International Coalition for Drug Awareness
A source for researching the dangers of many prescription drugs.

www.drugawareness.org

The Weston A. Price Foundation A wonderful source for education on nutrition, farming and the healing arts.

www.westonaprice.org

American Iatrogenic Association
Medical errors are the third leading cause of death in the United States. In fact, one out of every five drug prescriptions in the typical hospital is wrong. But medical errors are the not only way that consumers are harmed. The Centers for Disease Control and Prevention estimates that 2 million people annually acquire infections while hospitalized and 90,000 people die from those infections. This is a website promoting accountability for medical professionals and institutions and reporting of illness.

www.iatrogenic.org

Nutrition Education Resource
International Foundation for Nutrition and Health The International Foundation for Nutrition and Health is a non-profit educational organization reaching out to health care professionals. IFNH collects and disseminates unique information on nutrition and whole food concentrates. It is our belief that the research on nutrition and health prior to the 1940s was done with natural whole foods, whereas the research done after World War II has been done with synthesized chemical by-products. It is also our belief that there is no reason to re-invent the wheel, the answers to all our health needs are well stated and documented in many earlier works.

3963 Mission Blvd.
San Diego, CA 92109
Phone: 1-858-488-8932
Fax: 1-858-4880-2566

www.ifnh.org

390

Pathways to Health Publishing (PTH)

PTH
P.O. Box 457
Brookport, IL 62910

ORDER FORM

Ordered By (Billing Address):

Name _____

Company _____

Address _____

City, State ZIP _____

Phone _____

Ship To: (if Different than Billing Address)

We Are Unable to Ship to a P.O. Box

Name _____

Company _____

Address _____

City, State ZIP _____

Phone _____

QTY	Item#	DESCRIPTION	UNIT PRICE	TOTAL
	RLRJ Wellness Companion to Glyconutrients and Meridians	Book "Remarkable Life Remarkable Journey" ISBN: 0-9770984-0-0 (S&H $7.00 first book; $4.00 ea. additional book).	$49.00	

Visa ☐   MasterCard ☐

Credit
Card#   _____

Expiration
Date   _____   3 Digit Code on
Back of Card _____

SUBTOTAL	
IL res 7.5% Sales Tax	
SHIPPING & HANDLING	
OTHER	
TOTAL	

1. **Send Check or Fax Credit Card Information to above address.**
2. **Make Checks payable to PTH**
3. **Web Ordering:**
   www.mannatext.com
4. **Volume discounts call;**
   800-930-6851
5. **Order by Phone; 800-930-6851 or Fax to: 800-930-6851**

AUTHORIZED SIGNATURE

_____

Printed in the United States
33923LVS00001B/33-142

9 780977 098408